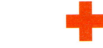

Australian Red Cross

First Aid

RESPONDING TO EMERGENCIES

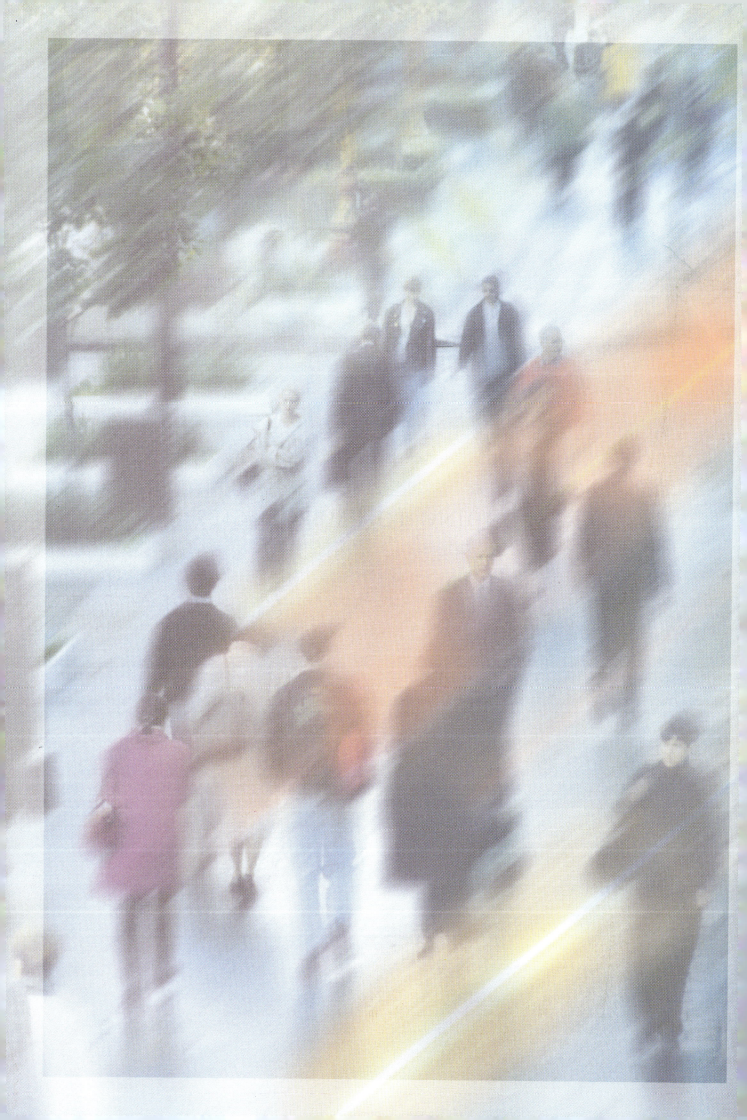

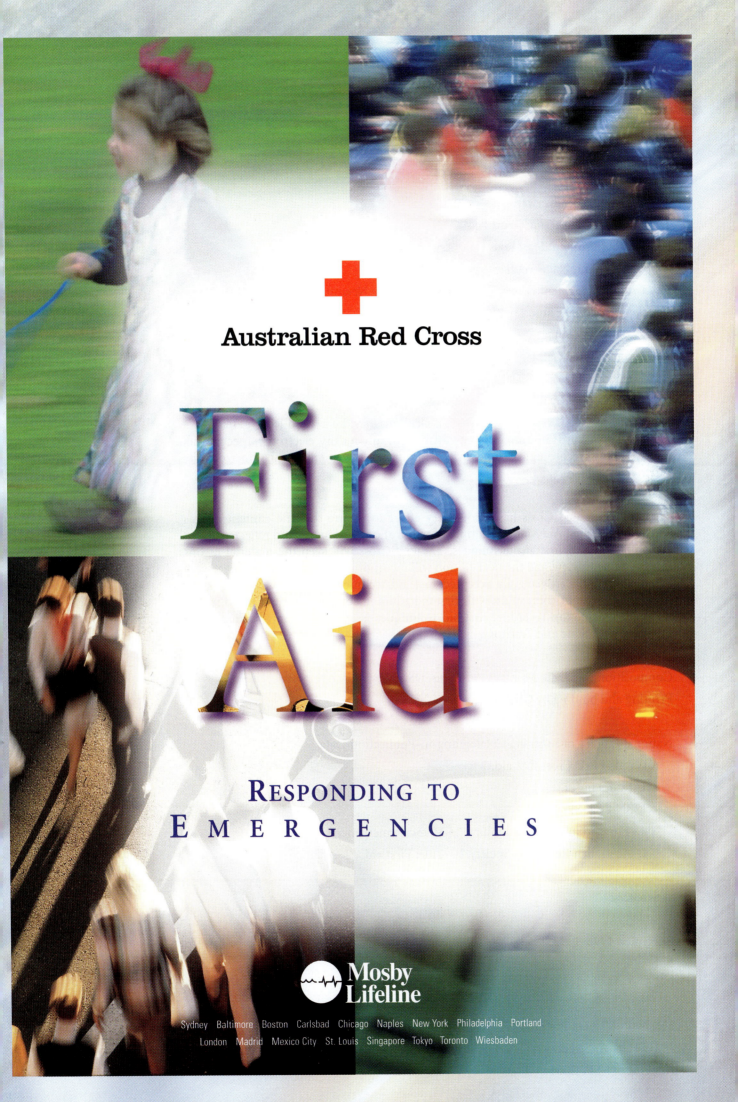

Australian Red Cross

First Aid

RESPONDING TO EMERGENCIES

Mosby Lifeline

Sydney   Baltimore   Boston   Carlsbad   Chicago   Naples   New York   Philadelphia   Portland
London   Madrid   Mexico City   St. Louis   Singapore   Tokyo   Toronto   Wiesbaden

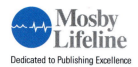

Publisher: David Culverwell

Director, TMIP, Australia: Geoff Hasler

Associate Aquisition Editor: Ross Goldberg

Managing Editor: Nada Madjar

Red Cross Development Committee: June Cullen, Judy Newnham, Di Treble, Ella Tyler

Development Editor: Tom Lochhaas

Design: Studio Montage

Photography: Jerry Galea

Copyright © 1995 by Australian Red Cross

All rights reserved. No part of this publication may be reproduced, stored in a retrieval system or transmitted, in any form or by any means, electronic, mechanical, photocopying, recording, or otherwise, without prior written permission from the Australian Red Cross.

The Australian Red Cross has made every effort to ensure that the content of this edition of the First Aid Manual, at time of publication, is accurate and reflects current generally accepted first aid techniques. The Red Cross will keep the material in this manual under review, and the next edition will incorporate any amendments necessary to reflect changes in generally accepted first aid techniques. This manual has been prepared for use in connection with first aid training courses. First aid training and updated information regarding first aid techniques is available from the Red Cross offices in each State and Territory.

Composition by Studio Montage, St. Louis, USA.

Printing and binding by Griffin Press

National Library of Australia Cataloguing-in-Publication Data

    Australian Red Cross first aid.

      Includes index.

      ISBN 1 875897 01 1.

        1. First aid in illness and injury. 2. Medical emergencies.

        I. Australian Red Cross Society. II. Title: First aid.

    616.0252

Reprinted 1996, 1997, 1998.

Mosby Publishers Pty Ltd

19/39 Herbert Street

Artarmon, NSW 2064

This textbook is dedicated to the many volunteers and staff of the Australian Red Cross who contribute their time and talents teaching first aid and life saving skills.

CONTENTS

ACKNOWLEDGMENTS

This first aid manual has been developed and produced through a joint effort of the Australian Red Cross and Mosby Lifeline. Some of the materials used in this manual have been adapted from the *Australian Red Cross First Aid Manual* (1993), and the American Red Cross have kindly authorised the use of some of the material from their manual *Responding to Emergencies* (1994).

The development team at the Australian Red Cross responsible for developing and compiling the manual consisted of: June Cullen (HASE Director, ACT), Judy Newnham (Training Development Officer, Vic.), Ella Tyler (National First Aid Advisor, SA) and Di Treble (National HASE Co-ordinator, National Office).

External review was provided by: David Aldous (Victorian College of Agriculture and Horticulture, Burnley, Vic.), Robyn Andrew (Royal Botanical Gardens, Melbourne, Vic.), Bill Berryman (CFA, Vic.), John Dolinas (National Injury Surveillance Unit, SA), Jenny Ginis (Australian Hearing Services, Vic.), Greg Jarvis (G. and L. Jarvis Sports Medicine and Rehabilitation Equipment, Vic.), Anne Learmonth (QUIT Campaign, Vic.), Robert Ryan (Royal Flying Doctor Service, SA), Peter May (Emergency Management Australia, ACT), Heather Wood (CFA, Vic.), Phil Goulding (Royal Childrens Hospital, Vic.), Robin McKeown (Drugs and Poisons Information, ACT), Diabetes Australia, Epilepsy Foundation of Vic., Freemasons Hospital, Vic., Mercy Maternity Hospital, Vic. and National Heart Foundation.

The Australian Red Cross also wishes to acknowledge the efforts of its many volunteers and staff involved in the development of this manual, without whom this project would not have been possible. Special thanks are due to the members of the National HASE Advisory Committee, in particular the Chair, Kaye Hogan, and Professor Tess Cramond.

The Mosby Lifeline team included: David Culverwell, Ross Goldberg, Geoff Hasler, Kathy Metcalfe and Nada Madjar.

Special thanks to Studio Montage (Design and Electronic Production), Tom Lochhaas (Developmental Editor) and Jerry Galea (Photographer).

Australian Red Cross gratefully acknowledges the financial support of the Broken Hill Proprietary Company Limited in the production of this manual.

Why You Should Complete a First Aid Course

People need to know what to do in an emergency before medical help arrives. Because you, the first aider, are the person most likely to be first on the scene you need to know how to recognise an emergency and how to respond. A first aid course will prepare you to make appropriate decisions regarding first aid care and to act on those decisions.

The first critical step in any emergency depends on someone being there who will take appropriate action. After completing a Red Cross First Aid course, you should be able to:

- recognise when an emergency has occurred
- follow the step-by-step plan of action for any emergency
- provide care for injuries or sudden illnesses until professional medical help arrives

First aid training will clarify for you when and how to call for emergency medical help, eliminating the confusion that can occur in any emergency.

How You Will Learn

Course content is presented in various ways. This manual, which is recommended reading for everyone undertaking this first aid training, contains the information that will be discussed in class. Videos and transparencies will support this information, as well as discussions and other class activities. The audiovisual materials will emphasise the key points you will need to remember when making decisions in emergencies and will help you provide appropriate care. They also present skills that you will practice in class. Participating in all class activities will increase your confidence in your ability to respond to emergencies.

The course has been designed to enable you to evaluate your progress in terms of skills competency, knowledge and decision-making. Certain chapters in the manual include practice sessions which are designed to help you learn specific first aid skills. Some of the practice sessions require practice on a manikin, while others give you the opportunity to practice with another person. This will give you a sense of what it would be like to care for a real victim in an emergency situation and help reduce any concerns you may have about giving care. Your ability to perform specific skills competently will be checked by your instructor during the practice sessions.

Several written self-assessments are provided for you to evaluate your level of knowledge and understanding at particular points in the course. These assessments build on previously presented material and will help you prepare for the final examination.

Your ability to make appropriate decisions when faced with an emergency will be enhanced as you participate in the class activities. Periodically, you will be presented with scenarios which will provide you with the opportunity to apply the knowledge and skills you have learned. These scenarios will also provide an opportunity for you to discuss with your instructor the many different situations you may encounter in an emergency.

The Manual

The manual has been designed to facilitate your learning and understanding of the material presented in it. It includes the following features:

Key Terms

At the beginning of each chapter is a list of key terms with definitions. You will need to know these terms to understand the contents of each chapter. Some key terms are listed in more than one chapter because they are essential to each of those chapters and your understanding of the contents.

The pronunciation of certain medical and anatomical terms is provided. In the text of each chapter, key terms are printed in bold the first time they appear.

For Review

This section indicates what you need to know to understand the chapter you are about to read. For example, reviewing the information about the nervous system helps you better understand the chapter on head and spinal injuries.

Feature Articles

Feature articles highlighted in the boxes add to the information in the main body of the text. They appear in all chapters and are easily recognised in coloured boxes. They present a variety of material ranging from historical information and accounts of actual events to everyday application of the information in the text. You will not be tested on the information contained in these boxes.

Tables

Tables, on a blue background, are included in many chapters. They concisely summarise important concepts and information and may aid study.

Application Questions

Application questions throughout each chapter challenge you to apply the information you have learned. The answers are included at the end of each chapter.

Study Questions

At the end of each chapter you will also find study questions which have been designed to test your memory and understanding of chapter content. Answering these questions will help you evaluate your understanding of the material and prepare you for the final written examination. The answers are in Appendix A. If you wish, you may write the answers directly in your manual.

Practice Guides

Learning the skills you need to give first aid is an important part of first aid training. Illustrated practice guides, at the end of relevant chapters give step-by-step directions for performing each skill.

Appendices

Appendix A at the end of this manual provides the answers to the study questions, while the remaining appendices include additional information on certain topics. For example, Appendix B gives detailed information on first aid and disease transmission.

Glossary

The glossary defines all the key terms, as well as other words that may be unfamiliar to the trainee. A pronunciation guide is also included.

How to Use this Manual

To gain the most from this manual, follow these steps for each chapter:

1. Review the recommended information listed under "For Review" before reading the chapter.

2. Answer the application questions as you read each chapter, and check your answers with those at the end of the chapter. If you cannot answer or do not understand the answer given, ask your instructor for assistance.

3. Answer the study questions at the end of each chapter. Mark or write your answers in the manual to help you with your review and study. Answer as many questions as you can without looking back in the chapter, then review the information covering any questions you were unable to answer and try them again. Check your answers against the correct answers in Appendix A. If you have not answered a question correctly, read that part of the chapter again to ensure that you understand why the answer is correct. This will help you see how much information you are retaining and which areas you need to review. If after rereading that part of the chapter, you still do not understand, ask your instructor for help.

Requirements for First Aid Certification

When you complete an accredited first aid course, you will be eligible for a Red Cross certificate or attendance card. But first you must:

- perform specific first aid skills competently and demonstrate the ability to make appropriate decisions for care

- demonstrate competence in cardiopulmonary resuscitation (CPR) on a manikin

- pass a final theory test with a score of at least 75 per cent

- attend 80 per cent of the course

If you do not pass any one of these 4 sections, you may resit the part you have not passed after participating in an appropriate retraining session.

Some courses do not require certification, and a card which acknowledges attendance will be given. Attendance cards may also be awarded to students in certificated courses who are not required or do not wish to undertake the examination.

Course Completion Standards

Red Cross endeavours to provide services to a population with diverse needs. Individuals should not be denied full and equal participation in Red Cross programs, goods, services, facilities, advantages or accommodations on the basis of real or perceived disabilities.

In the maintenance and implementation of standards in first aid training, the Australian Red Cross follows the policies of the Australian Resuscitation Council. It is the position of the Australian Red Cross that all reasonable accommodations should be made to provide first aid training to anyone who desires it. It is understood, however, that not everyone will be able to meet the requirements for certification of a course. Such individuals include, but are not limited to, those with physical disabilities that prevent inflation of a manikin or victim, those unable to perform adequate chest compressions, and those with chronic infections. This may create a dilemma for an individual whose workplace requires a First Aid certificate.

Whether an infected person can care for others adequately and safely must be determined on an individual basis. This decision may be made in conjunction with the person's own doctor, the employing agency and its medical advisers.

It is not the role of the Australian Red Cross to lower course completion standards to accommodate, for purposes of employment, individuals unable to meet these standards. This issue must be resolved by the employer and the employee. The employer must decide whether to waive the first aid course completion requirement. The more important issue for someone who is unable to complete the desired course is whether that person is able to work in a situation that requires competent administration of first aid.

Since the beginning of public training in CPR (cardiopulmonary resuscitation), the Australian Red Cross has trained over 1 million people in these lifesaving skills.

The Australian Red Cross follows widely accepted guidelines for the cleaning and decontamination of training manikins including the recommendations of the Australian National Council on Aids and the Australian Resuscitation Council. If these guidelines are consistently followed and basic personal hygiene is practised, the risk of any kind of disease transmission during CPR training is extremely low.

There are some additional health precautions and guidelines to be followed if you have an infection or a condition that would increase the risk to you or other participants.

GUIDELINES TO FOLLOW DURING TRAINING

To protect yourself and other participants from infection, you should adhere to the following guidelines:

- Wash your hands thoroughly before working with the manikin, and repeat handwashing before each new contact with the manikin.
- Do not eat, drink, use tobacco products or chew gum during classes when manikins are used.
- Only simulate clearing a student partner's airway of foreign material; do not insert fingers into a colleague's mouth.
- Practise mouth-to-mouth and mouth-to-mask techniques of ventilation on the manikin, not on other members of the class.
- Following use, scrub the manikin's face or mouth-nose pieces with a nailbrush using a solution of soap and water. Rinse the pieces in clean water and dry them before disinfecting.
- Discard lung bags and other disposable items into an appropriate container; do not contaminate the manikins or the surrounding area with used equipment.

Physical Stress and Injury

CPR requires strenuous activity. If you have a medical condition or disability that prevents you from participating fully in the practice sessions, let your instructor know.

Damage to Manikins

To avoid damaging the manikins, do the following before you begin to practise:

- Remove pens and pencils from your pockets.
- Remove jewellery.
- Remove lipstick.
- Remove chewing gum or food from your mouth.
- Wash your hands.

FUNDAMENTAL PRINCIPLES OF THE RED CROSS AND RED CRESCENT MOVEMENT

All aspects of Red Cross work are guided by seven Fundamental Principles.

Humanity

The International Red Cross and Red Crescent Movement prevents and alleviates suffering. Its purpose is to protect life and health and to ensure respect for the human being. It promotes mutual understanding, friendship, co-operation and lasting peace amongst all people.

Impartiality

The Movement makes no discrimination on the basis of nationality, race, religious beliefs, class or political opinions.

Neutrality

The Movement does not take sides in hostilities, or engage in controversies of a political, racial, religious or ideological nature.

Independence

The Movement is independent. It must have autonomy to be able to take action that is in accordance with the Fundamental Principles of the Movement.

Voluntary service

The Movement is a voluntary relief organisation, not prompted in any way by desire for gain.

Unity

There can only be one Red Cross or Red Crescent Society in any one country—it must be open to all.

Universality

The International Red Cross and Red Crescent Movement is a worldwide institution. All National Societies have equal status and share equal responsibilities and duties in helping each other.

There are three components that together make up the International Red Cross and Red Crescent Movement.

The International Committee of the Red Cross (ICRC)

The ICRC is the founding body of the Red Cross, with its headquarters in Geneva, Switzerland. The ICRC acts as a neutral intermediary in armed conflict and disturbances. Under the terms of the Geneva Conventions and Red Cross statutes, it protects and assists both civilian and military victims.

The International Federation of Red Cross and Red Crescent Societies (IFRC)

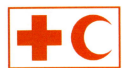

The Federation supports the development of humanitarian activities of National Societies, co-ordinates relief operations for victims of natural disasters, encourages the development of initiatives in social welfare programs, cares for refugees outside conflict areas and, in so doing, promotes peace.

National Societies

Today there are over 160 National Red Cross and Red Crescent Societies throughout the world, of which the Australian Red Cross is one. Each is an independent body which co-ordinates programs designed to assist its own people. Through networks of volunteers and staff, the National Societies carry out a vast range of humanitarian activities. First aid training is one of these.

The Australian Red Cross

In 1914 the Australian Red Cross was formed as a branch of the British Red Cross. In 1941 it became a Society in its own right. Today, it has a National Office in Melbourne, an office in each State and Territory and a network of over 1500 local units and branches throughout Australia. The National Office co-ordinates major activities on the national level. It also liaises with the Red Cross Headquarters in Geneva and with other National Societies. When requested by the Federation and the ICRC, the National Office recruits medical, paramedical, administrative and other field personnel and places them on international assignments. The state and territory offices are responsible for membership,

fundraising, formation of local units, relief assistance and Red Cross services within their own territory.

Since 1914, the Australian Red Cross has served the Australian community, responding to needs and protecting human life through the provision of services such as:

- Blood transfusion service.
- First aid training.
- Community services.
- Red Cross Youth.
- Disaster relief.
- National Tracing Agency.
- International Humanitarian Law.
- International relief and development programs.

Thousands of volunteers help Red Cross care for the community by assisting the sick, the elderly, the disabled and the housebound and by running youth activities. The Australian Red Cross relies on the kindness of these people who are prepared to give their time and talents to assist those in need.

Use of the Emblem

Many people believe that the red cross on a white background is a universal symbol for first aid or medical assistance. This is not entirely true. The red cross emblem is primarily a symbol of protection in times of armed conflict, used, as is the red crescent emblem, to protect the sick and wounded. Specifically, the two emblems are used by civilian and military medical units, religious personnel and Red Cross delegates in times of conflict. They are internationally recognised and protected under Geneva Conventions.

In times of peace, the red cross emblem can also be used by National Societies for identification purposes. In Islamic countries, most National Societies use the red crescent, which has the same status as the red cross emblem.

In Australia, it is a crime under the Commonwealth Geneva Conventions Act 1957 to use the emblem without the written authority of the Minister of Defence. The Australian Red Cross is the only body so authorised, and use of the emblem by any other person or body is a criminal offence.

The recognised symbol for first aid within Australia is a white cross on a green background. It is used on all workplace first aid kits and first aid directional signs.

Introduction to First Aid

EMERGENCIES can happen at any time, even when you feel you have done everything you can to prevent them. When an emergency does occur, you need to know the correct procedures to follow.

This chapter outlines how to recognise and respond to different emergencies, how to overcome the barriers that commonly keep people from acting, and what procedures to follow. When you give first aid based on your up-to-date training, you have nothing to fear legally in helping another person.

This chapter includes the reasons for learning first aid and how to summon assistance when necessary.

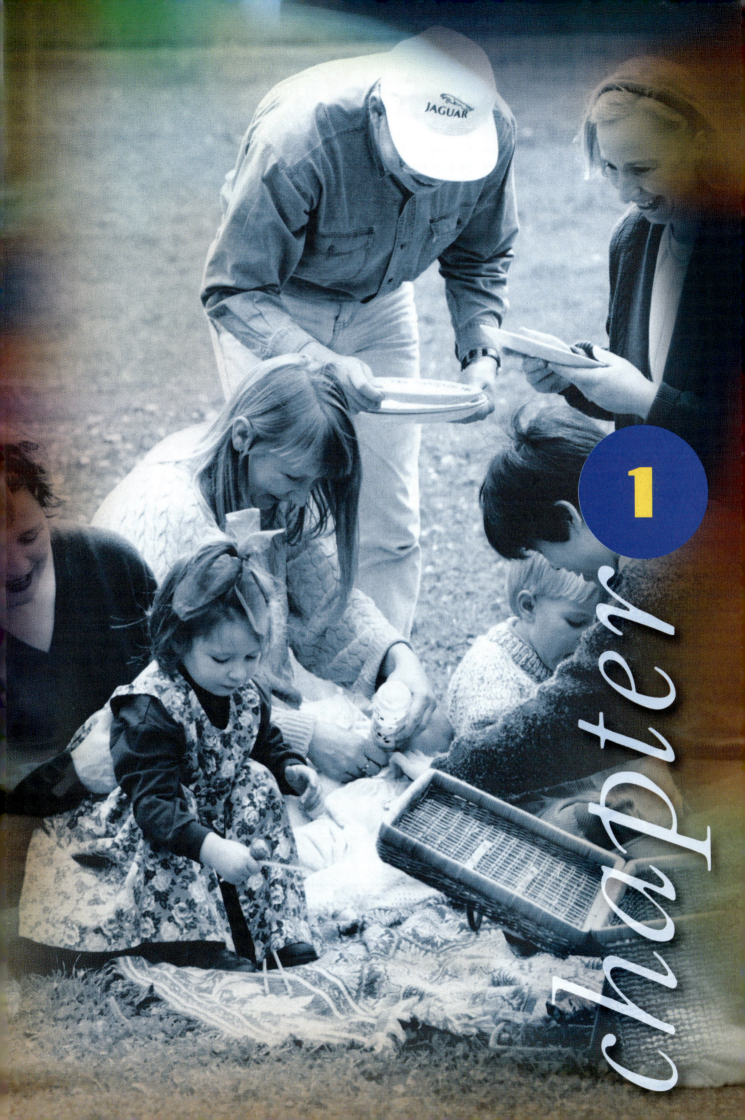

chapter

1

Key Terms

Emergency: A situation requiring immediate action.

First aid: Immediate care given to a victim of injury or sudden illness until more advanced care can be provided or recovery occurs.

First aider: A person trained in first aid, who voluntarily gives first aid when needed.

Injury: Damage that occurs when the body is subjected to force such as a blow, a fall or a collision.

Medical emergency: A sudden illness requiring immediate medical attention.

Poisons Information Centre: A centre staffed by medical professionals to give information about how to care for victims of poisoning.

Signs: Details observed about a sick or injured person using the five senses.

Symptoms: Sensations felt by the sick or injured person which are described to the first aider or health professional.

Victim: A person experiencing illness or injury and in need of medical assistance or first aid.

You and several friends are driving home after a football game. While stopped at an intersection, you see a car hit another car head-on. To your horror, one of the drivers crashes against the windscreen. Glass is everywhere and the injured driver slumps over the steering wheel, motionless.

On a Saturday afternoon you enter the garage and find your father lying on the floor. He seems barely conscious and is clutching at his chest.

In each of the cases above, what would you do? What help could you give?

As a **first aider** you are being trained to give **first aid** in an emergency. You may find yourself in a situation where someone suffering from an injury or sudden illness needs help until more advanced care can be provided. The aim of a first aid course is to train you in the basics of first aid to help you recognise and respond appropriately to any **emergency.** Your response may help save a life.

AIMS OF FIRST AID

First aid is given to a victim in an emergency for four purposes:

- To preserve life.
- To protect the unconscious victim.
- To prevent the condition from worsening and to relieve pain.
- To promote recovery.

RECOGNISING EMERGENCIES

Recognising an emergency is the first step in responding. An emergency is a situation requiring immediate action. A **medical emergency** is a sudden illness such as a heart attack, which requires immediate medical attention. An **injury** is damage to the body, such as a broken arm, which results from a violent force. Some injuries can be serious enough to be considered emergencies. The **victim** of an emergency can be anyone—a friend, family member, stranger or you. An emergency can happen anywhere—on the road, at home, work or play.

Table 1-1

RECOGNISING EMERGENCIES

Signs	Examples
Unusual noises	Screams, yells, moans or calls for help. Breaking glass, crashing metal, screeching tyres.
Unusual sights	Things that look out of the ordinary: • a stalled vehicle • an overturned saucepan • a spilled medicine container • broken glass • fallen high voltage electrical cables
Unusual smells	Smells that are stronger than usual. Unrecognisable smells.
Unusual symptoms and signs or behaviour	Unconsciousness. Difficult breathing. Clutching the chest or throat. Slurred, confused or hesitant speech. Unexplainable confusion, irritability or drowsiness. Sweating for no apparent reason. Uncharacteristic skin colour.

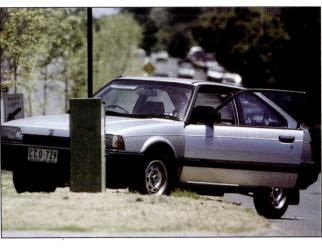

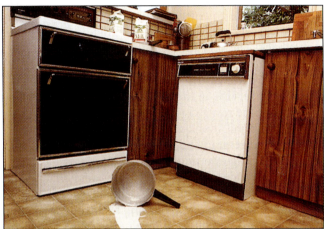

Recognising an emergency may be difficult at times. You may become aware of an emergency because of certain things you observe. Common indicators include unusual noises, sights, smells, symptoms and signs or behaviour. You will learn more about how to observe and interpret symptoms and signs in Chapter 3.

Unusual Noises

Noises are often the first thing that may call your attention to an emergency. Some noises that may indicate an emergency are:

- noises that indicate someone is in distress, such as screaming, yelling, moaning, crying and calling for help
- alarming identifiable noises, such as breaking glass, crashing metal or screeching tyres
- abrupt or loud noises that are not identifiable, such as collapsing structures or falling ladders

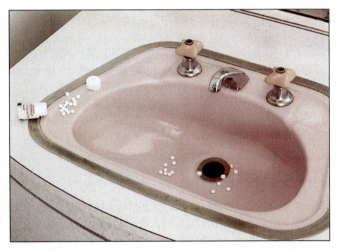

Unusual Sights

Unusual sights that indicate a possible emergency can go unnoticed by the unaware observer (Figure 1-1). Some examples of sights that may signal an emergency are:

- a stalled vehicle
- an overturned saucepan on the kitchen floor
- a spilled medicine container
- a fallen chair

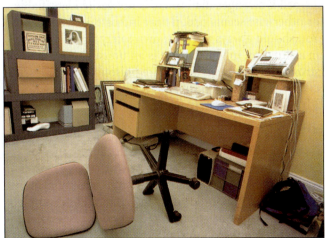

FIGURE 1-1 *Unusual sights may indicate an emergency.*

THE ROYAL FLYING DOCTOR SERVICE

Emergency medical services and first aid are especially crucial in our sparsely populated rural areas, which have few doctors or medical facilities. Here, people are likely to be engaged in such hazardous activities as riding, operating machinery or driving on poor roads. Tourists come to the outback for rock climbing, bush walking, camping, and other leisure activities that have the potential for mishaps requiring medical attention.

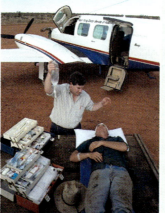

To provide emergency and other medical services for the people of the outback, The Very Reverend Dr John Flynn, a Presbyterian minister, founded the Royal Flying Doctor Service (RFDS), then called the Aerial Medical Service, in the 1920s. Flynn was able to bring together the relatively new technologies of flight and telecommunications, creating a network to provide medical care in the hope of preventing accidents from turning into tragedies.

Flynn's travels in the outback as a missionary convinced him of the need to serve these areas.

Flynn spent a decade working to introduce flying doctors and develop communication by wireless. His meeting with inventor Alfred Hermann Traeger in 1925 ultimately resulted in distribution of wireless sets to many rural areas, providing the necessary link with the flying doctors. Flynn contracted with the recently formed Qantas Airlines in March 1928 to provide an air ambulance covering 38,000 km.

The first flight of the Aerial Medical Service, under the auspices of the Australian Inland Mission of the Presbyterian Church, took place on May 15, 1928.

The de Havilland DH50A was piloted by Arthur Affleck, with Dr Kenyon St Vincent Welch accompanying him as the original Flying Doctor. A decade later, the newly named Australian Aerial Medical Service had assumed control of the program, which acquired its present title in 1955.

Today the RFDS has a staff of doctors, nurses, pilots and others, and with its clinics and fleet of about 40 aircraft it services 80 per cent of Australia, an area with 400,000 residents. A non-profit organisation, RFDS receives government and public funding. Health care is provided free of charge to residents and tourists alike.

In addition to responding to emergencies, RFDS has the following goals:

- To meet the health needs of specific rural communities.
- To create health care partnerships.
- To provide services for women, children, adolescents, Aborigines and those with diabetes.

RFDS has targeted specific health problems that are worse in rural areas because of limited access to doctors and facilities. These include:

- Road trauma.
- Youth suicide.
- Alcohol and substance abuse.

The exploits of RFDS have been chronicled on "The Flying Doctors", a television show increasing public awareness of the services provided. ■

Unusual Smells

Many smells are part of our everyday lives, for example, petrol fumes at petrol stations, the smell of chlorine at swimming pools or smoke from a fire. However, when a smell is stronger than usual, is not easily identifiable or otherwise seems odd, it may indicate an emergency. You should always put your own safety first if you are in a situation in which there is an unusual or very strong smell as many fumes are poisonous.

Unusual Symptoms and Signs or Behaviour

It may be difficult to tell if someone's appearance or behaviour is unusual, particularly when the person is a stranger. However, certain symptoms and signs or behaviours could indicate an emergency. For example, if you see someone collapse to the floor, that person obviously requires your immediate attention. However, you will not know if first aid is needed until you

approach the individual, who may have merely slipped and not be in need of any help. On the other hand, the person may be unconscious and need immediate medical assistance. Other symptoms and signs and behaviour that could indicate an emergency may be less obvious. They include:

- breathing difficulty
- clutching the chest or throat
- slurred, confused or hesitant speech
- confused or irritable behaviour
- sweating for no apparent reason
- uncharacteristic skin colour—pale, flushed or bluish skin

These and other signs may occur alone or together. For example, a heart attack may be indicated by chest pain alone, or chest pain may be accompanied by sweating and breathing difficulty.

RESPONDING TO EMERGENCIES

In an emergency, your involvement as a trained first aider may be crucial. Every year, countless first aiders and bystanders recognise and respond to emergencies. Some phone for help, some comfort the victim or family members, some give first aid to victims and others help keep order at the emergency scene (Figure 1-2). *There are many ways you can help, but in order to help, you must first decide to act.*

Barriers to Action

The involvement of trained first aiders and bystanders is the key to recognising an emergency and getting more advanced medical help to a victim. Sometimes people do not recognise that an emergency has occurred. At other times, people recognise an emergency but are reluctant to act. People have various reasons for hesitating or not acting. These are called barriers to action. Some are very personal. Common reasons people give for not acting include:

- presence of bystanders
- uncertainty about the victim
- nature of the injury or illness
- fear of disease transmission
- fear of doing something wrong

Thinking about these things now and mentally preparing yourself to act in an emergency will enable you to respond more confidently in an actual emergency.

Presence of Bystanders

The presence of bystanders can cause confusion at an emergency scene. It may not be easy to tell if anyone is providing first aid. Always ask if help is needed. Do not assume that, just because there is a crowd, someone is caring for the victim. The presence of other bystanders may make you reluctant to step forward and provide care. You may feel embarrassed about coming forward in front of strangers, but this should not deter you from offering help when needed. In fact, you may be the only one at the scene who knows first aid. Even if someone else is already giving care, offer your help.

Although you might not want to become the centre of attention, someone needs to act. Ensure that crowd members do not endanger themselves or the victim unnecessarily. Sometimes you may need to ask bystanders to back away and give the victim and rescuers ample space. At other times, bystanders can be of great help in an emergency. You can ask them to call for an ambulance, meet and direct the ambulance to the location, keep the area free of unnecessary traffic or help you to give care. You might send them for blankets or other supplies.

Bystanders may have valuable information about what happened or the location of the nearest phone. A friend or family member who is present may know if the victim has a pre-existing medical condition. Bystanders can also help comfort the victim and others at the scene.

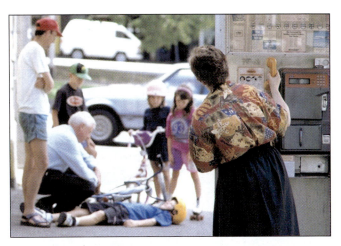

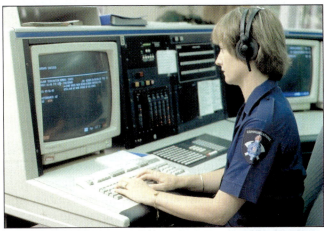

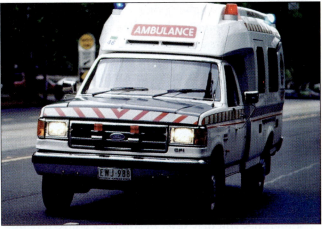

FIGURE 1-2 *Deciding to help means taking action. It includes calling the emergency switchboard number for assistance or giving first aid care at the scene until the arrival of the ambulance.*

Uncertainty about the Victim

As most emergencies happen in or near the home or workplace, you are more likely to give care to a friend or family member than you are to a stranger (Figure 1-3 on page 6). However, this is not always the case. You may not know the victim and may feel uncomfortable touching a stranger. Sometimes you may hesitate to act because the victim may be much older or much younger than you, be of a different gender or race, have a disabling condition or be a victim of crime. Sometimes you may have to reverse your usual role with the victim. For example, an employee may need to care for the boss, or a child may

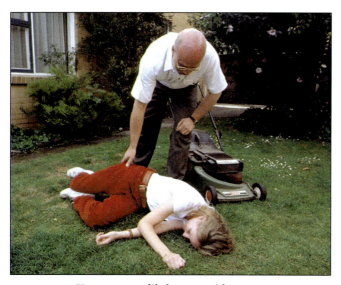
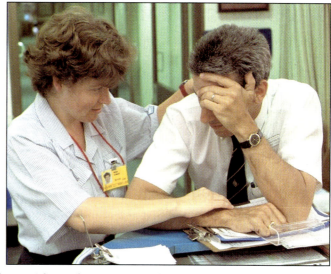

FIGURE 1-3 *You are most likely to provide care to someone you know either at home or at work.*

need to care for a parent or other adult. In an emergency, try to remember that you need to put these concerns aside and give the best care you can.

Sometimes victims of injury or sudden illness may act strangely or be unco-operative. The injury or illness, stress, or other factors such as the influence of alcohol or other substances, may make people act offensively. Do not take such behaviour personally. Remember, an emergency can cause even the nicest person to seem angry or unpleasant. If the victim's attitude or behaviour keeps you from giving first aid care, you can still help. Make sure someone has called for assistance, manage bystanders at the scene and try to reassure the victim until the ambulance arrives. If at any time the victim's behaviour becomes a threat to you, withdraw from the immediate area.

Nature of the Injury or Illness

Sometimes, an injury or illness may be very unpleasant to handle. The presence of blood, vomit, unpleasant smells or torn or burned skin is disturbing to almost everyone. You cannot predict how you will respond to these and other factors in an emergency situation.

Sometimes you may need to compose yourself before acting. If you must, turn away for a moment and take a few deep breaths before providing care. Remember that this is an emergency and your help is needed. If you are still unable to provide first aid because of the appearance of the injury, you can help in other ways. You can ensure your safety, the safety of victims and bystanders, call for help, reassure the victim and manage bystanders.

Fear of Disease Transmission

Fear of contracting a disease while giving first aid is a concern for some people. As a consequence of the AIDS epidemic, the fear of disease transmission has grown. This concern is understandable. Although there is a possibility of disease transmission in first aid care, the actual risk is far smaller than you may think.

In an emergency, you will not know what infection risks may be present. Although you should take steps to protect yourself against infection, you should also act to reduce the risk of disease transmission from you to the victim. This can occur through any cuts or open sores on your own skin. It is safest for you to assume that all contact with body fluids has a potential for disease transmission between the victim and rescuer. For example, controlling bleeding is such a situation.

Disease transmission in first aid is rare. Your intact skin protects you as you give first aid, but if the skin is broken by a small cut or sore, germs can enter the body. Germs also can enter the body through the membranes around the eyes and mouth. For these reasons, always take precautions to prevent direct contact with a victim's body fluids while giving first aid. Use protective barriers, such as disposable latex gloves, and always wash thoroughly as soon as possible after giving first aid (Figure 1-4). If you come into direct contact with a victim's body fluids while giving first aid, seek medical advice as soon as possible. Avoid unnecessary exposure to any hazards at the emergency scene. Appendix B (page 364) contains additional information on first aid and disease transmission.

1 *What conditions for disease transmission must be present for it to be possible for you to become infected with HIV (the virus that causes AIDS) when you give first aid?*

2 *Disease transmission is a possibility when giving first aid. Who faces the greater risk of infection— you or the victim? Why?*

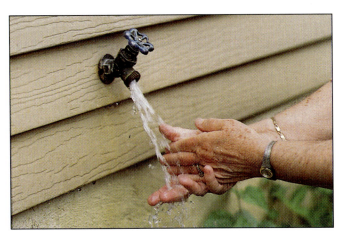
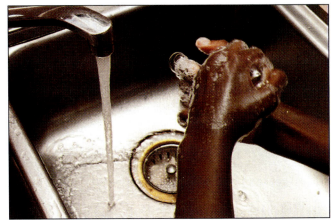

FIGURE 1-4 *Thorough handwashing after giving care helps protect you against disease.*

Table 1-2

YOU CAN ALWAYS DO SOMETHING TO HELP IN AN EMERGENCY

What to do	How to do it
Take appropriate safety precautions	Ensure the safety of the victim, yourself and bystanders. Be alert to possible dangers at the scene.
Call for help	Telephone your local emergency number.
Communicate effectively	Reassure the victim and others at the scene. Gather information from the victim, family, friends and bystanders. Provide necessary information to emergency personnel.
Manage bystanders	Organise bystanders to: • call the local emergency number • meet and direct the ambulance to the scene • comfort the victim and other bystanders • help obtain supplies • keep the area free of unnecessary traffic • help protect the victim from possible dangers.

Fear of Doing Something Wrong

We all respond to emergencies in different ways. Whether trained or untrained, some of us are afraid we will do the wrong thing and make the situation worse. If you are unsure about what to do, call for an ambulance. *The worst thing to do is to do nothing.*

LEGAL CONSIDERATIONS

People are sometimes afraid that in the stress of an emergency they may make mistakes when they give first aid and may thus cause harm to the victim. When giving first aid to a stranger, people may worry further that a mistake may lead to a legal problem or that they will be sued if they do the wrong thing.

Be reassured that in the eyes of the law, first aiders are not expected to be perfect, and not every emergency turns out perfectly. The general legal principle is that the first aider is expected to act reasonably and prudently with a genuine concern for the best interests of the victim. When your first aid follows that principle, you should not worry about being sued. See Appendix C (page 366) for more information on the legal implications of first aid.

The first aider has nothing to fear as long as he or she acts reasonably, with caution, and follows accepted teaching and protocols, such as the Australian Resuscitation Council policies.

PREVENTING EMERGENCIES

Being responsible means that you take reasonable precautions to prevent emergencies from occurring. Injuries remain the leading cause of death and disability in children and young adults. Thousands of Australians die each year as a result of injuries (Figure 1-5, on page 8). No one knows for sure how many of these victims die needlessly from preventable incidents.

Emergencies also occur as a result of unhealthy lifestyles. For example, your exercise and dietary habits influence the health of your heart. Unhealthy habits, such as overeating, smoking and lack of exercise, can increase your chances of heart attack.

3 *As you approach the scene of a car crash, you see blood on the car windscreen and hear people crying in pain. You begin to feel faint and nauseated and are not sure if you can proceed. How can you still help?*

4 *Knowing that most injuries can be prevented, list three things you can do to reduce the chance of being injured.*

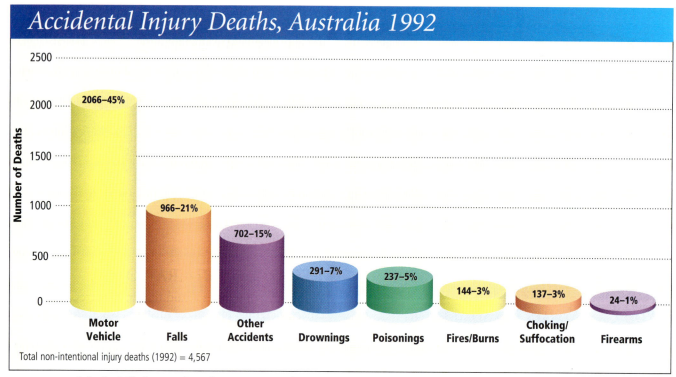

Accidental Injury Deaths, Australia 1992

Number of Deaths

- Motor Vehicle: 2066–45%
- Falls: 966–21%
- Other Accidents: 702–15%
- Drownings: 291–7%
- Poisonings: 237–5%
- Fires/Burns: 144–3%
- Choking/Suffocation: 137–3%
- Firearms: 24–1%

Total non-intentional injury deaths (1992) = 4,567

FIGURE 1-5 *Injuries kill thousands each year. No-one knows how many people die needlessly from preventable injuries.* (Source: National Injury Surveillance Unit, 1994.)

PREPARING FOR EMERGENCIES

Emergencies can and do happen, regardless of attempts to prevent them.

If you are prepared for unforeseen emergencies, you can help ensure that care begins as soon as possible—for yourself, your family and friends, and others in your community. First aid training provides you with both the knowledge and skills necessary to respond confidently to emergency situations. Your training will help you to focus on the most important aspects of care by giving you a basic plan of action that can be used in any emergency. By knowing what to do, you will be better able to manage your fears and overcome barriers to action. Your training will enable you to respond more effectively in your role as a first aider, provided you keep your skills up to date.

You can be ready for most emergencies if you do the following things *now*:

- Keep important information about you and your family in a handy place such as on the refrigerator door and in your car's glove compartment (Figure 1-6). Include everyone's date of birth, medical conditions, allergies and prescriptions and dosages. List doctors' names and phone numbers.

- Keep medical and insurance records up to date.

- Find out if your community is served by an emergency 000 telephone number. If it is not, look up the numbers for police, fire department, ambulance service and the Poisons Information Centre (see Chapter 10). As soon as they are old enough to use the telephone, teach your children how to call for help.

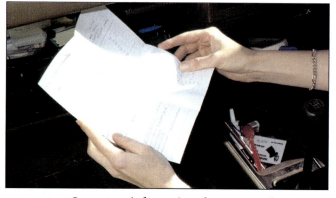

FIGURE 1-6 *Important information about you and your family should be readily available.*

- Keep emergency telephone numbers listed in a handy place such as by the telephone and in your first aid kit. Include the home and office phone numbers of family members, friends or neighbours who can help. Be sure to keep both the list and the telephone numbers current.

- Make sure your house or unit number is easy to read. Numerals are easier to read than spelled out numbers. Report any missing street signs to the proper authorities.

- Wear a medical alert tag if you have a potentially serious medical condition such as epilepsy, diabetes, heart disease or allergies (Figure 1-7). A medical alert tag, usually worn on a necklace or bracelet, or a personal medical ID card provides important medical information if you cannot communicate. Contact the Australian Medic Alert Foundation on 008-882-222.

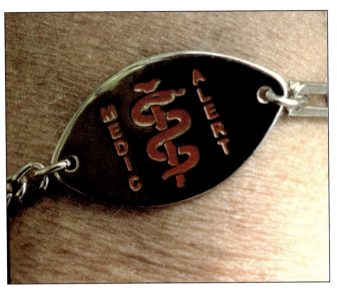

FIGURE 1-7 *Medical alert tags can provide important medical information about a victim.*

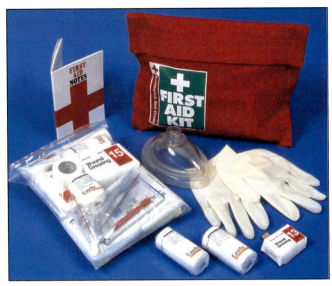

FIGURE 1-8 *Be prepared for emergencies with a well-stocked first aid kit.*

- Keep a first aid kit readily available in your home, car, workplace and recreation area (Figure 1-8). Store each kit in a dry place and replace used contents regularly. Different first aid kits are required for various circumstances. State and Territory laws govern what workplace first aid kits should contain. There are Australian standards for portable first aid kits and kits for the car. First aid kits contain a variety of dressings and bandages together with scissors, forceps and other items. See Chapter 13 for a detailed listing of the recommended contents.

Summary

- With your first aid training, you can help save the life of a victim of injury or sudden illness.

- First, use all your senses to note anything unusual and recognise that an emergency has occurred; immediately call your emergency number.

- Don't let the common barriers to action keep you from acting in an emergency and giving first aid until help arrives.

- Legally you have nothing to fear when you act with reason and caution and follow the protocols you will learn in a first-aid course.

- Take steps both to prevent emergencies and to be prepared when they occur.

In the following chapters you will learn how to manage emergencies. You will learn a plan of action that you can apply to any emergency and how to give first aid for both life-threatening and less serious emergencies.

Answers to Application Questions

1. You can become infected with HIV only through cuts or open sores that come into contact with infected body fluids.

2. There is a risk of infection for both you and the victim. The degree of risk depends on the situation and the health status of the people involved. Disease can be transmitted as easily from you to the victim as from the victim to you. Follow the guidelines in this chapter to protect yourself and the victim.

3. Although you may feel ill and be incapacitated by the sight of blood or cries of pain, you can still help. If necessary, turn away for a moment and try to control your feelings. If you are still unable to proceed, make sure the emergency number has been called. Then find other ways to help, such as asking bystanders to assist you or help to keep the area safe.

4. You can do many things to reduce your chance of injury. Do not drive under the influence of alcohol or other substances or ride with people under the influence of alcohol or other substances. Always wear a safety belt. Know the possible dangers in and around your home, neighbourhood and workplace. Know your own limitations when you do something that is physically demanding.

Study Questions

1. **Match each term with the correct definition.**

   a. Bystander.
   b. Emergency services personnel.
   c. Ambulance officer and paramedic.
   d. Hospital care providers.
   e. Emergency operator.

   _____ Often the first trained person on the scene, such as a police officer, fire officer or ambulance officer.

   _____ A field extension of the doctor; provides the highest level of pre-hospital care such as administering medication or intravenous fluids.

   _____ The person who answers the emergency call and determines what help is needed at the scene.

   _____ The professionals who strive to return victims to their previous state of health.

   _____ Someone who recognises an emergency and decides to act; the first link in the chain of survival.

2. **List the four aims of first aid.**

3. **List four indicators of an emergency and give one example of each.**

4. **List five barriers to action.**

5. **List three ways bystanders can help in an emergency.**

6. *List four ways to prepare for an emergency.*

7. *Match each term with the correct definition.*

  a. First aid.
  b. Calling emergency personnel.
  c. Medical emergency.
  d. Barriers to action.
  e. Indicator of an emergency.
  f. First aid response.
  g. Emergency.

  _____ A situation that requires immediate action.
  _____ The immediate care given to a victim of injury or sudden illness until more advanced care can be obtained.
  _____ The most important action you can take in a life-threatening emergency.
  _____ A sudden illness requiring immediate medical attention.
  _____ An unidentifiable or exceptionally strong smell.
  _____ Recognising an emergency and deciding to act.
  _____ Reasons for not acting or for hesitating to act.

8. *List five indicators of an emergency found in this scenario.*

On your way to the supermarket from the carpark you hear the loud screech of tyres and the crash of metal. You turn around and head in the direction of the sound. As you reach the corner of the carpark, you notice that across the street a car has struck a telephone pole, causing it to lean at an odd angle. Cables are hanging down from the pole. Another vehicle is stalled in the middle of the street.

9. *What might have happened along these links in the chain of survival to cause this delay in reaching the victims and getting them to the hospital?*

A recent newspaper account of a multiple vehicle freeway collision reported that the approximate time of the incident was 4.50 pm, that ambulance help did not arrive until 5.25 pm, and that the last victim did not arrive at the hospital until 6.30 pm.

Answers are in Appendix A (page 360).

Body Systems

AS A FIRST AIDER you need a basic understanding of what the human body consists of and how it works. The body is a series of systems which are made up of organs and other structures especially adapted to perform specific functions. Body systems do not work independently but rely on other systems to function properly. When you understand the position of major organs within the body and how they work, you can better understand what is happening in the body when illness or injury causes something to go wrong.

This chapter discusses different body systems, how they are inter-related, and how they are affected in different kinds of emergencies.

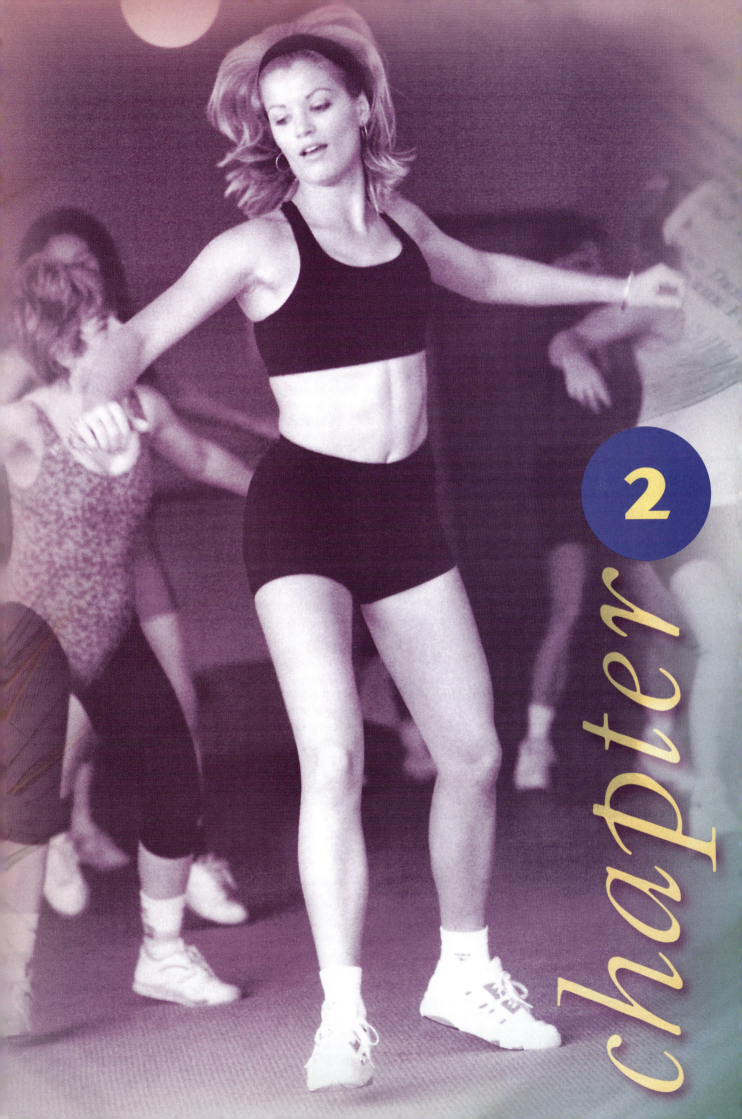

chapter **2**

Key Terms

Airway: The pathway for air from the mouth and nose to the lungs.

Alimentary *(al-i-men-ta-ry)* **canal:** The long passage through which food passes and is digested and absorbed; it extends from the mouth to the anus.

Alveoli *(al-vee-o-ly)* **:** The air sacs of the lungs in which the exchange of oxygen and carbon dioxide takes place.

Arteries: Large blood vessels that carry oxygen-rich blood from the heart to all parts of the body.

Bone: A dense, hard tissue that forms the skeleton.

Bronchi *(bron-kee)* **:** The large passages through which air passes to and from the lungs.

Cells: The basic units of all living tissue.

Cyanosis *(sy-a-no-sis)* **:** A bluish discolouration of the skin, tongue and lining of the mouth.

Epiglottis *(ep-i-glot-is)* **:** A small flap of tissue which covers the windpipe when food or liquids are swallowed.

Infection: Condition caused by disease-producing micro-organisms in the body.

Large intestine: Part of the alimentary canal where water and some minerals are absorbed from the digested material entering from the small intestine, and where waste products are prepared for elimination.

Lymph *(limf)* **:** A fluid containing white cells that flows through body tissues to help the body fight infections.

Muscle: A fibrous tissue that lengthens and shortens to create movement.

Nerve: A part of the nervous system which carries impulses to and from the brain and all body parts.

Oesophagus *(ee-sof-a-guss)* **:** The tubular structure which carries food and liquids from the mouth into the stomach; also known as the gullet.

Pulse: The beat felt in arteries near the skin's surface with each contraction of the heart.

Respiration: The breathing process of the body that takes in oxygen and eliminates carbon dioxide and other waste gases.

Skin: The tough, supple membrane that covers the entire surface of the body.

Small intestine: Part of the alimentary canal where digested food substances from the stomach are absorbed into the blood.

Spinal cord: A bundle of nerves extending from the brain at the base of the skull to the lower back, protected by the spinal column.

Stomach: The major organ of digestion, where partly processed food and liquid are broken down into substances the body can use.

Tissue: A collection of similar cells that act together to perform specific body functions.

Trachea *(tra-kee-a)* **:** The tube from the upper airway to the lungs; also called the windpipe.

Veins: Blood vessels that carry blood low in oxygen from all parts of the body to the heart.

The human body is a miraculous machine. It performs many complex functions, each of which helps us live. The body is made up of billions of cells that are microscopic in size. A cell is the basic unit of all living tissue. There are many different types of cells, each of which contributes in a specific way to keep the body functioning normally. A collection of similar cells is a tissue.

Different cells and tissues working together make up organs (Figure 2-1). Organs have specialised functions. For example, the heart is an organ; its job is to pump blood throughout the body. Vital organs are those organs whose function is essential for life— they include the **heart, lungs** and **brain**.

A body system is a group of organs and other structures which are especially adapted to perform specific body functions. They work together to carry out functions needed for life. For example, the heart, blood and blood vessels make up the circulatory system, which keeps all parts of the body supplied with oxygen-rich blood.

For the body to work properly, all the different systems must work well together. The following body systems are covered in this chapter:

- respiratory
- circulatory
- lymphatic
- nervous
- digestive
- musculoskeletal
- the skin

You do not need to be an expert on body systems to give first aid to someone who needs it. However, knowing how the body works will help you better understand when something is wrong. You will learn that the different body systems depend on each other. Just as different body systems work together well when you are healthy, an injury or illness that affects one body system can affect others. For instance, a head injury may affect the nervous system; this in turn can affect the respiratory system and cause breathing to stop.

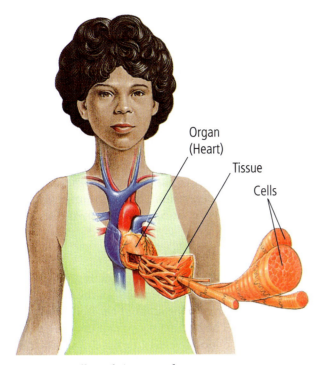

FIGURE 2-1 *Cells and tissues make up organs.*

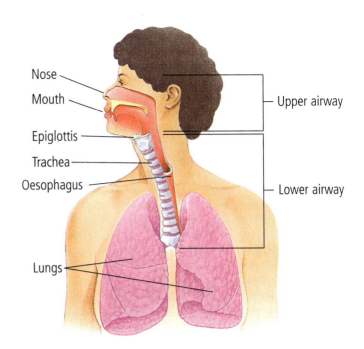

FIGURE 2-2 *The respiratory system includes the mouth, nose, epiglottis, trachea and lungs.*

RESPIRATORY SYSTEM

The body must have a constant supply of oxygen to stay alive. The respiratory system supplies the body with oxygen through breathing. When you **inhale**, air fills the lungs and the oxygen in the air is transferred to the blood. The blood carries oxygen to all parts of the body. This same system removes carbon dioxide. Carbon dioxide is transferred from the blood to the lungs. When you **exhale**, air is forced from the lungs, expelling carbon dioxide and other waste gases. This breathing process is called **respiration**.

The respiratory system includes the airway and lungs. Figure 2-2 shows the parts of the respiratory system in detail. The airway begins at the nose and mouth, which form the upper airway. Air passes through the mouth and nose, then through the **trachea**, on its way to the lungs. The trachea is the windpipe, behind which is the oesophagus, otherwise known as the gullet. The oesophagus carries food and liquids from the mouth to the stomach. A small flap of tissue, called the epiglottis, covers the trachea when you swallow to keep food and liquids out of the lungs.

Air reaches the lungs through two tubes called bronchi. The bronchi (Figure 2-3A) branch into increasingly smaller tubes, known as bronchioles, which are like tree branches. These eventually end in millions of tiny air sacs called alveoli (Figure 2-3B). Oxygen and carbon dioxide pass into and out of the blood through the thin cell walls of the alveoli and capillaries.

Air enters the lungs when you inhale and leaves the lungs when you exhale. When you inhale, the chest muscles and the diaphragm contract. This expands the chest and draws air into the lungs. When you exhale, the chest muscles and diaphragm relax, allowing air to

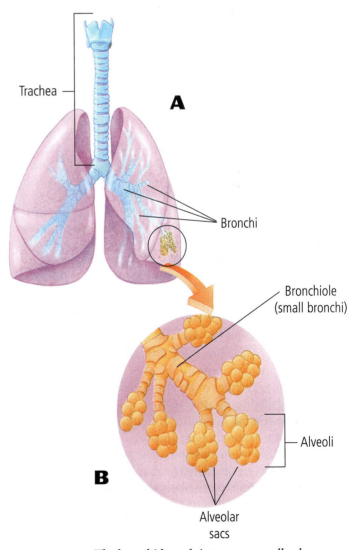

FIGURE 2-3 A *The bronchi branch into many small tubes.* **B** *Oxygen and carbon dioxide pass into and out of the blood through the cell walls of alveoli.*

INHALATION

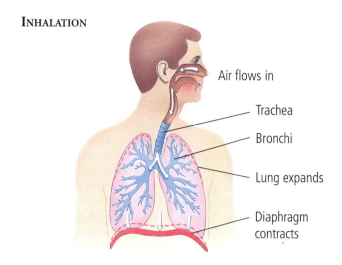

Air flows in

Trachea

Bronchi

Lung expands

Diaphragm contracts

EXHALATION

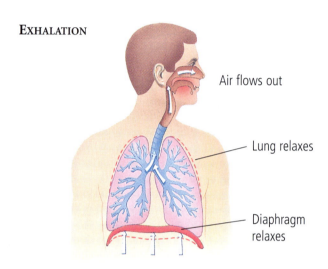

Air flows out

Lung relaxes

Diaphragm relaxes

FIGURE 2-4 *In the breathing process, the diaphragm and chest muscles contract and relax during inhalation and exhalation.*

exit the lungs (Figure 2-4). An adult breathes about 500 ml of air per breath. The average resting adult breathes about 15 to 20 times per minute. This ongoing breathing process is involuntary and is controlled by the brain.

Problems that Require First Aid

Because of the body's constant need for oxygen, you need to recognise breathing difficulties and give first aid immediately. Some causes of breathing difficulties are asthma, allergies or chest injuries. Breathing difficulty is called respiratory distress.

If a person has breathing difficulties, you may see or hear noisy breathing or gasping. The victim may be conscious or unconscious. The conscious victim may be anxious or excited or may feel short of breath. The victim's skin, particularly the lips and under the nails, may have a blue tint. This is called **cyanosis** and occurs when the tissues do not get enough oxygen.

If a person stops breathing, it is called respiratory arrest. Respiratory arrest is a life-threatening emergency. Without the oxygen obtained from breathing, other body systems fail to function. For example, if the

brain does not receive oxygen, it cannot send messages to the heart to beat. The heart will soon stop beating.

Respiratory problems require immediate attention. Making sure the airway is open and clear is an important first aid step. You may have to breathe for the non-breathing victim or give chest thrusts to someone who is choking. Breathing to ventilate the lungs of a non-breathing victim is called expired air resuscitation. These resuscitation skills are discussed in Chapter 4.

Because it is vital for the respiratory system to keep functioning, one of the first aider's priorities is to make sure the victim is breathing. The victim must always have adequate oxygen, or other systems will fail.

CIRCULATORY SYSTEM

The circulatory system works with the respiratory system to carry oxygen to every cell in the body. It also carries other nutrients throughout the body and removes waste. The circulatory system includes the heart, blood and blood vessels. Figure 2-5 shows this system in detail.

The heart is a muscular organ behind the sternum, or breastbone. The heart pumps blood throughout the body through **arteries** and **veins**. Arteries are large blood vessels which carry oxygen-rich blood from the heart to the rest of the body. The arteries subdivide into smaller blood vessels and ultimately become tiny capillaries. The capillaries transport blood to all the cells of the body and nourish them with oxygen. After the

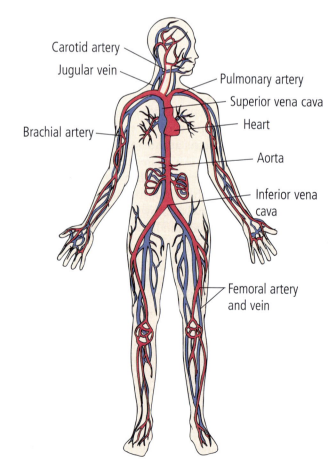

Carotid artery

Jugular vein

Pulmonary artery

Superior vena cava

Brachial artery

Heart

Aorta

Inferior vena cava

Femoral artery and vein

FIGURE 2-5 *The circulatory system.*

oxygen in the blood is given to the cells, veins carry the blood low in oxygen back to the heart. The heart pumps this blood to the lungs to pick up more oxygen, before pumping it to other parts of the body. This cycle is called the circulatory cycle. The cross-section of the heart in Figure 2-6 shows how blood moves through both sides of the heart to complete the circulatory cycle.

The pumping action of the heart is called a contraction. Contractions are controlled by the electrical system within the heart, which makes the heart beat regularly. You can feel the heart's contractions in the arteries that are close to the skin, for instance, at the neck or the wrist. The beat you feel with each contraction is called the **pulse**. You feel for the carotid pulse at the neck and the radial pulse at the wrist (Figures 2-7 and 2-8). The heart must beat regularly to deliver oxygen to body cells to keep the body functioning properly.

If an injury results in external or internal bleeding, the body reacts in several ways to minimise the blood loss. A damaged blood vessel contracts to slow or stop the leakage of blood which is escaping from the wound. Clots will form to plug the vessel and stop further bleeding (Figure 2-9). With heavier bleeding, the blood pressure is lowered so that blood escapes more slowly from the wound. Finally, with a large wound the arteries carrying blood to the muscles and skin constrict to keep more blood available for circulation to the vital organs such as the heart and brain. Later bodily processes include healing of the wound and defences against **infection.**

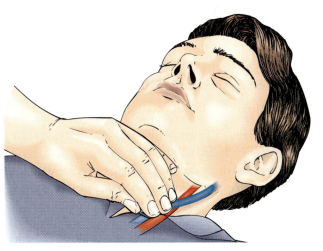

FIGURE 2-7 *The carotid artery.*

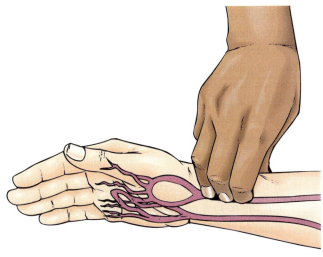

FIGURE 2-8 *A side view of the radial artery where a pulse can be felt.*

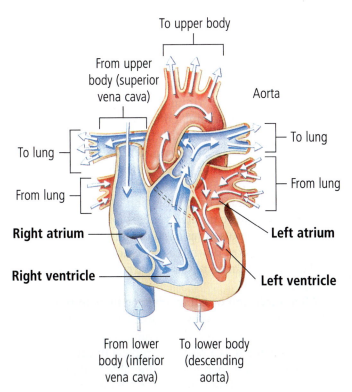

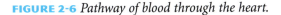

Oxygen-poor blood pumped from the body to the lungs.

Oxygen-rich blood pumped from the lungs to the body.

FIGURE 2-6 *Pathway of blood through the heart.*

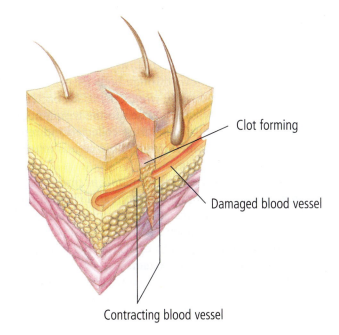

FIGURE 2-9 *Cross-section of damaged skin showing the body's reaction to minimise blood loss.*

Problems that Require First Aid

The following problems threaten the delivery of oxygen to body cells:

1. Blood loss caused by severe bleeding (example: a severed artery).

2. Impaired circulation (example: a blood clot).

3. Failure of the heart to pump adequately (example: a heart attack).

Body tissues which do not receive oxygen are damaged beyond recovery. For example, when one of the arteries supplying the brain with blood is blocked, brain tissue is damaged, resulting in a stroke. Likewise, when one of the arteries supplying the heart with blood is blocked, heart muscle tissue is damaged, resulting in a heart attack.

When someone has a heart attack, the heart functions irregularly and may stop. If the heart stops, breathing will also stop. When the heart stops beating, it is called cardiac arrest. Victims of heart attack or cardiac arrest need immediate first aid. Cardiac arrest victims need to have circulation maintained artificially by receiving external cardiac compressions and expired air resuscitation to maintain oxygen levels. This combination is called cardiopulmonary resuscitation, or CPR. You will learn more about the heart and how to perform CPR in Chapters 4 and 8.

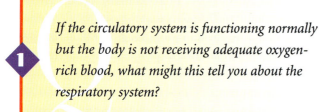

1 *If the circulatory system is functioning normally but the body is not receiving adequate oxygen-rich blood, what might this tell you about the respiratory system?*

LYMPHATIC SYSTEM

The lymphatic system consists of lymph, lymph vessels, lymph nodes and the spleen. **Lymph** is a fluid containing white cells which flows through body tissues to help the body fight infection. The white cells attack bacteria and move through the lymph vessels to the lymph nodes, where the infectious bacteria are collected and removed from blood and tissues. Lymph fluid is then returned to the general circulation.

Lymph nodes are grouped mainly in three body areas: the neck, armpits and groin area (Figure 2-10). Lymph is slow moving, and the lymphatic system circulates only approximately 2.5 litres of fluid per day, compared to the 10,000 litres of fluid per day moved through the circulatory system.

The spleen is also considered part of the lymphatic system because it contains lymph nodes.

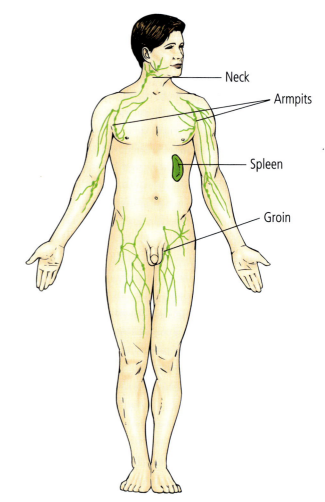

FIGURE 2-10 *The lymph nodes are grouped mainly in three areas of the body.*

Problems that Require First Aid

The lymphatic system responds to significant infection within the body. The lymph glands typically swell and become tender or painful. Often you can feel swollen lymph nodes in the neck with your fingers. Whenever the lymph glands are swollen or tender, the body is fighting an infection and the person should seek medical attention.

In first aid, an important function of the lymphatic system is to remove injected venoms following a bite or sting from a poisonous animal. The aim of first aid therefore is to slow down the movement of lymph and delay its eventual return to the circulation (see Chapter 10).

After a collision or fall involving a blow to the abdomen, the spleen may be damaged. Bleeding can be severe enough to be life-threatening. The spleen may become enlarged as a result of tropical infections, such as malaria, and is then more vulnerable to injury. First aid for bleeding is covered in Chapter 5.

The lymph system is also involved in the body's immunological functions. A disease such as AIDS (acquired immunological deficiency syndrome) also weakens the lymphatic system. Other diseases, such as some kinds of cancer, attack the lymph glands directly.

NERVOUS SYSTEM

The nervous system is the most complex and delicate of all body systems. The brain, the centre of the nervous system, is the master organ of the body. It regulates all body functions, including the respiratory and circulatory systems. The primary functions of the brain can be divided into three categories. These are the sensory, motor and integrated functions of consciousness, memory, emotions and use of language. The brain transmits and receives information through a network of **nerves**. Figure 2-11 shows the nervous system in detail. The **spinal cord**, a large bundle of nerves, extends from the brain through a canal in the spine, or backbone. Nerves extend from the brain and spinal cord to every part of the body.

Nerves transmit information as electrical impulses from one area of the body to another. Some nerves conduct impulses from the body to the brain. This allows you to see, hear, smell, taste and touch. These are the sensory functions. Other nerves conduct impulses from the brain to the muscles to control the motor functions, or movement (Figure 2-12).

The integrated functions of the brain are more complex. One of these functions is consciousness. Normally, when you are awake, you are conscious. Being conscious means that you know who you are, where you are, the approximate date and time and what is happening around you. There are various degrees, or levels, of consciousness. Your level of consciousness can vary from being highly aware in certain situations to being less aware during periods of relaxation or sleep.

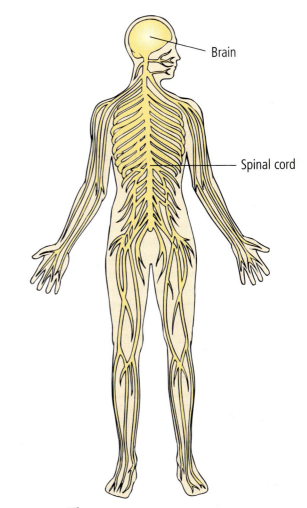

FIGURE 2-11 *The nervous system.*

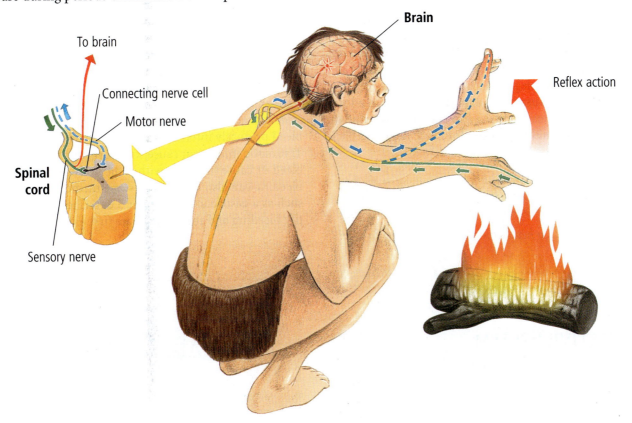

FIGURE 2-12 *Messages are sent to and from the brain along the nerves. A reflex action bypasses the normal pathway to give a quicker response to danger.*

If the body experiences a harmful stimulus, such as when one's hand touches a hot stove, the body's reflex action tries to move that body part away from the danger directly and quickly by bypassing the path of nerves to and from the brain. Similarly, coughing and swallowing are two vital reflexes that protect the airway.

Problems that Require First Aid

Unlike other body cells, brain cells cannot regenerate. Once brain cells are damaged, they are not replaced. Brain cells may be damaged by disease or injury. When a particular part of the brain is diseased or injured, the body functions controlled by that area of the brain may be lost forever. For example, if the part of the brain that regulates breathing is damaged, respiratory functions can be lost and the person may stop breathing.

A person's conscious state may be altered as a result of illness or injury. It may be affected by emotions, in which case the victim may be intensely aware of what is going on. At other times the victim's mind may seem to be dull, hazy or cloudy. Illness or injury affecting the brain can also alter memory, emotions and the ability to use language.

A head injury can cause a temporary loss of consciousness. Any head injury resulting in a loss of consciousness could cause brain injury and should be considered serious. These injuries require medical evaluation because injury to the brain can cause blood to pool within the skull. This puts pressure on the brain and limits the supply of oxygen to the brain cells. Without oxygen, brain cells die.

Injury to the spinal cord or a nerve can result in a permanent loss of feeling and movement below the injury. This loss of movement is called paralysis. For example, a lower back injury can result in paralysed legs (paraplegia); a neck injury can result in paralysis of all four limbs (quadriplegia). A broken **bone** or a deep wound can also cause nerve damage, resulting in a loss of sensation or movement. In a first aid course, you will learn about first aid techniques for head, neck and back injuries.

2 *How could a head injury cause breathing to stop?*

DIGESTIVE SYSTEM

The digestive system provides the body with substances needed to produce energy to keep all body cells alive and functioning. The two main functions of the digestive system are to take in and break down food into simple substances that can be absorbed into the blood to reach body tissues and to remove waste products.

Digestion begins in the mouth, where chewing and saliva start the process of breaking down food. Throughout the digestive system, digestive juices are secreted by glands to assist in continuing this process. From the mouth, food and liquid move through the **oesophagus** (also called the gullet) to the **stomach**, where it is partly digested by gastric juices. It then moves to the **small intestine**, which completes the digestive process. Here, the final substances, or nutrients, are absorbed into the blood.

The material remaining after digestion, including dietary fibre, moves to the **large intestine**. Here water and certain minerals are absorbed. The remaining waste is eliminated from the body through the rectum in the form of stools (faeces). The entire passage through which food passes, from the mouth to the anus, is called the **alimentary canal**.

Several other organs assist also in the digestive process. The liver and kidneys filter and remove unwanted substances. The gallbladder and pancreas assist with additional secretions important in the digestive process.

Figure 2.13 shows the main organs of the digestive system.

Problems that Require First Aid

The digestive system can be affected by many different illnesses. However, most of these do not occur suddenly or require immediate first aid. Two of the most serious first aid problems involving the gastrointestinal system are poisoning and bleeding.

Poisons are substances with toxic effects which enter the body. Poisons which are swallowed can be absorbed into the bloodstream quickly and produce a range of effects throughout the body, including organ damage or death. Chapter 10 describes in detail poisoning and the appropriate first aid.

Bleeding can occur at any point in the gastrointestinal system. Many organs, such as the liver and stomach, are richly supplied by blood vessels and can bleed profusely internally or externally if injured. Traumatic injury can cause some organs to burst and bleed or cause infection within the body. Internal bleeding can also occur from some medical conditions such as a gastric ulcer. Chapter 5 describes how to identify bleeding and the appropriate first aid to give.

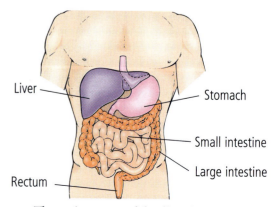

FIGURE 2-13 *The main organs of the digestive system.*

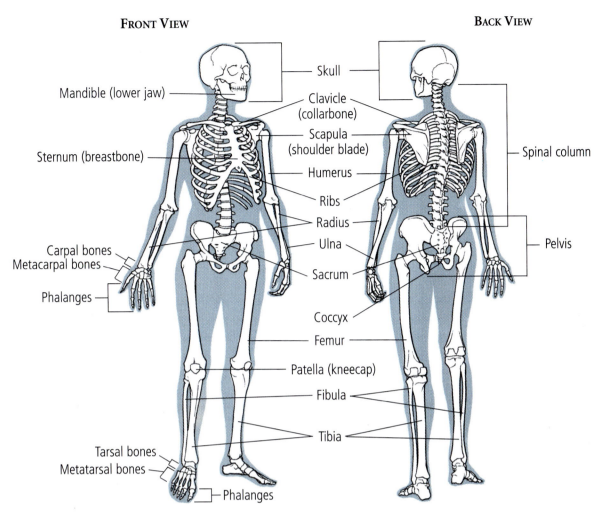

FRONT VIEW

BACK VIEW

- Skull
- Mandible (lower jaw)
- Clavicle (collarbone)
- Scapula (shoulder blade)
- Sternum (breastbone)
- Humerus
- Ribs
- Radius
- Spinal column
- Carpal bones
- Metacarpal bones
- Ulna
- Phalanges
- Sacrum
- Pelvis
- Coccyx
- Femur
- Patella (kneecap)
- Fibula
- Tibia
- Tarsal bones
- Metatarsal bones
- Phalanges

FIGURE 2-14 *The skeleton.*

MUSCULOSKELETAL SYSTEM

The musculoskeletal system consists of the bones, muscles, ligaments and tendons. This system performs several functions:

- Supporting the body.
- Protecting internal organs.
- Allowing movement.
- Storing minerals and producing blood cells.
- Producing heat.

Bones and Ligaments

The body has over 200 bones. Bone is hard, dense tissue that forms the skeleton. The skeleton forms the framework that supports the body (Figure 2-14). Where two or more bones join, they form a joint. Figure 2-15 shows a typical joint. Bones are usually held together at joints by fibrous bands called ligaments. You will notice that bones vary in size and shape. This variation allows bones to perform specific functions.

The bones of the skull protect the brain. The spine is made of bones called vertebrae that protect the spinal cord. The ribs attach to the spine and to the breastbone, forming a protective shell for vital organs such as the heart and lungs.

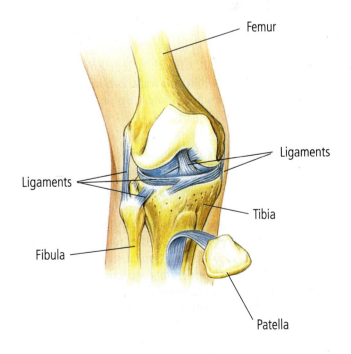

- Femur
- Ligaments
- Ligaments
- Tibia
- Fibula
- Patella

FIGURE 2-15 *A typical joint consists of two or more bones held together by ligaments.*

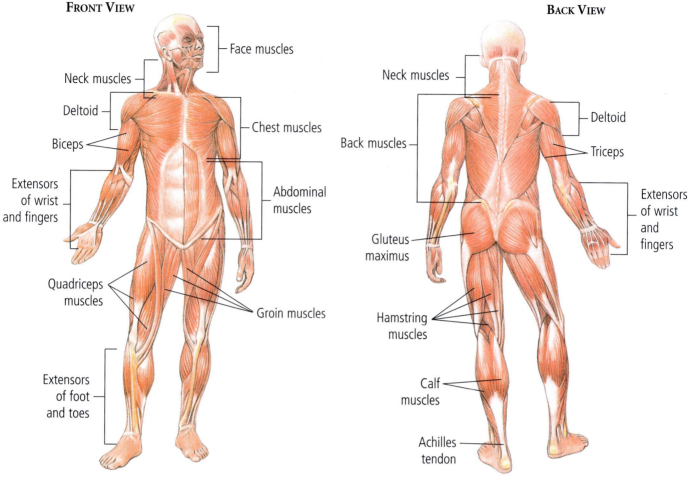

FRONT VIEW

Face muscles

Neck muscles

Deltoid

Biceps

Chest muscles

Extensors of wrist and fingers

Abdominal muscles

Quadriceps muscles

Groin muscles

Extensors of foot and toes

BACK VIEW

Neck muscles

Back muscles

Deltoid

Triceps

Extensors of wrist and fingers

Gluteus maximus

Hamstring muscles

Calf muscles

Achilles tendon

FIGURE 2-16 *The muscular system.*

In addition to supporting and protecting the body, bones aid movement. The bones of the arms and legs work like a system of levers and pulleys to position the hands and feet so they can function. Bones of the wrist, hand and fingers are progressively smaller to allow for fine movements such as writing. The small bones of the feet enable you to walk smoothly. Together they work as shock absorbers when you walk, run or jump.

Bones also store minerals and help produce blood cells.

Muscles and Tendons

Muscles are made of special tissue that can lengthen and shorten, resulting in movement. Figure 2-16 shows the major muscles of the body. Tendons are tissues that attach muscles to bones. Muscles band together to form muscle groups, which work together to produce movement (Figure 2-17). Working muscles produce heat. Muscles also protect underlying structures such as bones, nerves and blood vessels.

Muscle action is controlled by the nervous system. Nerves carry information from the muscles to the brain. The brain processes this information and directs the muscles to move by way of the nerves. Figure 2-18 (see page 23) shows how the brain sends signals to muscles, directing them to move.

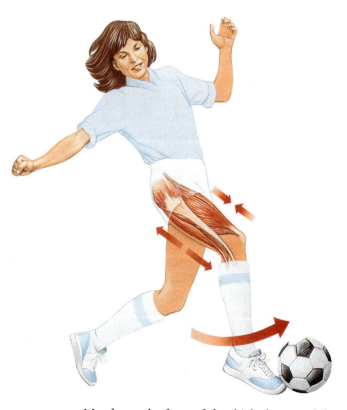

FIGURE 2-17 *Muscles at the front of the thigh shorten while muscles at the back of the thigh lengthen, allowing the lower leg to swing forward.*

HOW DO YOU CATCH A SOFTBALL?

The softball flies through the air, spinning back in your direction. In a few seconds, it is in your glove and you are preparing to throw it back. But what really happens? How do you catch a softball?

1. The left and the right eye each transmit the softball's image to the brain through electrical impulses that travel at a speed of up to 100 metres per second.

2. The brain receives the image and then calculates the softball's path and the speed at which it is travelling.

3. The brain also transmits electrical impulses to muscles in your arms and legs to reposition. As you reach for the softball, the pelvis and vertebral column move to compensate for the change in balance. Tiny muscles and bones in the hand move the glove into position and tighten it around the ball as it falls into the pocket. ■

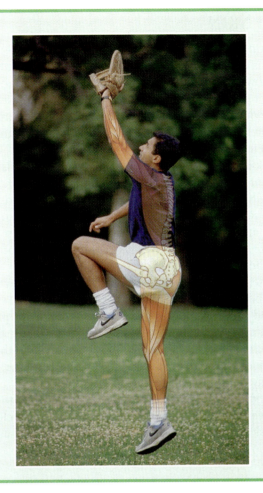

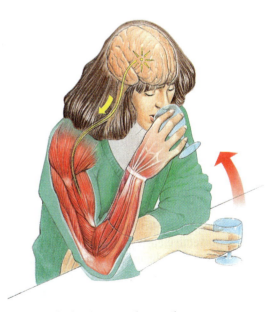

FIGURE 2-18 *The brain controls muscle movement.*

Muscle actions may be involuntary or voluntary. Involuntary muscles, such as the heart, diaphragm and intestines, are automatically controlled by the brain. You don't have to think about making them work. For example, the heart beats between 60 and 80 beats per minute without any direction from you. Voluntary muscles, such as leg and arm muscles, are under your conscious control.

Problems that Require First Aid

Injuries to bones and muscles include fractures, dislocations, strains and sprains. A fracture is a broken bone. Dislocations occur when bones of a joint are moved out of place. Strains are injuries to muscles and tendons, whereas sprains are injuries to ligaments. Although injuries to bones and muscles may not look serious, nearby nerves, blood vessels and organs may be damaged. Regardless of how they appear, these injuries may cause lifelong disabilities or become life-threatening emergencies. For example, torn ligaments in the knee can limit activities, and broken ribs can puncture the lungs and threaten breathing.

When you give first aid, you should remember that injuries to muscles and bones often result in additional injuries. You will learn how to provide first aid for musculoskeletal injuries in Chapter 14.

 Describe how a fractured leg could be a life-threatening emergency.

THE SKIN

The skin, along with the hair and nails (Figure 2-19), protects the body and helps keep fluids in. It prevents infection by keeping disease-producing micro-organisms, or germs, out. The skin is made of tough, elastic fibres which stretch without easily tearing, preventing the skin from injury. The skin also helps make vitamin D, and it stores minerals.

The outer surface of the skin is made of dead cells which are continually rubbed away and replaced by new cells. The skin contains the hair roots, oil glands and sweat glands. Oil glands help to keep the skin soft, supple and waterproof. Sweat glands and pores help regulate body temperature. The nervous system monitors blood temperature and causes you to sweat if blood temperature rises even slightly. Sweat often evaporates before you even see it on the skin.

Blood supplies the skin with nutrients and helps provide skin with its colour. When blood vessels dilate, the blood circulates close to the skin's surface, making the skin appear flushed, or red, and feel warm. However, you may not be able to recognise this reddening in people with darker skin. On the other hand, when the blood vessels constrict, there is not as much blood close to the skin's surface. As a result, the skin looks pale and feels cool.

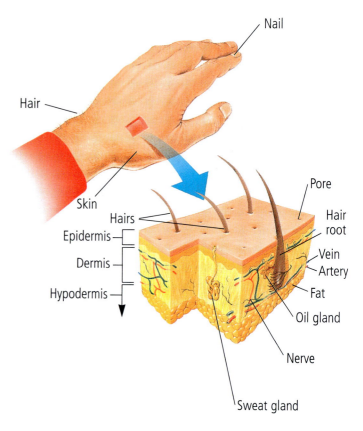

FIGURE 2-19 *The structures of the skin, hair and nails.*

TOO MUCH OF A GOOD THING

Contrary to what some people believe, being tanned is not healthy—in fact, it is a sign of skin damage. Although some sun stimulates your skin to produce vitamin D for healthy bones, prolonged exposure can cause problems such as skin cancer and premature ageing.

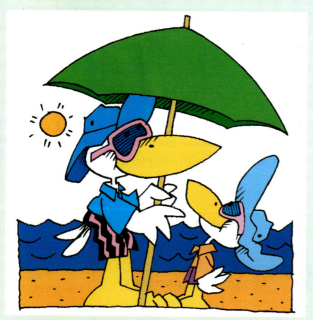

(Sid Seagull and "slip, slop, slap" are reproduced with the kind permission of the Anti-Cancer Council of Victoria.)

Sunlight has two kinds of ultraviolet light rays in it. Ultraviolet beta rays (UVB) cause sunburns and skin cancer. These rays damage the skin's surface. Ultraviolet alpha rays (UVA) have been considered safe by many, but they, too, are dangerous. UVA rays more readily penetrate the deeper layers of the skin, which increases the risk of skin cancer, skin ageing and eye damage and contributes to skin changes that lessen the skin's ability to fight disease.

To be safe, begin by limiting your exposure. Avoid the sun between 10 am and 2 pm (11 am to 3 pm during daylight saving time), even on cool or cloudy days. Wear protective clothing, including a broad-brimmed hat, and apply an SPF 15+ broad-spectrum sunscreen to all remaining areas of exposed skin.

Wearing close-fitting sunglasses that conform to the Australian Standard AS 1067 (check the tag before you purchase them) will help protect your eyes, especially where there is strong glare or reflected light, such as in the snow or near water.

By following these simple guidelines, you can avoid exposure to radiation and significantly reduce your risk of skin cancer and premature ageing of the skin.

The next time the sun beckons, *slip* on a shirt, *slop* on a protective sunscreen and *slap* on a hat. Then go outside and have a great time! ■

Nerves in the skin make it very sensitive to sensations such as touch, pain and temperature. Therefore, the skin is also an important part of the body's communication network.

Problems that Require First Aid

Although the skin is tough, it can be injured. Sharp objects may puncture, slice or tear the skin. Rough objects can scrape it, and extreme heat or cold may burn or freeze it. Burns and skin injuries that cause bleeding may result in the loss of vital fluids. Germs may enter the body where there are breaks in the skin, causing infection, which may become a serious problem.

In later chapters, you will learn how to care for wounds, burns and heat and cold emergencies.

After vigorous exercise, your skin is flushed, you perspire profusely and you breathe heavily, that is, your musculoskeletal and respiratory systems work harder during exercise. Explain why your skin becomes flushed and why you perspire profusely. Give specific reasons for these conditions.

If someone experiences difficulty in breathing, what other body systems might be affected? Explain why?

Table 2-1

SUMMARY OF BODY SYSTEMS

System	Major structures	Primary functions	How the body system works with other body systems
Respiratory system	Airways and lungs	Supplies the body with the oxygen it needs through breathing.	Works with the circulatory system to provide oxygen to cells; is under the control of the nervous system.
Circulatory system	Heart, blood vessels and blood	Transports nutrients and oxygen to body cells and removes waste products.	Works with the respiratory system to provide oxygen to cells; works with the urinary and digestive systems to remove waste products; helps give skin colour; is under the control of the nervous system.
Lymphatic system	Lymph, lymph nodes and spleen	Fights infection.	Works with the circulatory system to remove infectious material from tissues and blood.
Nervous system	Brain, spinal cord and nerves	One of two primary regulatory systems in the body; transmits messages to and from the brain.	The brain regulates all body systems through networks of nerves.
Digestive system	Oesophagus, stomach, small and large intestines	Breaks down food and liquids into substances the body can use.	Works with the circulatory system to absorb nutrients into the blood.
Musculoskeletal system	Bones, ligaments, muscles and tendons	Provides body's framework; protects internal organs and other underlying structures; allows movement; produces heat; manufactures blood components.	Muscles and bones provide protection to organs and structures of other body systems; muscle action is controlled by the nervous system.
Skin	Skin, hair and nails	Skin is an important part of the body's communication network; prevents infection and dehydration; assists with temperature regulation; aids in production of certain vitamins.	Skin helps to protect the body from disease-producing organisms; together with the circulatory system, helps to regulate body temperature under the control of the nervous system; communicates sensation to the brain by way of the nerves.

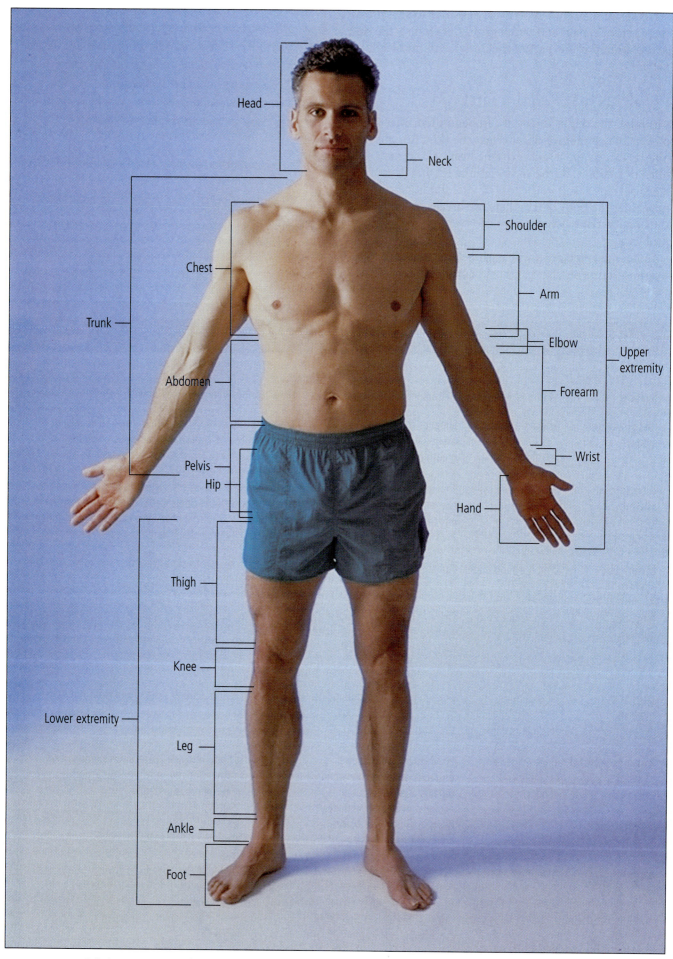

FIGURE 2-20 *It is important to refer correctly to the parts of the body.*

HOW BODY SYSTEMS WORK TOGETHER

Each body system plays a vital role in survival. Body systems work together to help the body maintain a constant healthy state. When the environment changes, body systems adapt to the new conditions. For example, because your musculoskeletal system works harder when you exercise, your respiratory and circulatory systems must also work harder to meet your body's increased oxygen demands.

None of the body systems works independently. The impact of an injury or a disease is rarely isolated to one body system, especially when the brain is affected. For example, a broken bone may result in nerve damage that will impair movement and feeling. Injuries to the ribs can make breathing difficult. If the heart stops beating for any reason, breathing will also stop.

In any significant illness or injury, body systems may be seriously affected. This may result in a progressive failure of body systems. This failure is called shock. Shock is caused by the inability of the circulatory system to provide adequate oxygen-rich blood to all parts of the body, especially the vital organs.

Generally, the more body systems involved in an emergency, the more serious the emergency. Body systems depend on each other for survival. In cases of serious injury or illness, the body may not be able to keep functioning. In these cases, regardless of your best efforts, the victim may die.

REFERENCING PARTS OF THE BODY

When describing an injury or illness, it helps to use standard terms for body parts that health professionals will understand. Examine Figure 2-20 to learn the exact parts of the body to which these standard terms refer.

Summary

- The body includes a number of systems, all of which must work together for the body to function properly.
- The brain controls all body functions, including those of the skin, circulatory, digestive, musculoskeletal, nervous and respiratory systems.

- An illness or injury that affects one body system can have a serious impact on another system.
- Basic first aid is usually all that is needed to support injured body systems until more advanced care can be given.

Answers to Application Questions

1. If the circulatory system is pumping blood but is still unable to deliver oxygen-rich blood to the body, there may be a problem with the respiratory system. It could be an oxygen supply problem. The airway could be blocked or injured, or an illness that affects the lungs might be preventing adequate oxygen from entering the circulatory system.

2. A head injury may result in a condition such as pooling of blood in the skull or a blood clot that would interrupt blood flow to brain cells. If oxygen flow to brain cells is interrupted, they can die from lack of oxygen and their functions may be lost forever. If a head injury interrupts the flow of oxygen to the brain cells that control respiration, it would cause breathing to stop.

3. A fractured leg could be a life-threatening emergency if the fracture caused other injuries or conditions such as a severed artery, blood clot, internal bleeding, severe bleeding, infection, shock or unconsciousness.

4. For working muscles to function, they require increased amounts of oxygen. Therefore, your respiratory system works harder to meet the demands of the muscles. As more oxygen is brought into the body, blood flow increases and blood vessels dilate to deliver it. Your skin is flushed because of the increased blood flow near the skin's surface. In addition to demanding more oxygen, your working muscles produce heat and cause body temperature to rise. Sweating is your body's way of cooling off and thus regulating body temperature.

5. Breathing difficulty may affect any or all other body systems because a lack of oxygen results in tissue dysfunction and eventually tissue death. Furthermore, once the oxygen supply to the brain is limited, the brain may become unable to control body functions. The functions of the nervous, musculoskeletal and all other body systems will be severely impaired or will fail.

Study Questions

1.   *Complete the table with the correct system, structures or function(s).*

System	Structures	Function(s)
a. _____	b. _____	Supplies the body with the oxygen it needs through breathing.
c. _____	Heart, blood, blood vessels.	d. _____
Skin	e. _____	f. _____
Musculoskeletal	g. _____	h. _____
i. _____	j. _____	Regulates all body functions; a communications network.

2.   *Match each term with the correct definition.*

  a.   Airway.
  b.   Arteries.
  c.   Cell.
  d.   Bone.
  e.   Muscle.
  f.   Skin.
  g.   Nerve.
  h.   Infection.
  i.   Pulse.
  j.   Spinal cord.
  k.   Lungs.
  l.   Respiration.
  m.   Brain.
  n.   Shock.
  o.   Veins.

_____ Blood vessels that carry oxygen-poor blood to the heart.

_____ Dense, hard tissue that forms the skeleton.

_____ Process of breathing.

_____ Regulates all body functions.

_____ Conducts impulses between the brain and all parts of the body.

_____ Basic unit of living tissue.

_____ A pair of organs in the chest that provides the mechanism for taking in oxygen and removing carbon dioxide during breathing.

_____ Beat created by each contraction of the heart; felt in arteries near the skin's surface.

_____ Pathway for air from the mouth and nose to the lungs.

_____ A tissue that lengthens and shortens to produce movement.

_____ Condition caused by germs in the body.

_____ A tough membrane that covers the entire surface of the body.

_____ A large bundle of nerves extending from the brain through the spinal column.

_____ Blood vessels that carry oxygen-rich blood to all parts of the body.

_____ The failure of the circulatory system to provide adequate oxygen-rich blood to body parts, especially vital organs.

In questions 3 to 6, circle the letter of the correct answer.

3. **Which of the following could result from breathing difficulty or other problems of the respiratory system?**

   a. Cardiac arrest.
   b. No delivery of oxygen to body parts via the circulatory system.
   c. Brain cell death.
   d. All of the above.

4. **The respiratory system works with other body systems to provide oxygen to all body cells. These systems include the:**

   a. circulatory and nervous systems
   b. nervous system
   c. musculoskeletal, nervous and circulatory systems
   d. musculoskeletal and circulatory systems

5. **A blood clot in the brain could cut off all blood flow to brain cells. Which body systems would fail to function?**

   a. Nervous system.
   b. All body systems.
   c. Circulatory and respiratory systems.
   d. Nervous and respiratory systems.

6. **The human body rapidly adapts to new environments. For example, when you step outside an airconditioned building on a hot summer day you immediately begin to sweat. Your body adapts to its 'new' environment. What systems work together to produce this specific adaptation?**

   a. Nervous and musculoskeletal systems.
   b. Skin and respiratory systems.
   c. Circulatory and respiratory systems.
   d. Skin and nervous systems.

7. **Why can an injury to the spinal cord or a nerve result in paralysis?**

Answers are in Appendix A (page 360).

Responding to Emergencies

WHEN YOU ENCOUNTER a victim who has been injured in an accident or suddenly becomes ill, you follow four basic emergency action principles regardless of the specific situation or the victim's condition. These principles are a guide to the first aid you give and they provide the victim with the best opportunity for recovery.

This chapter outlines how to follow the emergency action principles to ensure your safety and that of others in any emergency, to check for life-threatening situations and to provide care for the victim.

For Review

A review of how the respiratory and circulatory systems function will help your understanding of the chapter.

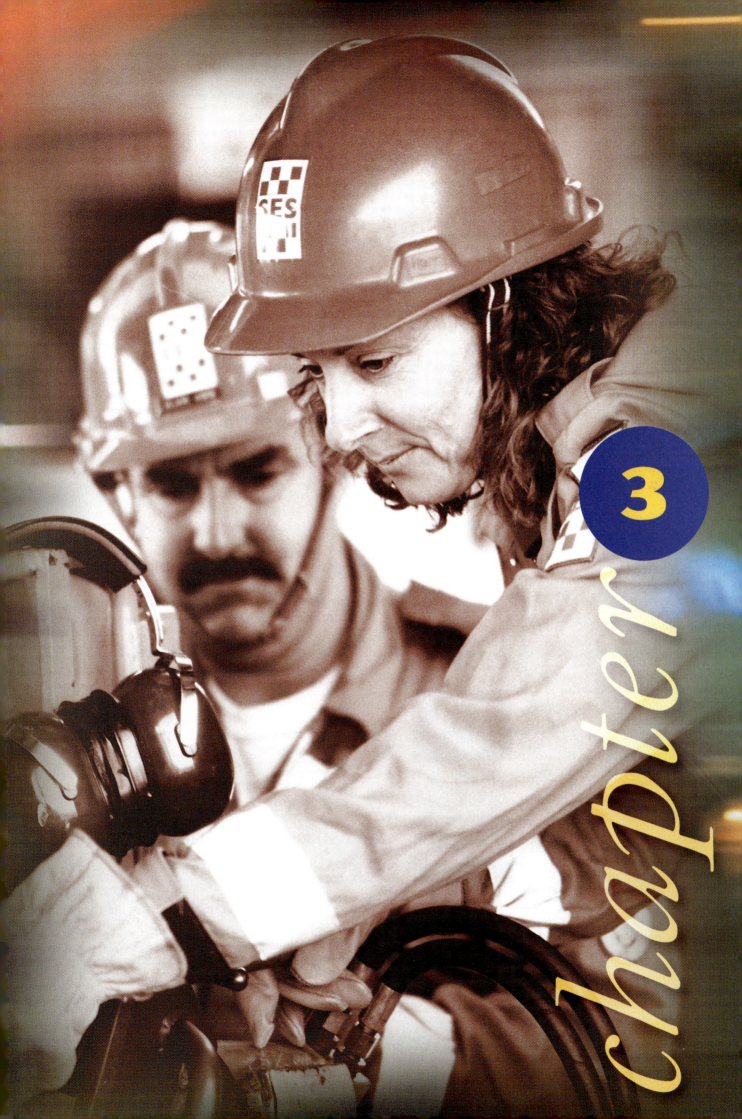

chapter

3

Key Terms

Carotid (*ca-rot-id*) **arteries:** Major blood vessels that supply blood to the head and neck.

Consent: Permission given by the victim to the first aider.

CPR: Cardiopulmonary Resuscitation.

EAR: Expired Air resuscitation.

ECC: External Cardiac Compression.

Emergency action principles: Four steps to guide your actions in any emergency.

Primary survey: A check for life-threatening conditions.

Radial arteries: Blood vessels near the surface of the skin at the wrist, where the pulse is commonly taken.

Secondary survey: A check for injuries or conditions that could become life-threatening if not cared for.

Vital signs: Important information about the victim's condition from checking breathing, pulse and skin characteristics.

On your way home, you notice that a car has veered off the road and landed in the ditch. You decide there may be an emergency. After surveying the scene and deciding it is safe, you approach the car. As you come closer, you see a woman lying on the ground, near the car. But you also notice a strong smell of petrol. What should you do? Is there a danger? Should you move her away from the car or try to care for her there?

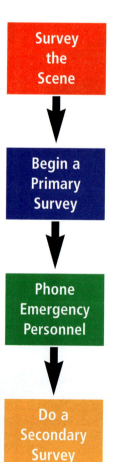

In Chapter 1 you learned that with your first aid training you can make a difference in an emergency—you may even save a life. You learned how to recognise an emergency, how to respond, and how to prevent and prepare for emergencies. Most importantly, you learned that your decision to act is vital to the victim's survival. You can always do something to help.

In this chapter, you will learn a plan of action to guide you through any emergency. When an emergency occurs, you may at first feel confused. But you can train yourself to remain calm and to think before you act. Ask yourself, "What do I need to do? How can I help most effectively?" The four **emergency action principles** answer these questions. They are your plan of action for any emergency.

EMERGENCY ACTION PRINCIPLES

The emergency action principles are:

1. Survey the scene.
2. Do a **primary survey** and care for life-threatening problems.
3. Call emergency personnel for help.
4. Do a **secondary survey,** when appropriate, and care for additional problems.

These actions, done in this order, can ensure your safety and that of the victim and other bystanders, and increase the victim's chance of survival.

Survey the Scene

Once you recognise that an emergency has occurred and decide to act, you must make sure the emergency scene is safe for you and any bystanders. Take time to survey the scene and answer these questions:

1. Is the scene safe?

2. What happened?

3. How many victims are there?

4. Can bystanders help?

When you survey the scene, look for anything that may threaten your safety and that of the victim and bystanders. Examples of dangers that may be present are fallen power lines, falling rocks, traffic, fire, smoke, dangerous fumes, extreme weather and deep or swift-moving water (Figure 3-1). *If any of these or other dangers are threatening, do not approach the victim. Call emergency personnel immediately for help.*

Nothing is gained by risking your own safety. An emergency that begins with one victim could end up with two if you are hurt. Leave dangerous situations for emergency professionals who have the training and proper equipment to handle them. If you suspect the scene is unsafe, wait and watch until emergency personnel arrive. If conditions change, you may then be able to approach the victim.

Find out what happened. Look around for clues about what caused the emergency and the type and extent of the victim's injuries. By looking around, you may discover a situation that requires your immediate action. As you approach the victim, take in the whole picture. Nearby objects, such as shattered glass, a fallen ladder or a spilled bottle of medicine, might tell you what happened. If the victim is unconscious, your survey of the scene may be the only way to tell what happened.

Look carefully for more than one victim because you may not spot everyone at first. For example, in a car crash, an open door may be a clue that a victim has left or was thrown from the car. If one victim is bleeding or screaming loudly, you may overlook another victim who is silent and unconscious. It is also easy to overlook an infant or small child. Ask anyone present how many people may be involved. If you find more than one victim, ask bystanders for help.

Look for bystanders who can help or who may be able to tell you what happened or help in other ways. A bystander who knows the victim may know of any

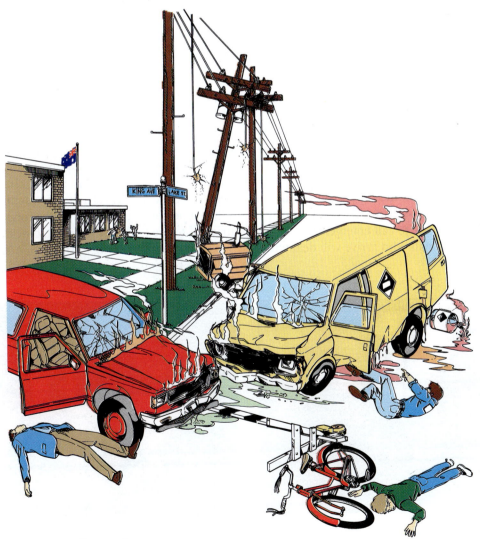

FIGURE 3-1 *Survey the scene.*

relevant medical problems or allergies. Bystanders may call emergency professionals for help, meet and direct the ambulance to your location, keep the area free of unnecessary traffic or help you provide care. If there is no one nearby, shout for help to summon someone who can help you.

Once You Reach the Victim

Once you reach the victim, quickly survey the scene again to see if it is still safe. At this point, you may see other dangers, clues to what happened, or victims and bystanders that you did not notice before.

As a rule, do not move a victim unless there is an immediate danger such as a fire, poisonous fumes or an unstable structure. In this case, try to move the victim as quickly as possible without making the situation worse. If there is no immediate danger, tell the victim not to move. Warn bystanders not to move the victim.

Identify yourself

When you approach, try not to alarm the victim. Try to position yourself close to the victim's eye level (Figure 3-2). Speak in a calm and positive manner. Identify yourself to the victim and bystanders. Ask if you can help. Tell them that you have some first aid training. This may provide some reassurance.

Before giving first aid, you must get a conscious victim's permission to give that person care, if the person is able to communicate. This permission is called **consent**. A conscious victim has the right to either refuse or accept care.

In an emergency where a person is unconscious or bleeding seriously and unable to communicate, the law will infer the consent of the injured person. However, the consent will apply only to conditions that threaten the life or the future health of that person.

With an infant or child, ask the supervising adult for consent. If a person refuses your help, stay nearby if possible and ask someone to call emergency personnel. The professionals who arrive will deal with the situation.

Perform a Primary Survey For Life-Threatening Conditions

In every emergency situation, you must first look for conditions that are an immediate threat to the victim's life. This second emergency action principle is called the primary survey. In the primary survey, you check each of the following:

- Conscious state.
- Airway.
- Breathing.
- Circulation.
- Severe bleeding.

The steps of the primary survey are summarised in the basic life support flow chart shown on page 35.

Determine if the Victim is Conscious

Begin the primary survey by determining if the victim is conscious by the "shake and shout" technique (Figure 3-3):

1. Shake the victim gently by the shoulders.
2. Ask: "What is your name?"
3. Give a simple command such as "Squeeze my hand, now let it go."

A victim who responds to you is conscious and breathing and has a pulse. Let a conscious victim adopt the position of greatest comfort. Once you are sure there are no life-threatening conditions needing attention, you can begin the secondary survey (page 38). Continue to observe the victim's conscious state and check that the condition remains stable. Preferably allow 10 to 15 minutes for recovery before letting the victim move.

A victim who does not respond is unconscious. If you are alone and the victim is unconscious, shout for help. Unconsciousness is a life-threatening condition. When a person is unconscious, the tongue relaxes and may fall to the back of the throat, blocking the airway. This can cause breathing to stop. Soon after, the heart will stop beating.

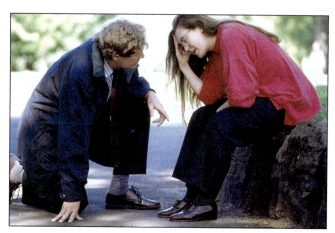

FIGURE 3-2 *When talking to the victim, position yourself close to the victim's eye level and speak in a calm and positive manner.*

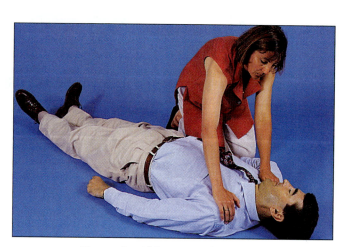

FIGURE 3-3 *Determine if the person is conscious.*

Basic Life Support Flow Chart

In the event of collapse, it is important that no time is wasted. Stay with the victim and follow the steps of the Basic Life Support Flow Chart:

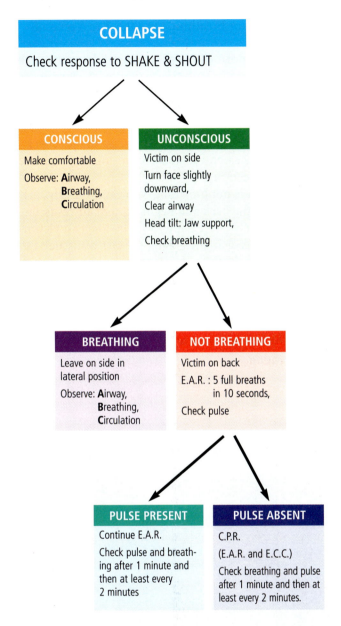

Source: Australian Resuscitation Council.

Unconscious victims cannot protect themselves from other dangers, such as oncoming traffic, hot road surfaces, fire or surf. The victim cannot maintain a clear airway, may stop breathing, or may die from uncontrolled bleeding. Skin and nerves may be damaged by pressure from hard objects.

If unconscious, position the victim on one side to maintain an open airway. Unconscious victims are at risk of choking because the ability to swallow and cough out any foreign objects is lost. This can lead to an obstructed upper airway, and material from the stomach may flow back up the oesophagus and enter the lungs.

Turning unconscious victims onto one side allows gravity to help drain any material from the mouth. You should remove any visible material with your fingers.

In addition to opening the airway and helping drain out foreign material, turning unconscious victims onto the side helps to:

- provide easy access to the airway
- minimise bending and twisting of the neck
- permit continuation of observation of the victim
- facilitate expansion of the chest.

With an unconscious victim, care of the airway takes precedence over any injury, including the possibility of a broken neck, but all unconscious victims must be handled gently with no twisting or forward movement of the head and neck.

If possible, have someone help you when you move the victim. This person should support the head.

Do not give an unconscious victim anything by mouth or attempt to make the victim vomit.

After positioning the unconscious victim on the side, next you must check the airway, breathing and circulation. Remembering these steps is easy. The three steps are called the ABC of the primary survey:

Remember:

A = *Airway.*

B = *Breathing.*

C = *Circulation.*

Check the Airway

When an unconscious victim is lying face-up, gravity lets the jaw drop backwards. The mouth falls open but this tends to block rather than open the airway. Because the victim is unconscious, the muscles are relaxed and the tongue falls against the back wall of the mouth and blocks air from entering and leaving the lungs. The soft palate, which is also made of muscle, may contribute to blockage of the airway. Turning the victim on the side prevents this obstruction.

In addition to the tongue and soft palate, other causes of upper airway obstruction include:

- Solid or semi-solid material such as food, vomit, blood or a foreign body.
- Laryngeal spasm.
- Swelling or injury of the airway.

When the victim is positioned on the side, quickly clear the mouth of any visible foreign material, using your fingers. Remove dentures only if they are broken or are so loose that they may block the airway. Do not probe down the throat with your fingers if you do not see anything to remove as you may accidentally push material further into the airway or cause damage inside the mouth.

Tilt the head backward by placing one hand on the top of the head. Support the jaw at the point of the chin with the other hand, without using force. Turn the victim's face slightly downwards to enable fluid or mucus to drain from the mouth.

Figure 3-4 shows this process of positioning the victim, clearing the mouth and tilting the head.

Jaw Support

You may need to support the victim's jaw to keep an open airway when the victim is on the side. Use a "pistol-grip" technique as follows:

1. Support the jaw at the point of the chin without putting any pressure on the soft tissues of the neck.

2. Support the point of the chin with the knuckle of your middle finger, with the little and ring fingers clear of the soft tissues of the neck. Keep your index finger along the line of the jaw.

3. Put your thumb along the front of the lower jaw between the lower lip and the point of the chin, using it to open the mouth slightly.

Check Breathing

After opening the airway, check for breathing. A conscious person who can speak, cough or cry is breathing. However, you may not know if an unconscious person is breathing until you check.

If the victim is breathing, the chest will rise and fall. However, chest movement by itself does not mean air is reaching the lungs. You must also listen and feel for signs of breathing. Position yourself so you can hear and feel air as it escapes from the nose and mouth. At the same time, watch the rise and fall of the lower chest and upper abdomen. Take the time to look, listen and feel for breathing for a full 3 to 5 seconds (Figure 3-5).

If breathing normally, keep the victim lying in a stable position on the side, with the head tilted backward, jaw supported and face pointed slightly downwards to keep the airway open. Ensure that someone calls for emergency help.

If the victim's breathing is noisy or laboured, check the airway very carefully. Noisy breathing may indicate a partial obstruction.

If the victim is not breathing, you must quickly turn the victim on the back and begin expired air resuscitation immediately (see Chapter 4). The longer a victim goes without oxygen, the greater the risk of tissue damage and/or death.

1 *Why is it necessary to look, listen and feel for breathing?*

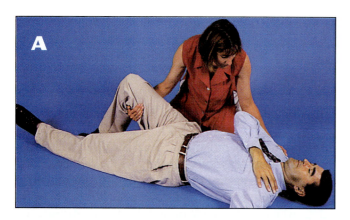

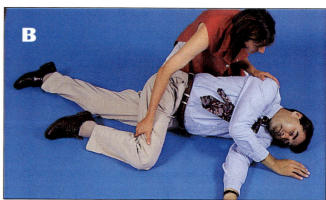

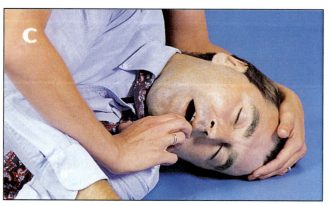

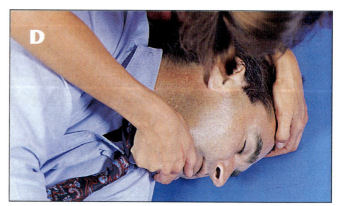

FIGURE 3-4 A *Prepare to turn the victim on the side.* **B** *The victim on the side in the lateral position.* **C** *Clear the mouth of any foreign matter using your fingers.* **D** *Tilt the victim's head to open the airway.*

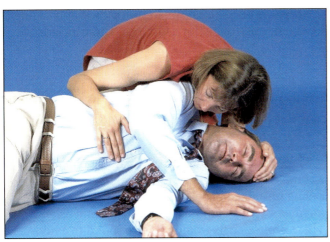

FIGURE 3-5 *To check for breathing, look, listen and feel for breathing for up to 5 seconds.*

Check Circulation

The last step in the primary survey is checking for the circulation of blood. If the heart has stopped, blood will not circulate throughout the body. If this happens, the victim will die in just a few minutes because the brain is not getting any oxygen. The victim will need cardiopulmonary resuscitation (CPR) to maintain life (see Chapter 4).

If a person is breathing, the heart is beating and is circulating blood. You determine the rate and rhythm of the heart by checking the radial pulse. This is covered in greater detail later in this chapter in the section on the secondary survey (page 38).

Check for severe bleeding

Checking circulation also means looking for severe bleeding. Bleeding is severe when blood spurts from the wound or cannot be controlled. Check for severe bleeding by looking quickly from head to toe for signs of external bleeding. Severe bleeding must be controlled as soon as possible. (Bleeding is dealt with in detail in Chapter 5.)

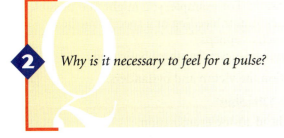

2 *Why is it necessary to feel for a pulse?*

3 *Why must severe bleeding be controlled as soon as possible?*

Summary of the Primary Survey

The primary survey lets you know of any life-threatening conditions that need to be cared for immediately. Check the conscious state, the airway, breathing and circulation. Call emergency personnel or send someone else to call as soon as you determine the victim is unconscious and have cleared and opened the airway.

The Practice Guide at the end of this chapter (on page 46) details the steps of the primary survey.

Call Emergency Personnel

The third emergency action principle is to get professional help to the victim as soon as you can. The ambulance service works more effectively if you can give information about the victim's condition when the call is placed. The information you provide will help to ensure that the victim receives proper medical care as quickly as possible. By calling the emergency number, you put into motion a response system that rushes the appropriate emergency care personnel to the victim.

Making the Call

You can ask a bystander to call the emergency number for you, stating the victim's condition. For example, say "Call the emergency number. Tell them the victim is a child with a leg injury." Sending someone else to make the call will enable you to stay with the victim to provide needed care (Figure 3-6).

When you tell someone to call for help:

1. Send a bystander, or possibly two, to make the call.
2. Tell the caller to ring 000. (In some remote areas, there may be a local number to call.)
3. Tell the caller to give the operator the necessary information. Most operators will ask for the following important facts:
   a. Give the exact address or location of the emergency and the name of the city or town. Give the names of nearby cross streets or roads,

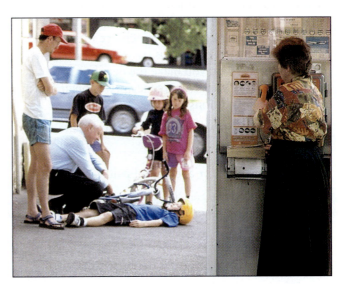

FIGURE 3-6 *Sending someone else to call the emergency number will enable you to stay with the victim.*

landmarks, the name of the building, the floor and the room number.

    b. Telephone number from which the call is being made.

    c. Caller's name.

    d. What happened—e.g., a car collision or fall.

    e. How many people are involved.

    f. Condition of the victim(s)—e.g., chest pain, trouble breathing, no pulse, bleeding.

    g. First aid being given.

4. Tell the caller not to hang up until the operator hangs up. Make sure the operator has all the information needed. The ambulance operator may also be able to give the caller instructions on how best to care for the victim until help arrives.

5. Tell the caller to report to you after making the call and tell you what the operator said.

If you are alone with the victim, shout for help. If the victim is unconscious and breathing and no-one comes at once to help you, you will need to get professional help fast. Turn the victim on the side and clear and open the airway. Find the nearest telephone as quickly as possible. Make the call and return to the victim promptly. Delay may result in death. On your return, immediately recheck the victim and give the necessary care. Do not leave a non-breathing victim.

With your first aid training, you can do two important things that can make a difference in the outcome of a seriously ill or injured person. You can give care for life-threatening problems and call emergency personnel as quickly as possible.

When to Call

At times, you may be unsure if emergency personnel are needed. For example, the victim may say not to call an ambulance because of embarrassment about creating a scene. Sometimes, you may be unsure if the severity of the victim's condition requires professional assistance. Remember, there is no charge for ambulance attendance unless the victim is transported. Your first aid training will help you make the decision.

As a general rule, call emergency personnel if any of the following conditions exist:

- Unconsciousness or altered conscious state.
- Breathing problems.
- Persistent chest or abdominal pain.
- Severe bleeding.
- Vomiting blood or passing blood.
- Poisoning.
- Seizures, severe headache or slurred speech.
- Injuries to head, neck or back.
- Possible broken bones.

There are also special situations that warrant calling emergency personnel for assistance. These include:

- Fire or explosion.
- The presence of poisonous gas.
- Fallen electrical wires.
- Car collisions with injured victims.
- Victims who cannot be moved easily.

These conditions and situations are by no means a complete list. Trust your instincts. Do not lose time calling untrained people such as friends or family members. Call an ambulance for help immediately. These professionals would rather respond to a non-emergency than arrive at an emergency scene too late to help.

As a trained first aider, one of your priorities is always to get professional help to the victim as soon as you can. With this in mind, why would you do a primary survey before calling emergency personnel?

Perform a Secondary Survey

If you find any life-threatening conditions during the primary survey, do *not* waste time with the secondary survey. Check the airway, breathing and circulation at regular intervals, and provide care only for the life-threatening conditions. Once you are certain that there are no life-threatening conditions needing attention you can begin the fourth emergency action principle, the secondary survey.

The secondary survey is a systematic method of finding other injuries or conditions that may need care. These are injuries or conditions that are not immediately life-threatening but could become so if not attended to. To establish a complete picture, you need to obtain the *history* of the incident, the *symptoms* described by the victim and any additional *signs* that you may observe. For example, you might find possible broken bones, minor bleeding or a specific medical condition such as epilepsy.

The secondary survey has three basic steps:

1. Question the victim and bystanders.

2. Check **vital signs.**

3. Do a head-to-toe examination.

It is useful to write down the information you find during the secondary survey to give to ambulance personnel when they arrive. If necessary, ask someone else to write down the information, which may help to decide the type of medical care the victim receives later.

In the workplace, it is important to write a report for any incident in which first aid is given. In a road accident or other emergency involving your home or family,

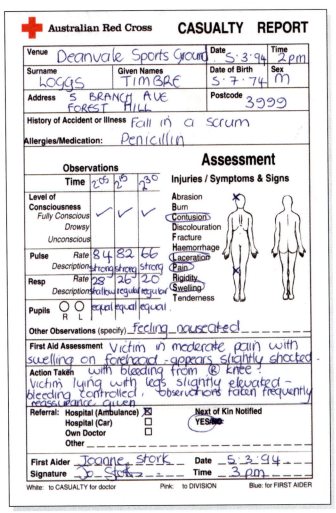

Australian Red Cross   CASUALTY   REPORT

| Venue | Deanvale Sports Ground | Date 5·3·94 | Time 2pm |

| Surname LOGGS | Given Names TIMBRE | Date of Birth 5·7·74 | Sex M |

| Address 5 BRANCH AVE FOREST HILL | Postcode 3999 |

History of Accident or Illness Fall in a scrum

Allergies/Medication: Penicillin

Assessment

Observations

| Time | 2·05 | 2·15 | 2·30 | **Injuries / Symptoms & Signs** |

Level of Consciousness
Fully Conscious ✓ ✓ ✓
Drowsy
Unconscious

Abrasion
Burn
Contusion
Discolouration
Fracture
Haemorrhage
Laceration
Pain
Rigidity
Swelling
Tenderness

| Pulse Rate | 84 | 82 | 66 |
| Description | strong | strong | strong |

| Resp Rate | 28 | 26 | 20 |
| Description | shallow | regular | regular |

Pupils O O equal equal equal
        R L

Other Observations (specify) feeling nauseated

First Aid Assessment Victim in moderate pain with swelling on forehead - appears slightly shocked

Action Taken with bleeding from ® knee : Victim lying with legs slightly elevated - bleeding controlled, observations taken frequently reassurance given

Referral: Hospital (Ambulance) ☒	Next of Kin Notified
Hospital (Car) ☐	YES/NO
Own Doctor ☐	
Other _____	

First Aider Joanne Stork   Date 5·3·94
Signature Jo Stork   Time 3pm

White: to CASUALTY for doctor   Pink: to DIVISION   Blue: for FIRST AIDER

FIGURE 3-7 *Example of a form to document first aid given to a sick or injured person.*

it is wise to make a few notes in case the police require further information. Figure 3-7 shows an example of a form used for reporting.

When you do the secondary survey, remember not to move the victim. Most injured people will adopt the most comfortable position for themselves. For example, a person with a chest injury who is having trouble breathing may be supporting the injured area. Let the victim stay this way. Do not suggest a change of position.

Question the Victim and Bystanders

Begin by asking the victim and bystanders simple questions to learn more about what happened and the victim's condition. This should not take much time.

If you have not done so already, remember to identify yourself and to get consent to help. Begin by asking the victim's name. Using the victim's name will make the person more relaxed and comfortable. Ask the following questions:

1. What happened?

2. Do you feel pain anywhere?

3. Do you have any allergies?

4. Do you have any medical conditions or are you taking any medication?

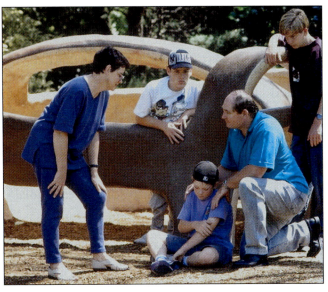

FIGURE 3-8 *Parents or other adults may be able to provide information for a child who is sick or injured.*

If the victim has pain, ask for a description. Ask when the pain started. Ask how bad the pain is. You can expect to get descriptions such as burning, throbbing, aching or sharp pain.

Sometimes the victim will be unable to provide you with the proper information. This is often the case with an infant or child. It may also be true for an adult who momentarily lost consciousness and may not be able to recall what happened. These victims may be frightened. Be calm and patient. Speak normally and in simple terms. Offer reassurance. Ask family members, friends or bystanders what happened because they may be able to give you helpful information (Figure 3-8). If parents or an adult guardian are present, ask for their help to calm the infant or child. Parents can also tell you if the child has a relevant medical condition.

Check Vital Signs

A person's conscious state, breathing, pulse and skin colour and appearance are called vital signs. These vital signs can give you information which tells you how the body is responding to injury or illness. Look for changes or any problems in breathing, pulse or skin appearance and temperature. Note anything unusual. Check these vital signs about every 5 minutes until ambulance personnel arrive.

Changes in breathing

A healthy person breathes regularly. Breathing should be effortless and quiet. Normal breathing for adults is 15 to 20 breaths per minute. Children and infants normally breathe faster. In the secondary survey, watch and listen for any changes in normal breathing. Abnormal breathing may indicate a potential problem. The features of abnormal breathing include:

- Gasping for air.
- Noisy breathing, including whistling sounds, crowing, gurgling.

- Excessively fast or slow breathing.
- Painful breathing.

In later chapters, you will learn more about what these changes in breathing may mean and what first aid to give.

Changes in pulse

With every heartbeat, a wave of blood moves through the blood vessels. This creates a beat called the pulse. You can feel it with your fingertips in arteries near the skin's surface, for example, with the **carotid** and **radial** arteries.

When the heart is healthy, it beats with a steady rhythm which creates a regular pulse. The normal pulse for an adult is 60 to 80 beats per minute. Children and infants normally have a faster pulse. If the heartbeat changes, so does the pulse. An abnormal pulse may indicate a potential problem. Signs of a problem include the following:

- Irregular pulse.
- Weak and hard-to-find pulse.
- Excessively fast or slow pulse.

With a severe injury or when the heart is not healthy, the heart may beat unevenly, generating an irregular pulse. Similarly, the pulse speeds up when a person is excited, anxious, in pain, losing blood or under stress. It slows down when a person is relaxed. Some heart conditions may also speed up or slow down the pulse rate.

These subtle changes may be difficult for a first aider to detect.

Checking a pulse involves placing two fingers on top of a major artery that is located close to the skin's surface. These include the carotid arteries in the neck and radial artery in the wrist (Figures 3-9 and 3-10).

A sick or injured person's pulse may be hard to find. It is easier to find the radial pulse if the palm is facing downward. Keep checking for a pulse periodically. Take your time. Remember, if a person is breathing, the heart is also beating. However, there may be a loss of pulse in an injured area. If you cannot find the pulse, check it over another major artery—in the other wrist or the neck.

In later chapters, you will learn more about what changes in pulse may mean and what first aid to give.

Changes in skin appearance and temperature

The appearance of the skin and its temperature often indicate something about the victim's condition. For example, a victim with a breathing problem may have a flushed, pale or bluish face.

Look at the victim's face. The skin looks red when the body is forced to work harder because the heart pumps faster to get more blood to the tissues. This increased blood flow causes reddened skin and makes the skin feel warm. In contrast, the skin may look pale or bluish and feel cool and moist if the blood flow is directed away from the skin's surface to increase the blood supply to vital organs. Determine the temperature of the skin by feeling it with your hand. In later chapters, you will learn more about what these changes may mean and what first aid to give.

Perform a Head-to-toe Examination

The last step of the secondary survey is the head-to-toe examination. This examination helps gather more information about the victim's condition. When you do the head-to-toe examination, use your senses—sight, sound and smell—to detect anything abnormal. For example, you may detect an unusual odour that could indicate that the victim has been poisoned or see a bruise or a deformed body part. *Listen carefully to what the victim may tell you.*

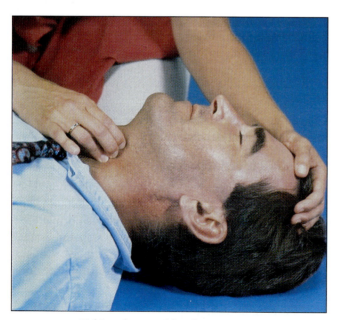

FIGURE 3-9 *Taking the carotid pulse.*

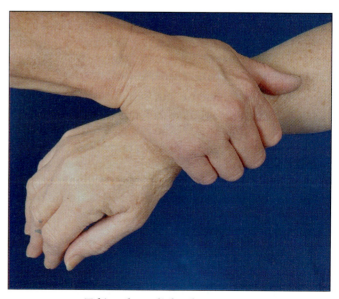

FIGURE 3-10 *Taking the radial pulse.*

Begin the head-to-toe examination by telling the victim what you are going to do. Ask the victim to remain still. A sick or injured person may move around but usually will not move a body part that is injured. Ask if any areas hurt and *avoid touching any painful areas or having the victim move any area in which there is discomfort.* Watch for facial expressions, and listen for a tone of voice that may reveal pain. Look for a Medical Alert tag on a necklace or bracelet. This tag may tell you what might be wrong, who to call for help and what care to give.

As you do the head-to-toe examination, think about how the body normally looks. Be alert for any sign of injuries—anything that looks or sounds unusual. If you are uncertain whether your finding is unusual, check the other side of the body.

To do a head-to-toe examination, visually inspect the entire body, starting with the head. You might see abnormal skin colour from bruising, a body fluid such as blood, or an unusual position of body parts. You may notice odd bumps or depressions. The victim may seem groggy or faint. Look for signs that may indicate a serious problem. If you see or suspect a condition that requires ambulance personnel, call right away if you have not already done so.

Next, if you do not suspect an injury to the head or spine, determine if there are any specific injuries by asking the victim to try to move each body part in which there is no pain or discomfort. To check the neck, ask if the injured person can slowly move the head from side to side (Figure 3-11). Check the shoulders by asking the person to shrug them. Check the chest and abdomen by asking the person to try to take a deep breath and then blow the air out. Ask if there is any pain in the abdomen. Check each arm by first asking the person to move the fingers and the hand. Next, ask if the arm can be bent (Figure 3-12). In the same way, check the hips and legs by first asking the person to move the toes, foot and ankle. Then determine if the leg can be bent (Figure 3-13). It is best to check only one extremity at a time.

If the victim can move all of the body parts without pain or discomfort and there are no other apparent signs of injury, encourage the person to rest for a few minutes in a sitting position. Continue to check the vital signs and monitor the airway, breathing and pulse. If no further difficulty develops, allow the victim to slowly stand when ready. Unless the victim can sit or stand unaided, maintain the resting position.

If the person is unable to move a body part or is experiencing dizziness or pain with movement, recheck the ABC. Help the person rest in the most comfortable position, maintain normal body temperature and provide reassurance. Determine what additional care is needed and whether to call an ambulance.

As you do this examination, keep watching the victim's conscious state, airway, breathing and skin colour. If any problems develop, *stop* whatever you are doing and give first aid *immediately.*

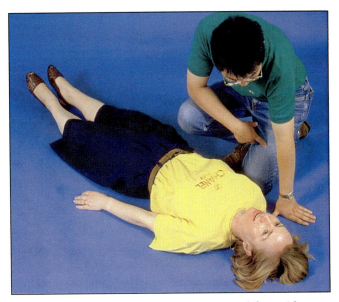

FIGURE 3-11 *Ask the victim to move her head from side to side to check the neck.*

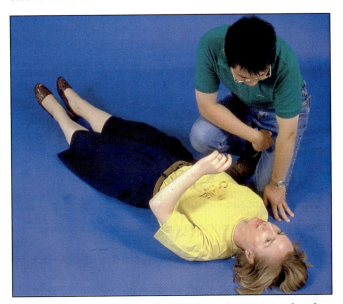

FIGURE 3-12 *Check the arms by asking the victim to bend her arms one at a time.*

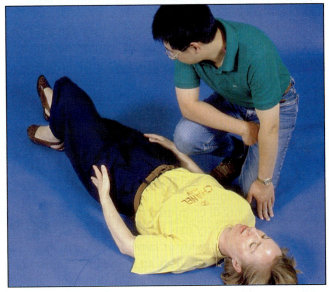

FIGURE 3-13 *Check the legs by asking the victim to bend her legs one at a time.*

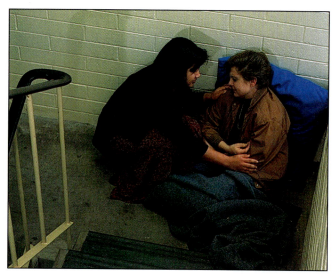

FIGURE 3-14 *Provide care for the victim until help arrives.*

Provide Care

Once you complete the secondary survey, provide care for any specific injuries you find (Figure 3-14).

To provide care for the victim until ambulance personnel arrive, follow these general steps:

1. Prevent further injury.
2. Monitor the ABC.
3. Help the victim to rest in the most comfortable position.
4. Maintain normal body temperature.
5. Reassure the victim.
6. Provide any specific care needed.

TRANSPORTATION OF THE VICTIM

In a remote area or in an unusual circumstance, you might consider transporting the victim to the hospital yourself if the victim's condition is not severe. This is an important decision. *Do not transport a victim with a life-threatening condition or one who has any chance of developing a life-threatening condition.* As a general rule, call for an ambulance because a car trip can be painful for the victim and may aggravate the injury or cause additional injury.

If you must transport the victim yourself, ask someone else to come with you. One person should drive while the other helps keep the victim comfortable. Be sure you know the quickest route to the nearest medical facility with emergency care capabilities. Pay close attention to the victim, and watch for any changes in the victim's condition.

Discourage any ill or injured person from driving to the hospital. An injury may restrict movement, or the victim may become giddy or faint. The sudden onset of pain may be distracting. Also, an injured or ill person may drive faster or more erratically than normal. Any of these conditions can make driving dangerous for the victim, passengers, pedestrians and other road users.

Emergency Action Principles

Survey the Scene
- Is it safe?

Begin a Primary survey
- Is the victim conscious?
- Does the victim have an open airway?
- Is the victim breathing?
- Does the victim have a pulse?
- Is the victim bleeding?

Phone Emergency Personnel
- Send someone to phone for an ambulance.

Do a Secondary Survey
- Interview the victim.
- Check vital signs.
- Perform a head-to-toe survey.

FIGURE 3-15 *Use the emergency action principles to make decisions in an emergency.*

If you find during the primary survey that the victim is conscious, has no difficulty breathing and has no severe bleeding, what should you do next? Why?

If you find during the primary survey that the victim is unconscious but breathing, and has no severe bleeding, what should you do next? Why?

Summary

- The four emergency action principles guide your actions in any emergency, provide for your safety and the safety of others, and ensure that urgent care is provided for life-threatening emergencies (Figure 3-15).

- First, survey the scene to ensure there are no dangers to you, the victim or bystanders.

- Second, do a primary survey of the victim. Check the conscious state and send someone to call for an ambulance immediately if the victim is unconscious. Determine if there are any problems with the airway, breathing or circulation, and care for them right away.

- Third, call for emergency help if needed. Try to send a bystander to call so that you can continue to provide care. Give the bystander the necessary information about the victim's condition.

- Fourth, if you find no life-threatening conditions, do a secondary survey to identify other symptoms and signs of injury or illness. Problems that are not an immediate threat to life could become serious if you do not give first aid.

Many variables exist when dealing with emergencies. You do not need to know exactly what is wrong with the victim to provide appropriate care. Use the emergency action principles as a tool to help you make decisions. Even though there may not always be a right or wrong answer, following the emergency action principles ensures that you take care of life-threatening emergencies first.

As you read the following chapters, remember to apply the emergency action principles to each injury or illness. They form the basis for providing care in any emergency.

Answers to Application Questions

1. The check for breathing is a crucial step in your evaluation of the victim's condition. It can mean the difference between life and death. Absence of breathing is a life-threatening emergency that requires immediate care. By using your senses to check for breathing, you can correctly determine the presence or absence of breathing and thus the care that is needed.

2. Checking for a pulse is another crucial step in your evaluation of the victim's condition. Changes in rate or rhythm may indicate the presence of severe bleeding.

3. Severe bleeding is defined as blood that spurts from the wound or cannot be controlled. Normally, oxygen taken into the body through breathing goes to the lungs, is distributed to the heart, and then circulated throughout the body. During severe bleeding, this is not the case. The injury that causes severe bleeding damages the circulatory system—particularly the blood vessels. This damage to the circulatory system impairs the delivery of oxygen-rich blood to all body tissues. Tissues that do not receive oxygen lose their ability to function and will soon die. If severe bleeding is not controlled, the vital organs will not receive the oxygen they need to function and will die. When vital organs fail to function, the victim will die.

4. As a person trained in first aid, you can provide care for life-threatening emergencies until ambulance personnel arrive. Doing a primary survey allows you to determine the victim's condition and thus the need for immediate lifesaving care. It also allows you to provide any immediate care that is needed while ambulance personnel are on their way. Further, giving information about the victim's condition and the situation helps the operator to dispatch the appropriate personnel.

5. When no apparent life-threatening emergencies exist, you should do a secondary survey to determine if there are other conditions present that require medical attention and/or ambulance personnel.

6. If you find during the primary survey that the victim is unconscious, you should place the victim on the side and clear and open the airway following the Basic Life Support flow chart, page 35. Send someone for help. Unconsciousness can be a life-threatening emergency.

Study Questions

1. **Match each emergency action principle with the actions it includes.**

    a. Survey the scene.
    b. Do a primary survey and care for life-threatening emergencies.
    c. Call emergency personnel.
    d. Do a secondary survey when appropriate.

    ____ Open the airway.
    ____ Look for bystanders who can help.
    ____ Interview the victim and bystanders.
    ____ Check for breathing.
    ____ Check vital signs.
    ____ Do a head-to-toe examination.
    ____ Dial 000 or the local emergency number.
    ____ Look for victims.
    ____ Check for severe bleeding.
    ____ Look for dangers.
    ____ Check for a pulse.
    ____ Look for clues to determine what happened.

2. **List the four emergency action principles.**

3. **List six conditions that require you to call emergency personnel immediately.**

4. **List four questions to be answered when surveying the scene.**

5. **List four important facts you should give emergency personnel when you call.**

6. *List the conditions you should check for in a primary survey.*

7. *Describe when and why you would do a secondary survey.*

8. *You walk into your boss's office for a meeting. You see a cup of coffee spilled on the desk. You find her lying on the floor, motionless. What should you do? Number the following actions in order:*

  a. Have someone call emergency personnel for help, if necessary.

  b. Check for breathing.

  c. Survey the scene.

  d. Check for pulse and severe bleeding.

  e. Check for consciousness.

  f. Turn her on the side, and clear and open the airway.

In questions 9 and 10, circle the letter of the correct answer.

9. *What should you do if you determine that the scene is unsafe?*

  a. Help anyway, this is an emergency—but, be careful.

  b. Get as close as you think is safe, try to see what happened, and then call emergency personnel for help.

  c. Do not approach; call emergency personnel for help immediately.

  d. Do not approach; wait for someone else to take action.

10. *Before beginning a primary survey, you should first:*

  a. Position the victim so that you can open the airway.

  b. Survey the scene.

  c. Check for consciousness.

  d. Call emergency professionals for help.

11. *As you walk to lunch, you notice a group of people gathered at the side of the street. As you come to the edge of the street, you see a car stopped in the street and a person lying immediately in front of it. It appears that the person has been struck by the car. Many people have gathered around, but no-one seems to be doing anything. What should you do? Should emergency personnel be called? What dangers may be present? How can bystanders help?*

Answers are in Appendix A (page 360).

Primary Survey

You find a person lying on the ground, motionless. You should survey the scene to see if it is safe and to get some idea of what happened. If the scene is safe, do a primary survey by checking the ABC.

Check conscious state

- Gently shake person.
- Shout, "Are you OK? Squeeze my hand; now let it go."

If person responds . . .

- Begin a secondary survey.

If person does not respond . . .

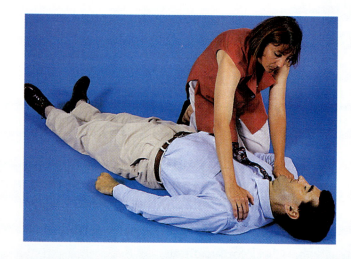

Roll the victim onto the side

- Kneel beside victim.
- Grasp thigh nearest to you, and lift at right angles to the trunk.
- Place near arm across the chest with fingers at opposite shoulder. Place the far arm at a right angle to the body.
- Lift under near shoulder and near thigh to roll victim away from you to lie on side.
- Keep thigh at right angle to trunk to prevent the victim from rolling onto face.
- Place upper arm across lower arm at elbow.

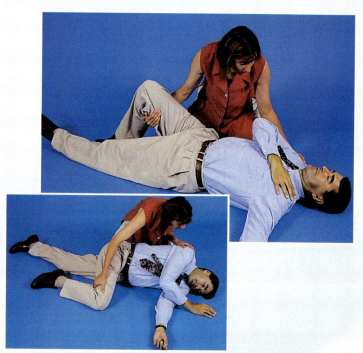

Clear airway

- Finger sweep mouth to clear foreign materials.

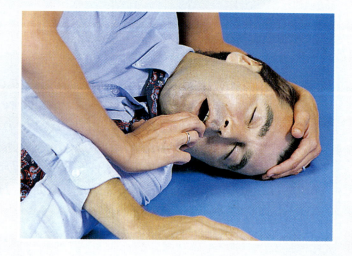

PRACTICE GUIDE

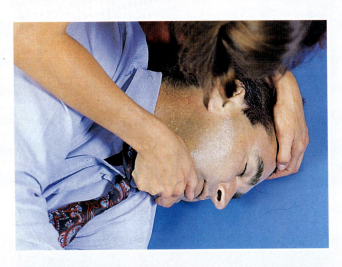

Open airway

- With hand on forehead, tilt head backwards.
- Support jaw with other hand.
- Keep victim's face turned downward for drainage.

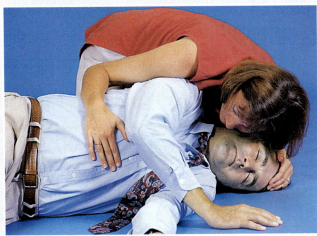

Check for breathing

- Look, listen and feel for breathing for 3 to 5 seconds.

If person is breathing . . .

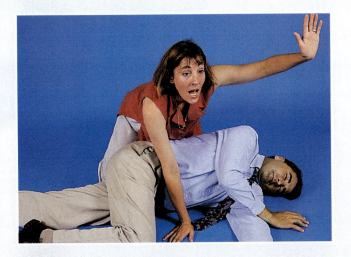

Shout for help

- Shout for help to attract attention.
- Send someone else to telephone emergency personnel, if possible.
- Keep airway open.
- Check for and control severe bleeding.

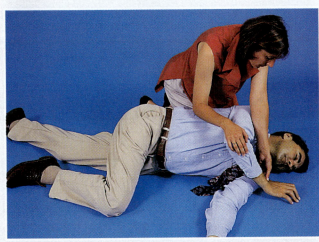

Check for pulse

- Find pulse at wrist.
- Slide fingers down into groove at base of thumb.
- Count for pulse for 5 to 10 seconds.
- Monitor ABC until ambulance personnel arrive.

PRACTICE GUIDE

Cardiopulmonary Resuscitation

THE FIRST FEW MINUTES in a life-threatening situation are vital. How you respond to the emergency is extremely important in helping the victim to recover and in preventing permanent disability. If the victim stops breathing, you can supply the oxygen to keep the brain alive; if the heart stops beating, you can help keep oxygenated blood circulating to reach the body's vital organs.

This chapter outlines the principles of expired air resuscitation and cardiopulmonary resuscitation, when to use these procedures and how to perform them.

For Review

A basic understanding of how the respiratory and circulatory systems function (Chapter 2) and a knowledge of the steps of the primary survey (Chapter 3) will help your understanding of the chapter.

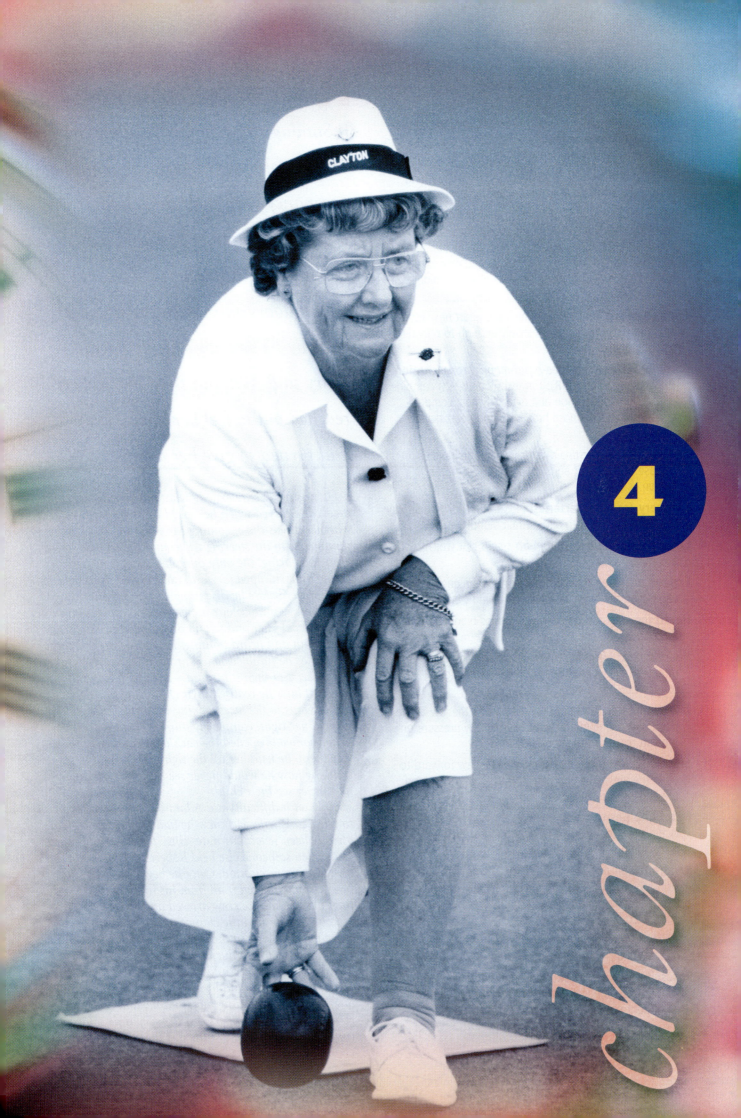

4

chapter

Key Terms

Aspiration: The contamination of the air passages of the lungs with foreign material such as blood, vomit, broken teeth or other foreign bodies.

Breathing emergency: Emergency in which breathing is so impaired that life is threatened.

Calipering: The method of locating the position on the chest for chest compressions, found by locating the notches at the upper and lower ends of the sternum with the index fingers of both hands and extending the thumbs an equal distance to meet in the middle of the sternum.

Cardiac arrest: Condition in which the heart has stopped or is too weak to pump effectively enough to provide a palpable pulse.

Cardiopulmonary *(car-dee-o-**pul**-mon-ry)* **resuscitation** *(re sus i tay shon)* **(CPR):** The technique which combines expired air resuscitation and external chest compressions for a victim whose breathing and heart have stopped.

Cardiovascular *(car-dee-o-**vask**-yoo-lar)* **disease:** Disease of the heart and blood vessels; commonly known as heart disease.

Coronary *(co-ron-ry)* **arteries:** Blood vessels which supply the heart muscle with oxygen-rich blood.

Coronary thrombosis *(throm-**bo**-sis)*: A clot which blocks a coronary artery.

Expired air resuscitation (EAR): The technique of ventilating the lungs of a non-breathing victim.

Heart: The muscular organ which pumps blood throughout the body.

Heart attack: A sudden illness involving damage to heart muscle tissue when it does not receive enough oxygen-rich blood.

Jaw support: The technique of supporting the jaw at the point of the chin in a way that avoids any pressure on the soft tissues of the neck.

Jaw thrust: The technique of moving the jaw forward to open the airway by applying forward pressure behind the angle of the jaw.

Pistol grip position: A position of the hand on the victim's jaw to support the jaw during expired air resuscitation.

Regurgitation *(ree-gur-ji-**tay**-shon)*: The passive flow of stomach contents into the mouth and airway, where it may be aspirated into the lungs; it is silent and may not be noticed by the first aider.

Respiratory arrest: Condition in which there is cessation of breathing.

Resuscitation face mask: A rigid or semi-rigid device which covers the victim's mouth and nose to provide an airtight seal during expired air resuscitation.

Robert and Mary Fowles were taking a Sunday afternoon drive along the coast. Mary was in her sixth month of pregnancy with their first child. It was a beautiful summer day, and they were looking for a café where they could sip tea outdoors and watch the sailboats glide by. "The baby's kicking again," Mary said. Without thinking, Robert reached out to feel her abdomen, and turned to give her a smile...

He was never sure exactly what happened—whether their car swerved when he looked away from the road or whether it was the oncoming car. After the shock of being slammed into the steering wheel and the terrible screech of metal tearing, the only thing he saw was his wife beside him, slumped forward, not moving. It seemed to take forever before he disentangled himself and reached her. There was no colour in her face, no movement in her body. He held her and felt no breathing, put his ear to her mouth and heard nothing. He could barely breathe himself as he fumbled to feel or hear her heart, to take her pulse, and then it hit him—she was dead. And a moment later he realised their child would be dead too.

Oblivious to the faces looking in through the windows, he held her tight, completely numbed by her death. When someone opened the car's doors and tried to separate them, he held her all the tighter. He could not stop thinking how he would never see her smile again, how he'd never see their child.

Only with difficulty did Adam Hazelton get Robert to release his wife. He knew he had to act fast—it had already been several minutes since the car crash, someone said. Then someone else held Robert back so Adam could give Mary resuscitation. Once he began, he was surprised how he remembered it all from his first aid class. And then the ambulance crew arrived and took over...

Robert never had the chance to meet or thank Adam Hazelton. He went in the ambulance with Mary and let them treat his own injuries once he saw Mary was breathing. In his pain and gratitude he forgot much of what happened around him. However, one of the nurses later told him the young man's name, and that he did remember. He remembers it still, every time someone comments what a pretty little girl their Hazel is.

In previous chapters, you learned what you can do to help in an emergency. You learned four emergency action principles which guide your actions in any emergency.

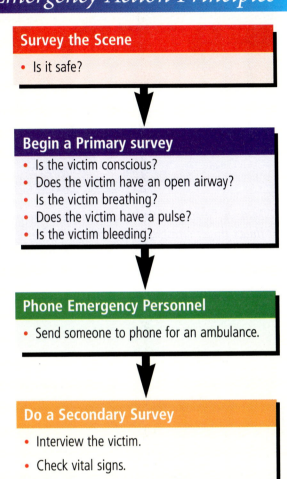

Emergency Action Principles

Survey the Scene
- Is it safe?

Begin a Primary survey
- Is the victim conscious?
- Does the victim have an open airway?
- Is the victim breathing?
- Does the victim have a pulse?
- Is the victim bleeding?

Phone Emergency Personnel
- Send someone to phone for an ambulance.

Do a Secondary Survey
- Interview the victim.
- Check vital signs.
- Perform a head-to-toe survey.

FIGURE 4-1 *The four emergency action principles.*

In this chapter, you will learn how to care for someone who has stopped breathing and whose heart may also have stopped beating. You will discover the presence of these life-threatening conditions when you assess the victim's condition in the primary survey.

As you learned in Chapter 3, first check that the scene is safe. Then check to see if the victim is conscious. Immediately put an unconscious victim on the side and

Remember:

A = *Airway.*

B = *Breathing.*

C = *Circulation.*

complete the primary survey by checking the ABC. As soon as possible, send a bystander to call for ambulance personnel.

Because oxygen is vital to life, you must always ensure that the victim has an open airway and is breathing. You should detect any **breathing emergency** during the primary survey. It occurs when someone's breathing has stopped or is so impaired that their life is threatened. A person who is having difficulty breathing is in respiratory distress (see Chapter 7). A person who is not breathing is in **respiratory arrest.** This person needs **expired air resuscitation (EAR).**

When a person is in respiratory arrest, the heart may still be beating. Without expired air resuscitation, the heart will stop beating soon after breathing stops. This is called **cardiac arrest.** In some instances the heart may stop beating first, and then breathing stops immediately.

The victim of cardiac arrest needs **cardiopulmonary resuscitation (CPR),** which combines expired air resuscitation with chest compressions to circulate the blood. Properly performed CPR can keep a victim's vital organs supplied with oxygen-rich blood until ambulance personnel arrive to provide advanced care.

Remember:

A victim in respiratory arrest whose heart is still beating needs only EAR. A victim in both respiratory and cardiac arrest needs both EAR and chest compressions. This chapter describes both of these techniques.

THE BREATHING PROCESS

Breathing requires the respiratory, circulatory, nervous and musculoskeletal systems to work together. As you read in Chapter 2, injuries or illnesses which affect any of these systems may impair breathing. For example, if the heart stops beating, the victim will stop breathing. Injury or disease in areas of the brain which control breathing may impair or stop breathing. Damage to muscles or bones of the chest and back can make breathing difficult or painful. All of these situations are, or could result in breathing emergencies. Chapter 7 covers in more detail the recognition and care of breathing emergencies.

The body requires constant oxygen for survival. When you breathe air into your lungs, the oxygen in the air is transferred to the blood. The circulatory system transports the oxygen-rich blood to the brain, organs, muscles and other parts of the body where it is used to provide energy. This energy allows the body to perform its many functions such as breathing, walking, talking, digesting food and maintaining body temperature. Different functions require different levels of energy and, therefore, different amounts of oxygen. For example, sitting in a chair requires less energy than jogging around the block. A body battling disease, even the common cold, uses more energy than a body in its normal healthy state

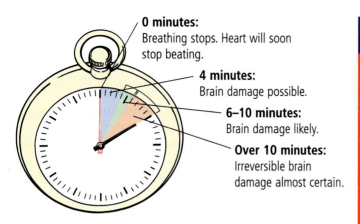

0 minutes:
Breathing stops. Heart will soon stop beating.

4 minutes:
Brain damage possible.

6–10 minutes:
Brain damage likely.

Over 10 minutes:
Irreversible brain damage almost certain.

FIGURE 4-2 *Time is critical in starting lifesaving procedures. Four minutes or less without oxygen generally causes brain damage.*

because it must carry out all the normal functions of life and simultaneously fight the disease. This explains why you are usually tired when you are sick.

Without oxygen, cells may begin to die in four minutes or less (Figure 4-2). Some tissues, such as the brain, are very sensitive to oxygen starvation. Unless the brain receives oxygen, brain damage or death will result.

Breathing emergencies can be caused by the following:

- An obstructed airway (choking).
- Illness (such as pneumonia).
- Respiratory conditions (such as asthma)
- Electrocution.
- Shock.
- Near-drowning.
- Heart attack or heart disease.
- Injury to the chest or lungs.
- Allergic reactions to foods, insect stings or chemicals.
- Drugs.
- Poisoning (such as inhaling or ingesting toxic substances).

The most serious consequence of a breathing emergency is **respiratory arrest.**

RESPIRATORY ARREST

Respiratory arrest is the condition in which breathing stops. It may be caused by illness, injury or an obstructed airway. The causes of respiratory distress, such as asthma, can also lead to respiratory arrest. In respiratory arrest, the person gets no oxygen to continue body functions. The body can function only for a few minutes without oxygen before body systems begin to fail. Without oxygen, the heart muscle stops functioning, causing the circulatory system to fail. When the heart stops, other body systems will start to fail. However, you can keep the person's respiratory system functioning with expired air resuscitation.

The Pistol Grip Position

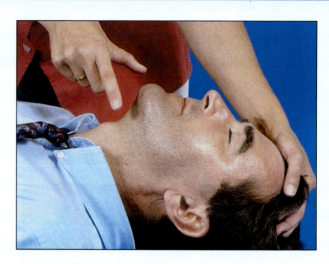

1. *Make a "pistol" of your hand by pointing the index finger straight out, cocking the thumb upward, and curling the other three fingers back into the palm.*

1   *Why do other systems fail when the heart fails?*

EXPIRED AIR RESUSCITATION

Expired air resuscitation (EAR) is a way of breathing air into someone to supply that person with the oxygen needed for survival. EAR is given to victims who are not breathing but still have a pulse.

EAR works because the air you breathe into the victim contains more than enough oxygen to keep that person alive. The air you take in with every breath contains about 21 per cent oxygen, but your body uses only a small part of that. The air you breathe out of your lungs and into the lungs of the victim contains about 16 per cent oxygen, which is enough oxygen to keep someone alive.

You will discover whether you need to give EAR during the first two steps of the ABC in the primary survey when you open the airway and check for breathing. If you cannot see, hear or feel any signs of breathing, you must begin EAR immediately.

EAR Technique

To give EAR, first turn the victim onto the back and keep the airway open with **head tilt and jaw support.** Place one hand on the top of the head and tilt the head back. Support the jaw with your fingers in a

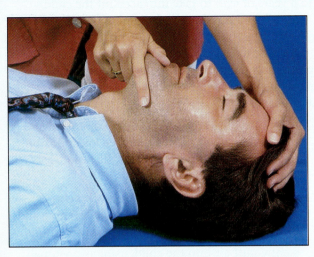

2. *Place your hand on the victim's jaw, with your index finger along the jaw line and the thumb between the lower lip and the point of the chin. Keep the fingers clear of the neck.*

"pistol grip" position (see box). Head tilt and jaw support not only open the airway by moving the tongue away from the back of the throat, but they also move the soft tissue flap, called the epiglottis, from the opening of the trachea.

If you know or see that the victim is wearing dentures, do not automatically remove them. Dentures can help the EAR process by supporting the victim's mouth and cheeks during mouth-to-mouth resuscitation. If the dentures are loose, the head-tilt and jaw-support technique may help keep them in place. Remove the dentures only if they are broken or become so loose that they block the airway or make it difficult for you to give breaths.

Begin the mouth-to-mouth method of EAR by giving 5 full breaths in 10 seconds (see box).

If you do not see the victim's chest rise and fall as you give each breath, you may not have the head tilted back far enough to open the airway adequately. Retilt the victim's head and try again to get air into the lungs. On the rare occasions that your breaths still do not go in, the victim's airway is obstructed. Therefore, you must give first aid for the obstructed airway (described in Chapter 7).

Remember:

- *Tilt the head and support the jaw.*
- *Seal the mouth and nose.*
- *Breathe into the victim.*
- *Look, listen and feel for the escape of air.*

Mouth-to-Mouth EAR

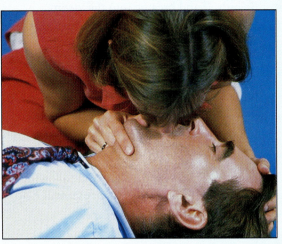

1. *Make a tight seal around the victim's mouth with your mouth. Close the victim's nostrils with your cheek.*

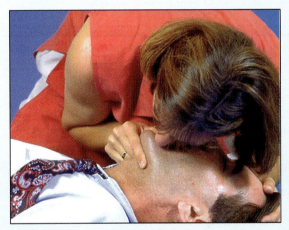

2. *Breathe into the victim until you see the chest rise. Each breath should last about 1 to 2 seconds, with a pause in between to let the air flow back out.*

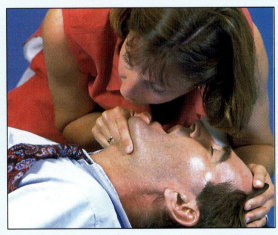

3. *Watch the victim's chest rise each time you breathe in to ensure that your breaths are actually going into the lungs, and watch as the chest falls.*

Check for a carotid pulse after giving the 5 full breaths (see box). If the victim has a pulse but is not breathing, continue EAR by giving 1 breath every 4 seconds. Take a breath yourself and breathe into the victim.

Do not stop EAR unless one of the following occurs:

- The victim begins to breathe unaided.
- The victim has no pulse. Begin CPR.
- Another first aider takes over for you.
- Ambulance personnel arrive on the scene and take over.
- You are physically unable to continue.

Practising EAR using a manikin and following the Practice Guide at the end of this chapter will help you to gain confidence.

Remember:

- *Breathe gently into the victim. Each breath should last about 1 to 2 seconds.*

- *After 1 minute of EAR (about 15 breaths), recheck the pulse to make sure the heart is still beating. If the victim still has a pulse but is not breathing, continue EAR at 15 breaths per minute.*

- *Recheck the pulse every 2 minutes.*

EAR for Children

The technique of EAR varies somewhat for a child (1 to 8 years of age) to take into account the child's underdeveloped physique and slightly faster breathing and heart rates. Be sure to turn the unconscious child onto the side to clear the airway (see upper box on opposite page) and then check for breathing. Follow the same sequence as for an adult, with the following exceptions:

1. Check for breathing with the jaw supported and the head in a neutral position (see lower box on opposite page). If necessary, tilt the head back slightly to open the airway.

2. Check breathing by looking for movement of the chest and upper abdomen while listening and feeling for air escaping from the nose and mouth.

3. Gently puff air into the child, using just enough pressure to make the chest rise.

4. If the breath does not go in, check that the airway is open. Sometimes gentle head tilt is needed to open the airway. The older the child, the more head tilt is needed to open the airway.

5. Because children breathe faster than adults, give a small breath or puff of air every 3 seconds (20 per minute) for a child.

If the child begins breathing unaided, turn the child onto the side and maintain an open airway.

Checking the Carotid and Brachial Pulses

CAROTID PULSE

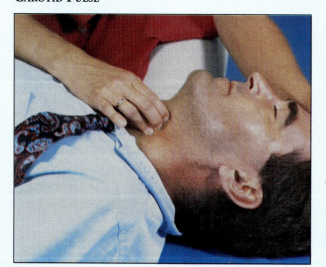

1. *With index and middle finger, feel the victim's windpipe and Adam's apple.*

2. *Slide fingers down into the groove of the neck on the side of the victim opposite you.*

3. *Feel for the pulse for 5 seconds, using the pads of your fingers.*

BRACHIAL PULSE

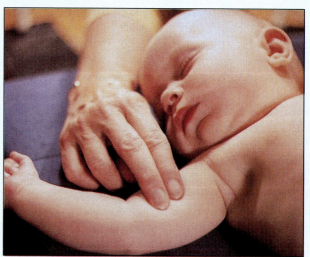

1. *With index and middle fingers, check the brachial pulse.*

2. *Feel for the pulse on the inside of the infant's arm, between the muscles.*

3. *Feel for the pulse for 5 seconds using the pads of your fingers.*

EAR for Children

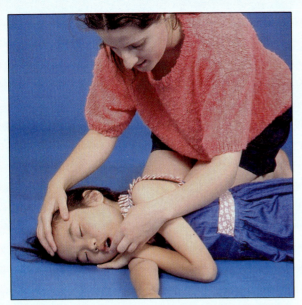

1. *Clear the airway quickly and check for breathing.*

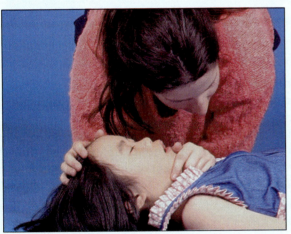

2. *Keep the victim's head in the neutral position and support the jaw while giving EAR.*

EAR for Infants

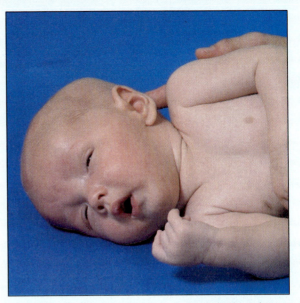

1. *Clear the airway quickly and check for breathing.*

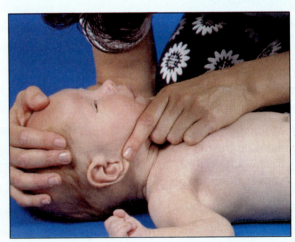

2. *Support the infant's jaw without tilting the head while giving EAR.*

EAR for Infants

An infant is defined as being under 1 year old. Because the infant's tongue is proportionally larger it is more likely to block the airway, so be sure the airway is open when you give EAR. The breathing rate is the same as for children: 1 puff every 3 seconds. The EAR technique is similar to that for children with the following differences:

- Steady the infant's head continuously because it is unstable.
- Do not tilt back the head, but support the jaw (see box above).
- Avoid putting any pressure on the soft tissues under the infant's chin because this could obstruct the airway.
- For EAR, cover both the infant's mouth and nose with your mouth.

- Use gentle puffs of air from your cheeks only. Use just enough pressure to make the chest rise to avoid distending the infant's stomach.
- After giving five puffs, check for the carotid pulse or the brachial pulse in the arm. Feel for the pulse on the inside of the infant's arm, between the muscles. (see box on page opposite).

> ## Remember:
> - *Breathe gently into the child or infant.*
> - *Recheck the carotid pulse every 2 minutes to make sure the heart is still beating.*
> - *If the child still has a pulse but is not breathing, continue EAR.*

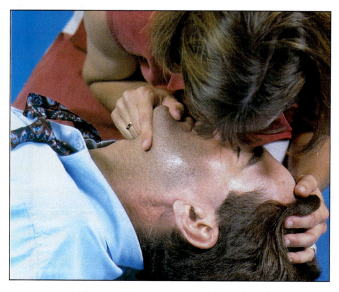

FIGURE 4-3 *For mouth-to-nose breathing, close the victim's mouth and seal your mouth around the victim's nose. Give full breaths, watching the chest rise to see that the air goes in.*

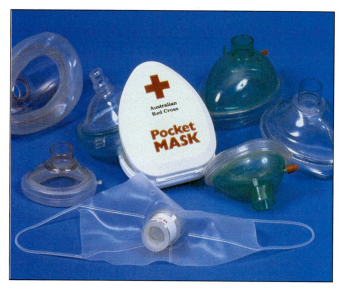

FIGURE 4-4 *Resuscitation face masks in common use.*

Mouth-to-Nose EAR

Sometimes you may not be able to make an adequate seal over a victim's mouth to perform EAR. For example, the person's jaw or mouth may be injured or the jaws clenched too tightly to open, or you may be rescuing the victim from deep water. If so, provide mouth-to-nose EAR as follows:

- Maintain the backward head tilt position with one hand on the top of the head. Use your other hand to close the victim's mouth, using jaw support with your hand in the pistol grip position.

- Open your mouth wide, take a deep breath, seal your mouth tightly around the victim's nose and breathe into the victim's nose (Figure 4-3). Peel back the victim's lips between breaths to let air come out.

EAR for Victims with Suspected Head, Neck or Back Injuries

You should suspect head, neck or back injuries in victims who have sustained a violent force, such as that which results from a car crash or a dive. Whether or not you suspect the victim has such an injury, you should try to minimise movement of the head and neck when opening the airway. If you suspect a neck injury, you should use jaw thrust (see box below), and not head tilt and jaw support.

The Jaw Thrust

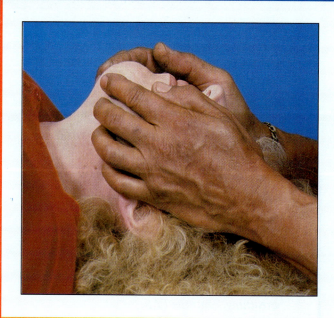

1. *Position yourself either at the top or side of the victim's head. Apply pressure behind the angle of the jaw to thrust the jaw forward, opening the airway. This may be enough to allow air to pass into the lungs.*

2. *If you attempt EAR and your breaths are not going in, you should tilt the head back very slightly. In most cases, this will be enough to allow air to pass into the lungs.*

3. *If air still does not go in, tilt back the head a little more. It is unlikely that this action will cause any additional injury to the victim. A person who is not breathing needs oxygen. Therefore, opening the airway is the primary concern.*

Remember:

Maintaining an open airway always takes precedence over other injuries, including the possibility of a fractured spine.

Mouth-to-Mask EAR

Mouth-to-mask expired air resuscitation avoids mouth-to-mouth contact between the first aider and the victim. A first aider who has a mask available may prefer this method for aesthetic reasons, or for personal comfort.

A resuscitation face mask is a rigid or semi-rigid device which covers the victim's mouth and nose, to provide an airtight seal for the first aider giving expired air resuscitation. Figure 4-4 shows a range of standard face masks for EAR. Use only an anaesthetic-type face mask which provides a good seal around the mouth and nose. Do not try to use the soft masks used to deliver oxygen to breathing victims (called "oxygen masks" or "therapy masks").

Use a face mask only if you have been trained in the use of that particular mask.

A face mask used for EAR should:

- be the smallest size that covers the victim's mouth and nose

- provide an airtight seal with or without an air cushion

- not contain a non-return valve.

The mask does not need to have a one-way (non-return) valve, because it may restrict the delivery of air to and escape of air from the victim. One-way valves do not protect the rescuer from droplet infection and frequently stick under pressure, therefore, they are not recommended. Use of a filter with a mask is unnecessary and is not recommended by the Australian Resuscitation Council.

Use the procedure shown in the box to give mouth-to-mask EAR. Note that because of the modified position required to give EAR, this technique should not be used for CPR by a solo rescuer.

Remember:

A mask is not essential for effective EAR, and you should never delay a resuscitation attempt to obtain a mask.

Mouth-to-Mask EAR

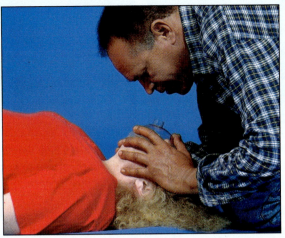

1. *Take a position behind the victim's head, facing the feet. Put the narrow end of the mask over the bridge of the nose.*

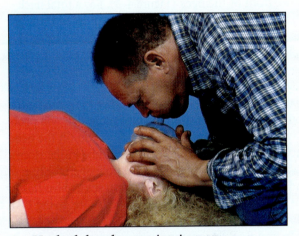

2. *Use both hands to maintain an open airway and seal the mask on the face. Maintain head tilt and use jaw thrust to pull up the jaw into the mask firmly enough to make a good seal. Blow through the mouthpiece of the mask to give EAR.*

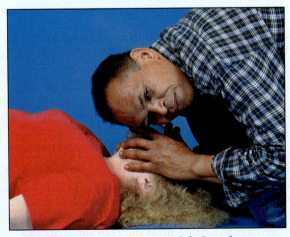

3. *Between breaths listen and feel at the mouthpiece for exhaled air.*

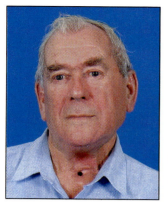

FIGURE 4-5 *You may need to perform EAR on a victim with a stoma.*

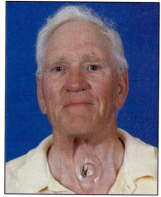

FIGURE 4-6 *There may be a tube in the stoma to help keep the airway open.*

Mouth-to-Stoma EAR

A laryngectomy is an operation which removes all or part of the upper end of the windpipe, that is, the person is a total or partial neck breather. After a laryngectomy the person must breathe through an opening called a stoma in the front of the neck (Figure 4-5). For a total neck breather, air passes directly into the windpipe through the stoma instead of through the mouth and nose. For a partial neck breather, some air may still enter through the mouth and nose.

Most people with a stoma wear a Medic Alert bracelet or necklace, or carry a card identifying their condition. You may not see the stoma immediately. You will probably notice the opening in the neck as you tilt the head back to open the airway. If you see a tube in the stoma, always keep it in place to keep the hole open for breathing and resuscitation (Figure 4-6). If you see a valve *closing* the tube, you must remove the valve before giving EAR to allow the air to enter.

To give EAR to someone with a stoma, you must give breaths through the stoma instead of the mouth or nose. Follow the same basic steps as for mouth-to-mouth breathing, except:

1. Look, listen and feel for breathing with your ear over the stoma (Figure 4-7).

2. Breathe into the stoma at the same rate as for mouth-to-mouth breathing.

Supporting the jaw with the head in a backward tilt makes it easier to seal your mouth over the stoma (Figure 4-8). If the victim's chest does not rise when you breathe in, make sure:

- your mouth is sealed around the stoma
- the stoma or tube is not blocked
- air is not escaping from the mouth and nose.

If air is escaping from the victim's mouth or nose, the victim is a partial neck breather, so you must put the palm of one hand over the victim's mouth and nose. Seal the nostrils with your index and middle fingers, and use your thumb to press the chin upwards and backwards (Figure 4-9). When the chest rises, lift your fingers sealing the nose and mouth, and listen for air coming out of the nostrils and stoma.

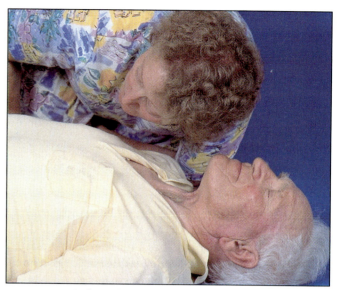

FIGURE 4-7 *When giving EAR to a victim with a stoma, check for breathing with your ear over the stoma.*

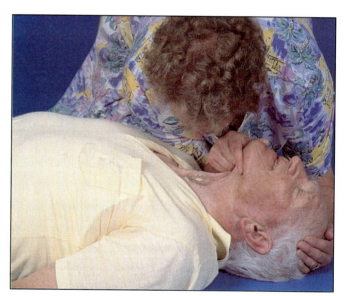

FIGURE 4-8 *Apply head tilt and jaw support when giving EAR to a victim with a stoma.*

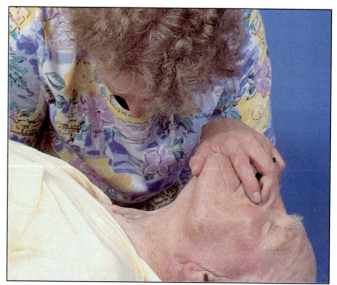

FIGURE 4-9 *Seal the nose and mouth of a victim with a stoma if air escapes from the nose or mouth.*

Special Considerations for EAR

Air in the Stomach

When you are giving EAR, air normally enters the victim's lungs. Sometimes, however, air may enter the victim's stomach instead. There are two main reasons why this could occur. Firstly, if the victim's head is not tilted back far enough, the airway will not open completely. As a result, you will tend to breathe more forcefully, causing air to enter the stomach. Secondly, over-inflating the lungs may force air into the stomach, so you must stop breathing into the victim when the chest has risen.

Distension of the stomach with air is a serious problem because it can lead to **regurgitation.** When an unconscious victim regurgitates, stomach contents may flow into the lungs, obstructing breathing. This is known as **aspiration,** or the contamination of the air passages of the lungs with foreign material such as blood, vomit, broken teeth or other foreign bodies. Aspiration can hamper resuscitation efforts and eventually may be fatal.

To avoid forcing air into the stomach, be sure to keep the victim's head tilted far enough back. Breathe gently into the victim, but enough to make the chest rise. Pause between breaths long enough for the victim's lungs to empty and for you to take another breath.

Regurgitation

When you give EAR the victim may regurgitate whether or not there is gastric distension. If this happens, roll the victim onto one side (Figure 4-10). This helps to prevent stomach contents from entering the lungs. Quickly clear the victim's mouth, reposition the victim on the back, and continue with EAR as before.

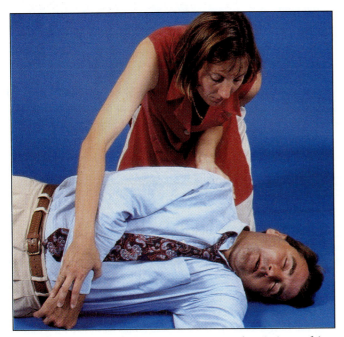

FIGURE 4-10 *If regurgitation occurs, turn the victim on his side and clear the mouth of any foreign material.*

MY BABY'S DROWNING

Connie Danson nearly collapsed when she saw her 18-month-old son in the pool. She pulled his limp, pale body from the water and hysterical, ran to the telephone to call 000 for an ambulance.

"My baby's drowned," she sobbed. "I think he's dead. He can't breathe,"

The ambulance operator sent an ambulance and then, speaking slowly, tried to calm Connie.

"There's an ambulance on the way," he said. "Where is the child now?"

"He's right here on the floor," Connie said.

"Put him on his side and open his mouth to clear out any foreign material. Look at his lower chest and tummy, and listen closely for any sounds," the operator said.

"He's not making any sounds and he's not moving at all," Connie cried.

"Connie, you're going to have to breathe for him; do you know how?"

"I learned it in a CPR program, but I'm not sure I remember," Connie said.

"Listen to me. Put him on his back. Put your mouth over his and seal his nose. Give 5 breaths and watch that his chest rises each time," the operator said.

"OK." Returning to the phone, Connie said, "OK, I did it."

"Now check for a pulse. Do you remember how to do that?" the operator asked.

"Yes," Connie said, leaning over to recheck her son. "He has a pulse, but he's still not breathing."

"Connie, you need to keep breathing for him. Give him one breath, count to three and breathe again. Do this for about a minute. I'll stay on the phone."

Connie listened as he reminded her what to do. Over and over, she gave a breath to her baby and watched his chest rise and fall.

Then she thought she heard him wheezing. She leaned closer and he began to cry.

Connie picked up the phone.

"Is that him?" the operator asked.

"Yes," Connie said tearfully.

"He sounds good," the operator said. "Is the ambulance there yet?"

"I hear the sirens outside," said Connie.

"OK. Hold on until they're inside. They'll take over now."

It is difficult to stay calm in an emergency. With the help of the ambulance operator, Connie provided lifesaving care for her baby. If you don't know what to do in an emergency, remember to call 000 for an ambulance immediately. ■

THE TECHNIQUE OF CARDIOPULMONARY RESUSCITATION

So far in this chapter you have learned how to recognise respiratory arrest and give expired air resuscitation when the victim has a pulse. In many cases where the victim has stopped breathing, the heart has also stopped and you need to give cardiopulmonary resuscitation (CPR), which includes external cardiac compressions (ECC) combined with EAR. Understanding the heart and circulation of blood will help you understand how CPR works and why it is needed.

THE HEART

The **heart** is a muscular organ about the size of your fist, which functions like a pump. It lies between the lungs, in the middle of the chest, behind the lower half of the sternum (breastbone). The heart is protected by the ribs and sternum in front and by the spine at the back (Figure 4-11). It is separated into right and left halves. Blood low in oxygen enters the right side of the heart and is pumped to the lungs, where it picks up oxygen. The now oxygen-rich blood returns to the left side of the heart, from which it is pumped to all parts of the body. One-way valves direct the flow of blood as it moves through the heart (Figure 4-12). For the circulatory system to be effective, the respiratory system must also work properly so that the blood can pick up oxygen in the lungs.

Like all living tissue, the cells of the heart need a continuous supply of oxygen. The **coronary arteries** supply the heart muscle with oxygen-rich blood. If heart muscle tissue is deprived of this blood, it dies. If enough tissue dies, the heart cannot pump effectively. When heart tissue dies, it is called a **heart attack.**

A heart attack interrupts the heart's electrical system. This may result in an irregular heartbeat and may therefore prevent blood from circulating effectively. Chapter 8 discusses in more detail the causes of heart attack and the risk factors, as well as what you can do to prevent heart attack or lower your risk.

CARDIAC ARREST

Cardiac arrest occurs when the heart stops beating or fails to beat regularly enough to circulate blood effectively. Breathing soon ceases. Cardiac arrest is a life-threatening emergency because the vital organs of the body are no longer receiving oxygen-rich blood. Every year, tens of thousands of heart attack victims die of cardiac arrest before reaching a hospital.

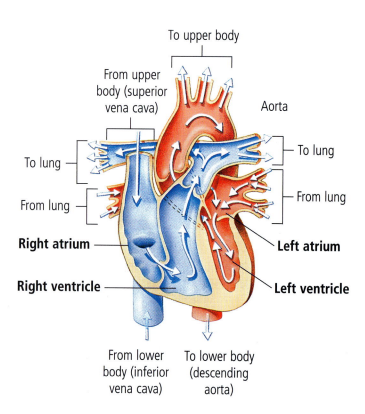

To upper body

From upper body (superior vena cava)

Aorta

To lung

From lung

To lung

From lung

Right atrium

Left atrium

Right ventricle

Left ventricle

From lower body (inferior vena cava)

To lower body (descending aorta)

Oxygen-poor blood pumped from the body to the lungs

Oxygen-rich blood pumped from the lungs to the body

FIGURE 4-12 *The heart is separated into right and left halves. The right side receives blood from the body and sends it to the lungs. The left side receives blood from the lungs and pumps it out through the body. One-way valves direct the flow of blood through the heart.*

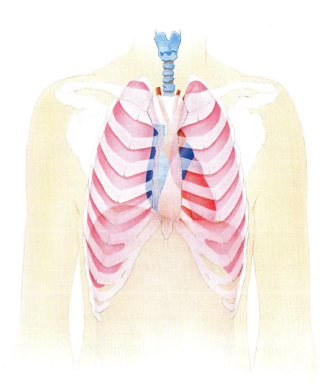

FIGURE 4-11 *The heart is located in the middle of the chest, behind the lower half of the sternum.*

Common Causes of Cardiac Arrest

Cardiovascular disease is the most common cause of cardiac arrest. The following conditions can cause the heart to stop:

- Near-drowning, suffocation and certain drugs can cause breathing to stop, which soon leads to cardiac arrest.
- Severe injuries to the chest or severe loss of blood.
- Electrocution disrupts the heart's own electrical activity.
- Stroke or other types of brain damage.

Whatever the cause, cardiac arrest is a life-threatening emergency requiring immediate action.

Signs of Cardiac Arrest

A victim in cardiac arrest is unconscious, not breathing, and without a pulse. The victim's heart has either stopped beating or is beating so weakly or irregularly that it cannot generate a pulse. The absence of a pulse in an unconscious, non-breathing person is the primary sign of cardiac arrest. No matter how hard you try, you will not be able to feel a pulse. If you cannot feel a carotid pulse, no blood is reaching the brain. The victim will be unconscious and breathing will have stopped.

Remember:

The three signs of cardiac arrest:

- *No response.*
- *No breathing.*
- *No pulse .*

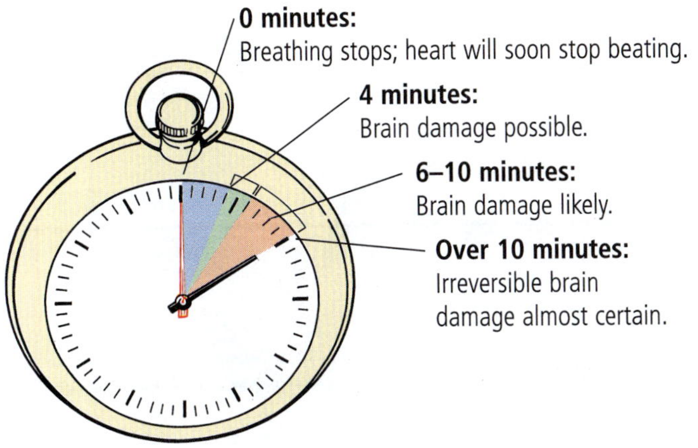

Care for Cardiac Arrest

A victim who is not breathing and has no pulse is considered clinically dead. However, the cells of the brain and other vital organs will continue to live for a short period of time until oxygen in the bloodstream is depleted. This victim needs cardiopulmonary resuscitation (CPR). The term "cardio" refers to the heart, and "pulmonary" refers to the lungs. CPR is a combination of EAR and external cardiac compressions (ECC). External cardiac compressions are a method of making the blood flow when the heart is not beating. Given together, EAR and ECC temporarily replace the functions of the lungs and heart. CPR increases a cardiac arrest victim's chances of survival by keeping the brain supplied with oxygen until advanced medical care can be given. Without CPR, the brain may begin to die within four minutes or less. The irreversible damage caused by brain cell death is known as biological death. Be aware, however, that even under the best of conditions, CPR only generates about one third of the normal blood flow to the brain (Figure 4-13).

Despite the best efforts of the first aider, CPR alone is not enough to help someone survive cardiac arrest. Advanced medical care is also needed, which is why it is so important to call an ambulance immediately. Trained ambulance personnel can provide some advanced life support (ALS) wherever they are called. In many parts of Australia, trained paramedics can administer medications or use a defibrillator (Figure 4-14). A defibrillator is a device which sends an electric shock through the chest to enable the heart to resume a functional heartbeat. Defibrillation given as soon as possible is the key to helping some victims survive cardiac arrest.

New, fully automatic defibrillators require little training and are now being placed on international aircraft, in some large factories, at major sporting venues and in other places where large numbers of people gather. Ongoing research may determine how widely automatic defibrillators are used in the future in Australia.

0 minutes:
Breathing stops; heart will soon stop beating.

4 minutes:
Brain damage possible.

6–10 minutes:
Brain damage likely.

Over 10 minutes:
Irreversible brain damage almost certain.

FIGURE 4-13 *Clinical death is a condition in which the heart and breathing stop. Clinical death may result in biological death, which is the irreversible death of brain cells.*

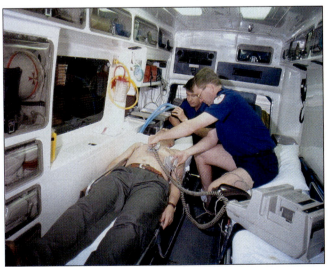

FIGURE 4-14 *Trained ambulance personnel using a defibrillator and other advanced measures may restore a heartbeat in a victim of cardiac arrest.*

It is very important to start CPR promptly and continue to provide CPR until ambulance personnel arrive. Immediate initiation of CPR by first aiders combined with early defibrillation administered by ambulance officers gives the victim of cardiac arrest the best chance for survival. As someone trained in first aid, you can help keep the victim alive until advanced care arrives.

REVIEW OF FIRST AID CARE FOR CARDIAC ARREST

As in any emergency, you care for cardiac arrest according to the emergency action principles. First aid for cardiac arrest always begins with airway care and 5 breaths of EAR. Take up to 10 seconds to check the pulse to be sure the heart is not beating. Chest compressions on a beating heart which are not needed may cause harm. If there is no pulse, begin CPR, and make sure someone calls for an ambulance immediately. If you are alone, begin CPR and shout for help to attract others.

It might help you to know that, even in the best of situations, when CPR is started promptly and ambulance personnel arrive quickly, many victims of cardiac arrest may not survive. Controlling your emotions and accepting death are not easy. Remember that any attempt to help is worthwhile. Because performing CPR and calling for help are only two of the several factors which determine whether a cardiac arrest victim survives, you should feel assured that you did everything you could to help.

EXTERNAL CARDIAC COMPRESSION

The theory most widely held today is that external cardiac compressions create raised pressure within the chest cavity which moves blood through the circulatory system.

Calipering for CPR Hand Position

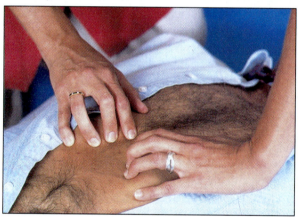

1. Find the lower edge of the victim's rib cage with your lower hand. Slide your index finger up the edge of the rib cage to the notch where the ribs meet the sternum. Leave your index finger on this notch.

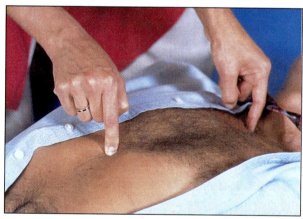

2. With the index finger of your upper hand, find the notch at the top of the sternum where the collar bones join it. Leave your index finger on this notch.

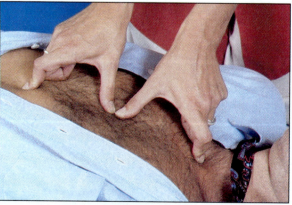

3. Caliper by extending both thumbs equally to find the middle of the sternum.

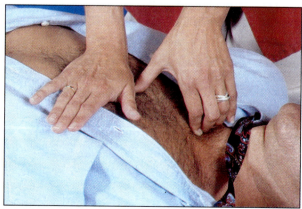

4. Place the heel of your compressing hand on the sternum just below the midpoint.

External Cardiac Compression Technique

For effective external cardiac compression (ECC), the victim should be lying flat on a firm surface. The victim's head should be kept on the same level as the heart. ECC is much less effective if the victim is on a soft surface, like a mattress or reclined car seat.

To give ECC, kneel beside the victim. Position yourself midway between the chest and the head in order to move easily between compressions and breaths.

Finding the Correct Hand Position

Using the correct hand position is important. It allows you to give the most effective compressions without causing injury. The correct position for your hands is over the lower half of the sternum (breastbone). At the lowest point of the sternum is an arrow-shaped piece of hard tissue called the xiphoid. You should avoid direct pressure on the xiphoid, which lies over the stomach, as pressure in this area can cause regurgitation and aspiration of stomach contents into the lungs.

Use the **calipering** method to locate the correct hand position for chest compressions (see box).

Once the heel of your hand is in position on the sternum, with your other hand grasp the wrist of the hand on the chest (Figure 4-15).

Use the heel of your hand to apply pressure on the sternum. Try to keep your fingers off the chest by holding them upward. Applying pressure with your fingers can lead to inefficient chest compressions or unnecessary damage to the chest wall.

The correct hand position provides the most effective compressions without the risk of complications.

The wrist grip position for the second hand is usually the best position to adopt for ECC. Alternatively, place your second hand directly on top of the hand on the chest (Figure 4-16). You can interlace the fingers so that the top fingers pull the bottom fingers off the chest during compressions. Use the position which allows you to deliver forceful compressions most smoothly and effectively.

The victim's clothing will not necessarily interfere with your ability to position your hands correctly to give chest compressions. If you can find the correct position without removing thin clothing, such as a T-shirt, do so. Sometimes a layer of thin clothing will help keep your hands from slipping, because the victim's chest may be moist with sweat. If you are not sure that you can find the correct hand position, uncover the victim's chest. You should not be overly concerned about being unable to find the correct hand position if the victim is obese, because fat does not accumulate as much over the sternum as it does elsewhere.

Position of the First Aider

Your body position is important when giving ECC. Compressing the chest straight down provides the best blood flow. The correct body position is also less tiring for you.

Kneel at the victim's chest with your hands in the correct position. Keep your shoulders directly over your hands (Figure 4-17, on the next page). When you press down in this position, you will be pushing straight down on to the sternum. If using the wrist grip technique, lock the elbow of the compressing arm. Locking the elbow keeps your arm straight and prevents you from tiring quickly. With the alternative hand grip, both elbows should be locked in a straight position.

Compressing the chest requires little effort in this position. When you press down, the weight of your upper body creates the force needed to compress the chest. Push with the weight of your upper body, not with the muscles of your arms. Push straight down. Do not rock back and forth. Rocking results in less effective compressions and wastes much needed energy. If your arms and shoulders tire quickly, you are not using the correct body position. After each compression, release the pressure on the chest without losing contact with it and allow the chest to return to its normal position before starting the next compression (Figure 4-18, on the next page).

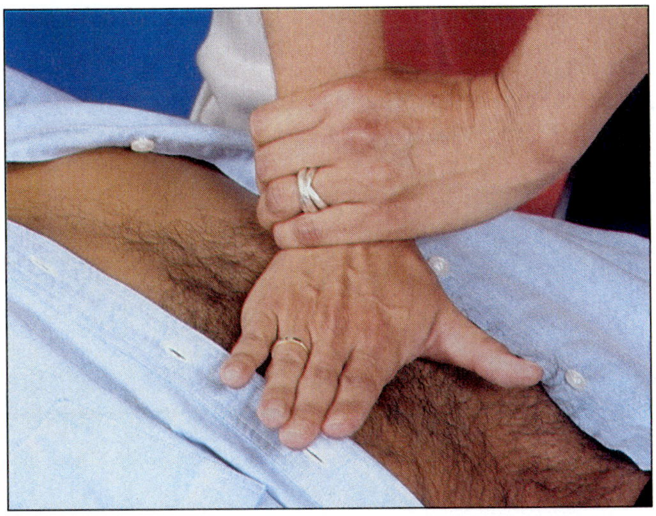

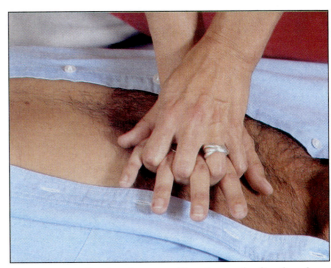

FIGURE 4-15 *After positioning the first hand on the chest, with your other hand grip the wrist. Use the heel of your bottom hand to apply pressure on the sternum.*

FIGURE 4-16 *Putting the second hand over the first hand positioned on the chest is an alternative hand position for giving chest compressions.*

With each compression, push the sternum down until you feel resistance. In a male weighing 80 kg this may be a compression of 5 cm, for example, whereas in a slender 50 kg woman it may be only 3.5 or 4 cm. The downward and upward movement should be smooth, not jerky. Maintain a steady down-and-up rhythm, and do not pause between compressions. Spend half of the time pushing down and half of the time coming up. When you press down, the chambers of the heart empty. When you come up to release all pressure on the chest, the chambers of the heart fill again with blood.

Keep your hands in their correct position on the sternum. If your hands slip, quickly find the notches as you did before and reposition your hands correctly.

Give compressions at the rate of 80 per minute. As you do compressions, count aloud, "One, two, three, four, five, six…" up to 15. Counting aloud will help you pace yourself. For an adult, do the 15 compressions in about 12 seconds. Even though you are compressing the chest at a rate of 80 times per minute, you will only actually perform 60 compressions in a minute. This is because you must take the time to do EAR, giving 2 breaths between groups of 15 compressions.

Compression/Breathing Cycles

When you give CPR, use cycles of 15 compressions and 2 breaths. For each cycle, give 15 chest compressions, then open the airway with head tilt and jaw support and give 2 full breaths (Figure 4-19). This cycle should take 15 seconds. For each new cycle of compressions and breaths, quickly recheck the correct hand position by finding the notch at the lower end of the sternum.

After doing 4 cycles of continuous CPR, which should take about 1 minute (Figure 4-20), tilt the victim's head to open the airway and check the carotid pulse. If there is no pulse, continue CPR. Check the pulse again every 2 minutes after giving EAR breaths. If you find a pulse, check for breathing. Continue EAR if necessary. If breathing recommences, keep the airway open by turning the victim on one side. Monitor breathing and pulse

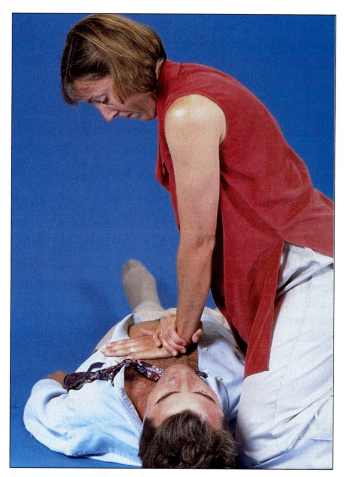

FIGURE 4-17 *With your hands in place, position yourself so that your shoulders are directly over your hands, arms straight and elbows locked.*

closely until ambulance personnel arrive. The Practice Guides at the end of this chapter provide step-by-step practice of CPR for adults, children and infants.

CPR FOR INFANTS AND CHILDREN

The technique of CPR for infants and children is similar to the technique for adults. Like CPR for adults, CPR

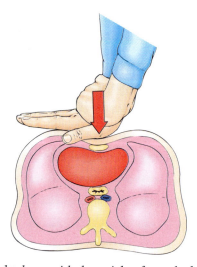
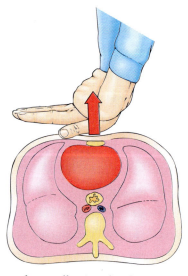

FIGURE 4-18 *Push straight down with the weight of your body then release, allowing the chest to return to the normal position. This allows the heart to refill after emptying.*

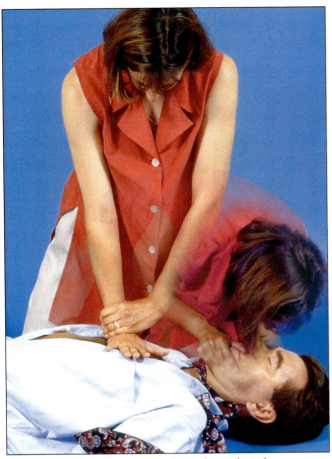

FIGURE 4-19 *Give 15 compressions, then 2 breaths.*

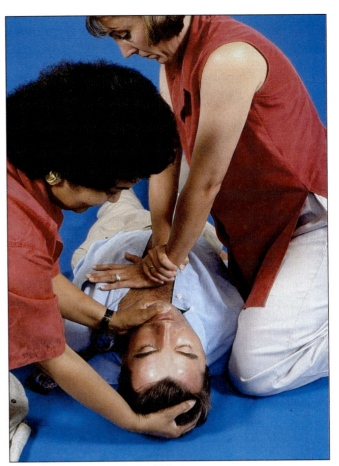

FIGURE 4-21 *Two-rescuer CPR.*

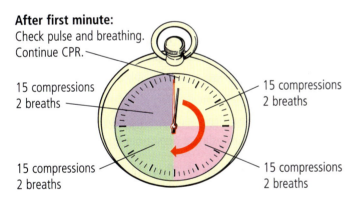

After first minute:
Check pulse and breathing.
Continue CPR.

15 compressions
2 breaths

15 compressions
2 breaths

15 compressions
2 breaths

15 compressions
2 breaths

FIGURE 4-20 *Check the pulse at the end of the fourth cycle of 15 compressions and 2 breaths.*

2 *Why are chest compressions and EAR both necessary for CPR to be effective?*

3 *Why would chest compressions alone not sustain the life of a person without a pulse?*

for infants and children consists of a series of alternating compressions and breaths. Infants and children have smaller bodies, and therefore they have faster heart and breathing rates. You must adjust the speed of your compressions and breaths as well as the pressure you use to give compressions.

For an adult, child or infant, CPR uses the same cycle of 15 compressions and 2 breaths. For a child or infant, use the same cycle at a faster rate: 15 compressions and 2 breaths in 10 seconds.

With a child, use only one hand for chest compressions. Position it in the same way as the first hand for an adult, but press on the sternum only with the heel of the first hand. Compress the sternum about 2 to 3 cm for an average-sized child. The depth of compression varies with the size of the child, so a range of 2 to 3 cm or more can be taken as a working guideline only.

With an infant, use only the index and middle fingers to give the compressions. Find the same position on the lower half of the sternum. On an average-sized infant, compress the sternum about 1 to 2 cm, varying the depth of compression according to the size of the infant.

MORE ABOUT CPR

Two-Rescuer CPR

When two first aiders trained in CPR are at the scene, you should both identify yourselves as CPR trained. One performs chest compressions while the other gives breaths (Figure 4-21). The first person should not pause

Chest Compression Technique for Adults, Children, Infants

	ADULT	CHILD	INFANT
HAND POSITION:	**Two hands** on lower 1/2 of sternum	**One hand** on lower 1/2 of sternum	**Two fingers** on lower 1/2 of sternum
COMPRESS:	about 4–5cm	about 2–3cm	about 1–2cm
BREATHE:	until chest rises	until chest rises	until chest rises
RATIO *ONE OPERATOR:*	15 compressions and 2 breaths in 15 seconds	15 compressions and 2 breaths in 10 seconds	15 compressions and 2 puffs in 10 seconds
RATIO *TWO OPERATORS:*	5 compressions and 1 breath (e.g. 60 compressions and 12 breaths per minute)	5 compressions and 1 breath (e.g. 100 compressions and 20 breaths per minute)	5 compressions and 1 puff (e.g. 100 compressions and 20 puffs per minute)

in the compressions, and the second gives one breath after each five compressions. The rescuer performing the compressions should count aloud up to five to help the second rescuer give synchronised breaths.

The rescuer giving breaths should also check for effective compression and for the return of a pulse. Check after the first full minute of CPR and then at least every 2 minutes. Follow these steps:

1. The rescuer giving breaths checks the carotid pulse while the first rescuer continues to give compressions.

2. If no pulse is felt, the rescuer giving compressions is advised that more effective compression is needed with improved technique.

3. If there is a pulse with each compression, then compressions are stopped so that the rescuer giving breaths can check for the return of a pulse. If no pulse is felt, CPR must continue.

4. If a spontaneous pulse has returned as indicated by a continuing pulse, compressions are stopped but EAR continues as long as it is necessary. The rescuer who is no longer giving compressions checks the radial pulse continuously; if this pulse cannot be felt, the carotid pulse is checked every

2 minutes. EAR is given until the victim is breathing unaided or ambulance personnel take over.

Change from One to Two Rescuers

When one trained rescuer has been giving CPR and a second trained rescuer arrives at the scene, the goal is to change to the two-operator method with minimal interruption to resuscitation. The rescuers should work on opposite sides of the victim. The first rescuer continues compressions and indicates readiness to make the change. Follow these steps:

1. The second rescuer feels for the carotid pulse to see if the compressions are effective.

2. If a pulse is felt with each compression, the first rescuer stops compressions long enough for the second rescuer to check for return of a spontaneous carotid pulse.

3. If there is no spontaneous pulse, the first rescuer gives a breath and the second rescuer begins compressions at a rate of 60 per minute without pausing for breaths. The first rescuer gives a breath after the fifth compression of one cycle and before the first compression of the next.

Change Over Between Two Rescuers

Trained rescuers may switch roles at the time of checking the pulse. The goal is to minimise any interruption in resuscitation.

The rescuer who has been giving EAR gives a breath and moves to the victim's side and prepares to take over compressions. The rescuer who has been giving compressions moves into position to give EAR. Resuscitation continues in the same pattern of one breath after every 5 compressions with regular pulse checks as before.

If an untrained person offers to help, the trained rescuer should explain the technique being used. When ready, the untrained person commences compressions under the guidance of the trained rescuer. An untrained person is unlikely to be capable of effective EAR, but can maintain compressions until other trained personnel arrive.

When to Stop CPR

Once you begin CPR, you should avoid interruption to the blood flow being created. However, there are several conditions under which you can stop CPR:

- If another trained person takes over CPR for you.
- If ambulance personnel arrive and take over care of the victim.
- If you are physically unable to continue.
- If the scene becomes unsafe.
- If the victim's heartbeat returns but there is still no breathing, continue giving EAR. If the victim begins to breathe again, turn the victim on the side, keep the airway open and check the vital signs closely until ambulance personnel arrive.

Summary

- For a victim who is not breathing, turn onto the back, open the airway with head tilt and jaw support, and give expired air resuscitation.
- For both EAR and CPR in children and infants, vary your technique appropriately.
- Immediate CPR helps keep the victim alive and the brain supplied with oxygen until the ambulance arrives.
- Follow these simple guidelines for CPR:
  — Find the correct position on the sternum, using the caliper method.
  — Use the correct hand position.
  — Compress and release smoothly.
  — Give 15 compressions in approximately 12 seconds.
  — Give 2 breaths.

  — Check for the return of a pulse after 1 minute.
  — If there is no pulse, continue CPR.
  — Recheck the pulse every 2 minutes.
  — If the victim's pulse returns, stop CPR and check to see if the person has started to breathe.
  — If the victim is still not breathing, continue EAR.

- Once you start CPR, do not stop unless the victim's heart starts beating, you are relieved by another trained person, you are unable to continue, or ambulance personnel arrive and take over.

In the next two chapters, you will learn how to care for bleeding and shock—two other life-threatening conditions you may find in the primary survey. Other breathing and cardiac emergencies are covered in Chapters 7 and 8.

Answers to Application Questions

1. When the heart fails, blood is not circulated to body tissues. Without the oxygen carried in the blood, tissues die and systems malfunction.

2. CPR is only effective if it replaces the circulatory and respiratory functions of the heart and lungs, respectively. Chest compressions function in place of the heart to circulate oxygen-rich blood to the body. EAR functions in place of the lungs, breathing air into the body.

3. A person without a pulse is not breathing. Although chest compressions deliver blood throughout the body, they cannot sustain life if oxygen is unavailable. CPR—the combination of EAR and ECC—not only provides the body with oxygen, but also delivers it to the body tissues.

Study Questions

1. *Match each term with the correct definition.*

   a. Face mask.

   b. Aspiration.

   c. Cardiac arrest.

   d. Head tilt and jaw support.

   e. EAR.

   f. Respiratory arrest.

   ____ The contamination of the air passages of the lungs with foreign material such as blood, vomit, broken teeth or other foreign bodies.

   ____ Process of ventilating the lungs of a non-breathing victim.

   ____ Device covering victim's mouth and nose during EAR, which separates the mouth of the rescuer from that of the victim.

   ____ Condition in which breathing stops.

   ____ Technique for opening the airway.

   ____ Condition in which the heart stops

2. *Which of the following statements about EAR is/are true:*

   a. EAR supplies the body with the oxygen required for survival.

   b. The airway must always be cleared and opened before commencing EAR.

   c. EAR is given to victims who are not breathing but still have a pulse.

   d. a and c.

   e. a, b and c.

3. *You discover the need for EAR during the primary survey when you determine the victim is:*

   a. unconscious

   b. unconscious and having difficulty breathing

   c. unconscious and not breathing

   d. all of the above

4. *After giving 5 breaths of EAR, you check the victim's pulse. The victim still has a pulse but is not breathing. You should:*

   a. continue EAR by giving 2 full breaths

   b. continue EAR giving 1 breath every 4 seconds

   c. stop EAR for 1 minute

   d. check vital signs

5. *Sequence the following actions for performing EAR from the time you discover that an adult victim is not breathing.*

   a. Turn victim on back.

   b. Check for pulse.

   c. Give 1 breath every 4 seconds.

   d. Give 5 full breaths.

   e. Recheck pulse after 1 minute.

6. *List the three signs of cardiac arrest.*

7. *List the conditions under which a first aider may stop CPR.*

8. *You know a person's heart is beating if the victim:*
   a. has a pulse
   b. is breathing
   c. is conscious
   d. is speaking
   e. all of the above

9. *The purpose of CPR is to:*
   a. keep a victim's airway open
   b. identify any immediate threats to life
   c. supply the vital organs with oxygen-rich blood.
   d. All of the above.

10. *CPR artificially takes over the functions of two body systems. They are the:*
   a. nervous and respiratory systems
   b. respiratory and circulatory systems
   c. circulatory and nervous systems
   d. circulatory and musculoskeletal systems

Use the following scenario to answer questions 11 and 12.

It is Saturday afternoon and you are at home with your parents watching a tennis match on television. During ads, you leave the room for 2 minutes. When you return, you find your father unconscious. You turn him onto his side, clear his airway and check his breathing. You find that he is not breathing. You give 5 breaths of EAR. You then find he has no pulse.

11. *Sequence the following actions you would now take to care for your father.*
   _____ Give 15 compressions.
   _____ Give 2 full breaths.
   _____ Locate the compression position.
   _____ Repeat cycles of 15 compressions and 2 breaths.
   _____ Recheck the pulse after 1 minute.

12. *After 1 minute of CPR, you recheck to see if your father has a pulse. He does not. What should you do next?*
   a. Stop CPR.
   b. Keep the airway open until the ambulance arrives.
   c. Check for breathing and begin EAR if needed.
   d. Continue CPR.
   e. None of the above.

Answers are in Appendix A (page 360).

PRACTICE GUIDE

Cardiopulmonary Resuscitation for an Adult

You find a person lying motionless on the ground. You should survey the scene to see if it is safe and to get some idea of what happened. If the scene is safe, do a primary survey by checking the victim's state of consciousness and the ABC.

Check conscious state

- Gently shake person.
- Shout, "Are you OK? Squeeze my hand; now let it go."

If person responds…

- Begin a secondary survey.

If the person does not respond…

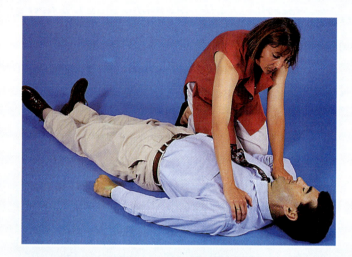

Roll person onto side

- Kneel beside victim.
- Grasp thigh nearest to you, and lift at right angles to the trunk.
- Place near arm across the chest with fingers at opposite shoulder.
- Lift under near shoulder and near thigh to roll victim away from you to lie on side.
- Keep thigh at right angle to trunk to prevent the victim from rolling onto face.
- Place upper arm across lower arm at elbow.

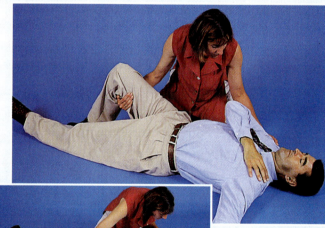

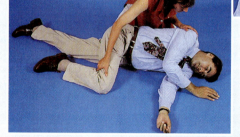

Clear airway

- Finger sweep mouth to clear foreign material.

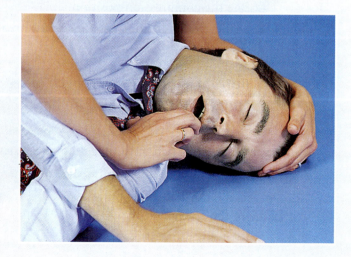

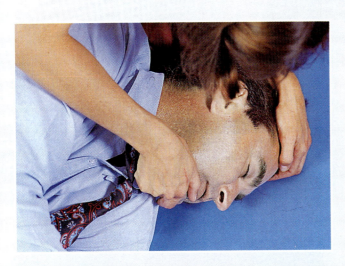

Open airway

- With your hand on top of the victim's head, tilt the head backwards.
- Support the victim's jaw with the other hand.
- Keep the victim's face turned slightly downwards for drainage.

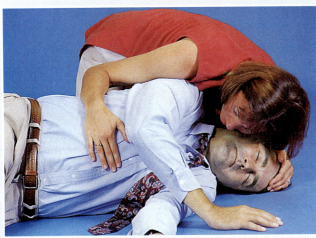

Check for breathing

- Look, listen, and feel for breathing for 3 to 5 seconds.

If the person is breathing. . .

- Leave the victim on the side

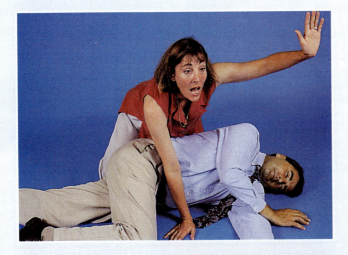

Shout for help

- Shout for help to attract attention.
- Send someone else to telephone emergency personnel, if possible.
- Keep airway open.
- Check for and control severe bleeding.
- Monitor ABC until ambulance personnel arrive.

If the person is not breathing, turn the victim onto the back...

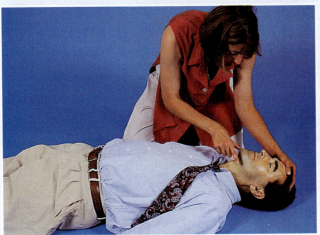

Give 5 full breaths

- Keep the victim's head tilted back with your hand on top of the head.
- Support the victim's jaw with a pistol grip.

- Seal your lips around the person's mouth.

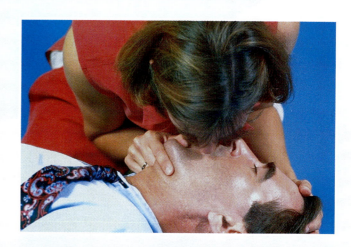

- Seal the victim's nose shut with your cheek.
- Give 5 full breaths in 10 seconds.
- Watch chest to see that it rises and falls.

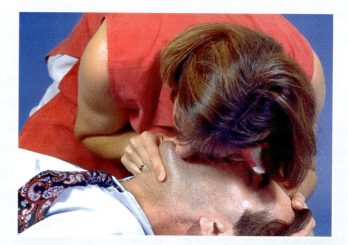

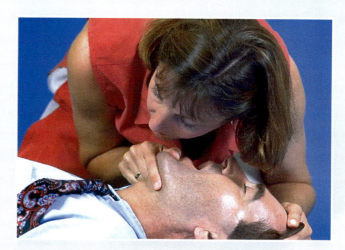

Check for pulse

- Keep the head tilted back.
- Locate the windpipe. (Adam's Apple).
- Slide your fingers down into the groove of the neck on the far side.
- Feel for pulse for up to 5 seconds.

If the person has a pulse...

- Continue EAR at a rate of 15 breaths per minute.
- Recheck pulse and breathing after one minute. Then keep checking both pulse and breathing after every two minutes.

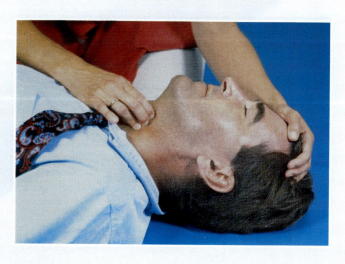

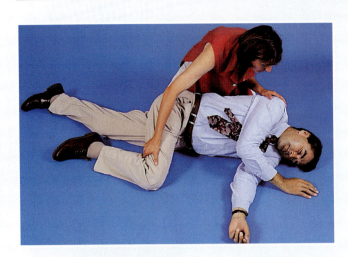

If breathing recommences…

- Roll the person onto the side.
- Support the victim's jaw, maintain an open airway and continue to monitor breathing and radial pulse at wrist.

If person does not have a pulse…

- Begin CPR.

Position hand for chest compression.

- Locate lower borders of the rib cage. Put index finger at the notch at lower end of sternum.

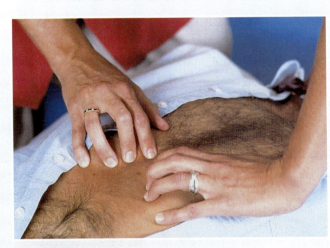

- Put other index finger on notch at top of sternum.

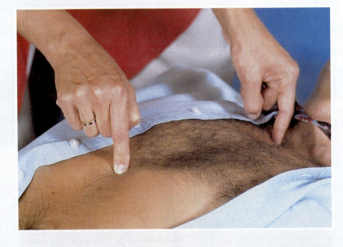

- Caliper with both hands to find the midpoint.

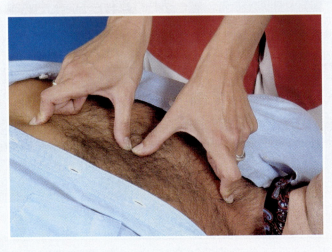

- Put the heel of compressing hand just below this point.

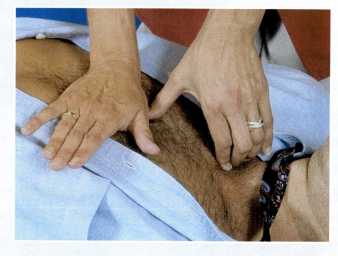

- Put other hand around wrist of compressing hand or on top of compressing hand.
- Keep your fingers off the victim's chest.

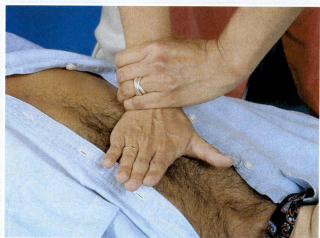

Give 15 compressions

- Position your shoulders over your hands.
- Compress the victim's sternum 4 to 5 cm.
- Give 15 compressions in approximately 12 seconds.
- Compress smoothly, keeping hand contact with the chest at all times.

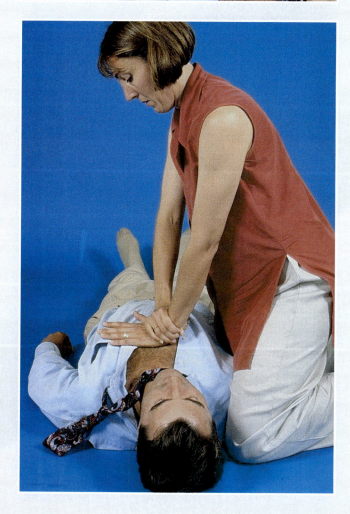

PRACTICE GUIDE

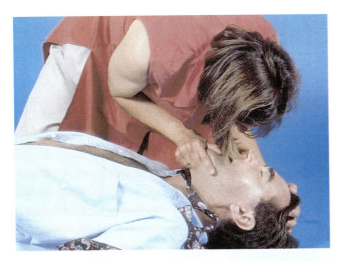

Give 2 full breaths

- Open airway with head-tilt and jaw-support.
- Seal your lips tightly around the person's mouth and seal the nose with your cheek.
- Give 2 full breaths, each lasting 1 to 2 seconds.
- Watch the victim's chest rise as your breaths go in and fall as breaths go out.

Repeat compression/breathing cycles

- Do 3 more cycles of 15 compressions and 2 breaths.

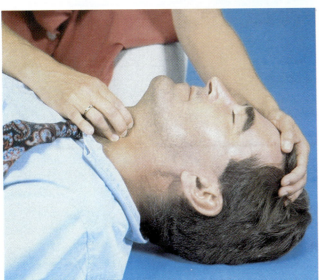

Recheck pulse and breathing

- Feel for pulse for up to 10 seconds.

If person has a pulse but is still not breathing...

- Continue EAR until ambulance officers arrive and take over.

If person does not have a pulse...

- Continue cycles of 15 compressions and 2 breaths
- Recheck pulse every 2 minutes
- Continue CPR until ambulance officers arrive and take over.

If a second person arrives

- If a second first aider arrives, ask for help with the compressions
- Change to a ratio of 5 compressions and 1 breath in continuous cycles.
- Recheck pulse and breathing every 2 minutes.

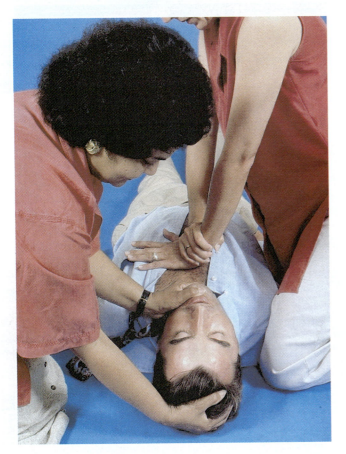

PRACTICE GUIDE

Cardiopulmonary Resuscitation for an Infant or Child

You find an infant or child lying motionless on the ground. After surveying the scene to make sure it is safe, do a primary survey by checking the state of consciousness and the ABC.

Check conscious state

- Tap or gently shake the infant or child.
- Shout, "Are you OK?"
- For a child, give a simple command: "Squeeze my hand; let it go."

If the infant or child cries or responds in any other way…

- Begin a secondary survey.

If the infant or child does not respond…

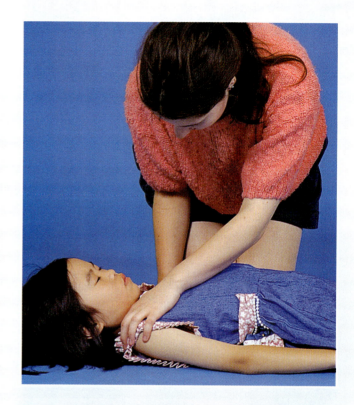

Roll the infant or child onto the side

- For an infant, support the head continuously.

Clear and open the airway

- Clear the mouth and nostrils of visible foreign matter.
- Support the jaw with the head in the neutral position, or tilted slightly back.

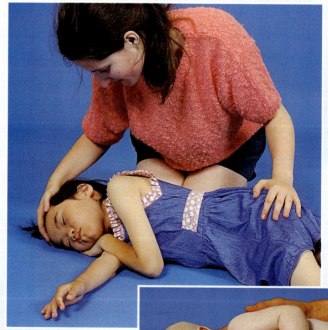

PRACTICE GUIDE

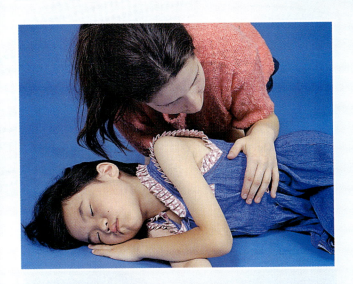

Check for breathing

- Look, listen and feel for breathing for 3 to 5 seconds.
- Remember to watch the lower chest and abdomen.

If the infant or child is breathing...

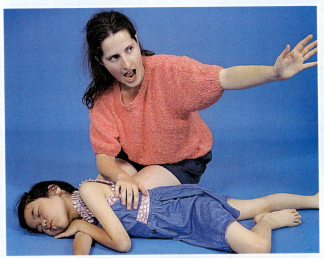

Call for help

- Call for help or send someone to call an ambulance.
- Leave the child or infant on the side.
- Keep airway open.
- Monitor breathing.
- Check and control severe bleeding.
- Await arrival of the ambulance.

If the infant or child is not breathing, turn the victim onto the back...

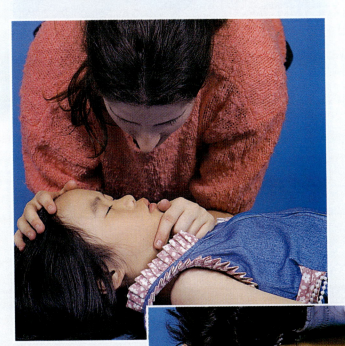

Give 5 breaths

Keep the head horizontal and jaw supported with the pistol grip.

- For a child, seal your lips around the child's mouth, seal the nose shut with your cheek and give 5 gentle breaths in 10 seconds.

- For an infant, seal your mouth around the infant's mouth and nose and give gentle puffs of air, just enough to make the chest rise.
- Watch the chest to see that it rises, and listen and feel for air being exhaled.

PRACTICE GUIDE

Check for a pulse

- For a child, check the carotid pulse.
- Keep the head horizontal.
- Locate the windpipe.
- Slide your fingers down into the groove of the neck on the far side.
- Feel for a pulse for up to 5 seconds.

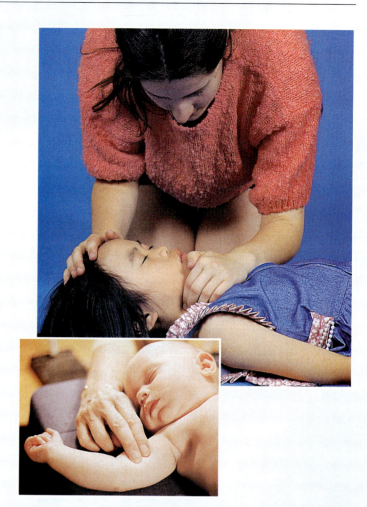

- For an infant, check the brachial pulse.
- Slide fingers over the upper arm of the child/infant, just above the elbow.
- Feel for pulse on the inside of the arm over the bone.

If the infant or child has a pulse but is still not breathing...

- Continue EAR at a rate of 20 breaths/puffs per minute.
- Recheck pulse and breathing after one minute. Then keep checking both pulse and breathing every two minutes.

If breathing recommences...

- Roll the infant or child onto the side.
- Support the jaw, maintain an open airway, and continue to monitor breathing and pulse.

If the infant or child does not have a pulse...

- Begin CPR.

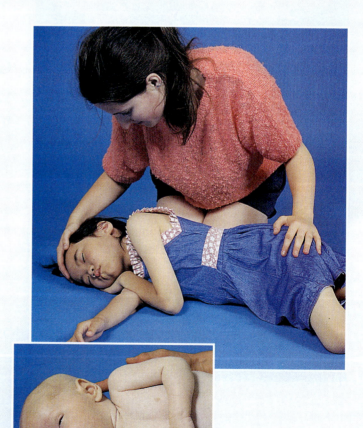

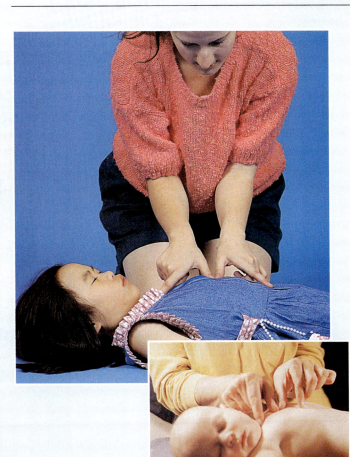

Position hand or fingers for chest compressions

- Locate the lower edge of the rib cage. Put your index finger on the notch at the lower end of sternum.

- Put your other index finger on the notch at top of the sternum.

- Caliper with both hands to find the midpoint.

- For a child, put the heel of one hand just below this point and keep your fingers off the chest. Use one hand only.

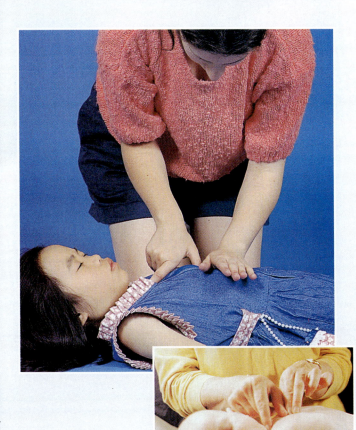

- For an infant, put 2 fingers below this point.

Give 15 compressions

- Position your shoulders over your hand.
- Compress the sternum about 2.5 cm for a child and about 1.5 cm for an infant.
- Give 15 compressions at the rate of approximately 90-100 per minute.
- Compress smoothly, keeping hand or finger contact with the chest at all times.

Give 2 breaths

- Open the airway with the head in the neutral position for an infant or tilted back very slightly for a child.
- Give 2 breaths/puffs, each lasting 1 to 2 seconds.
- Watch the chest rise as your breaths go in and fall as breaths go out.

Repeat compression/breathing cycles

- Give 5 more cycles of 15 compressions and 2 breaths.

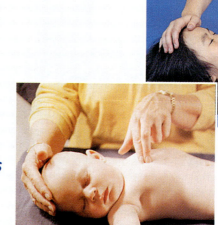

Recheck pulse and breathing.

- Feel for a pulse for up to 5 seconds.

If the infant or child has a pulse but is still not breathing...

- Continue EAR until ambulance officers arrive and take over.

If the infant or child does not have a pulse...

- Continue CPR until ambulance officers arrive and take over.

Continue compression/breathing cycles

- Continue cycles of 15 compressions and 2 breaths every 10 seconds.
- Recheck pulse every two minutes.

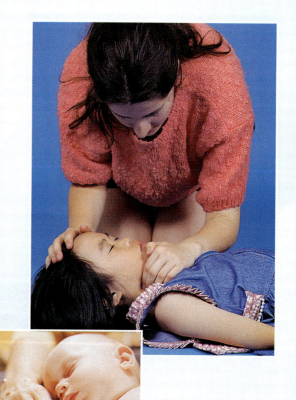

PRACTICE GUIDE

Basic Life Support Flow Chart

In the event of collapse, it is important that no time is wasted. Stay with the victim and follow the steps of the Basic Life Support Flow Chart:

COLLAPSE

Check response to SHAKE & SHOUT

CONSCIOUS

Make comfortable

Observe: **A**irway,
　　　　　Breathing,
　　　　　Circulation

UNCONSCIOUS

Victim on side

Turn face slightly downward,

Clear airway

Head tilt: Jaw support,

Check breathing

BREATHING

Leave on side in lateral position

Observe: **A**irway,
　　　　　Breathing,
　　　　　Circulation

NOT BREATHING

Victim on back

E.A.R. : 5 full breaths
　　　　　in 10 seconds,

Check pulse

PULSE PRESENT

Continue E.A.R.

Check pulse and breathing after 1 minute and then at least every 2 minutes

PULSE ABSENT

C.P.R.
(E.A.R. and E.C.C.)

Check breathing and pulse after 1 minute and then at least every 2 minutes.

Source: Australian Resuscitation Council.

Bleeding

BLEEDING is the loss of blood from blood vessels anywhere in the body. Bleeding may occur externally or within the body where it cannot be seen. Severe bleeding interferes with the circulation, causing damage to tissues and major organs, which can result in the death of the victim. As you have learned in previous chapters, you check for bleeding during the primary survey after checking the victim's pulse.

This chapter outlines how to recognise and care for both external and internal bleeding (wound care is covered in Chapter 12).

For Review

A review of how the circulatory system functions and how it interacts with other body systems (Chapter 2), and a revision of the emergency action principles (Chapter 3) will help your understanding of the chapter.

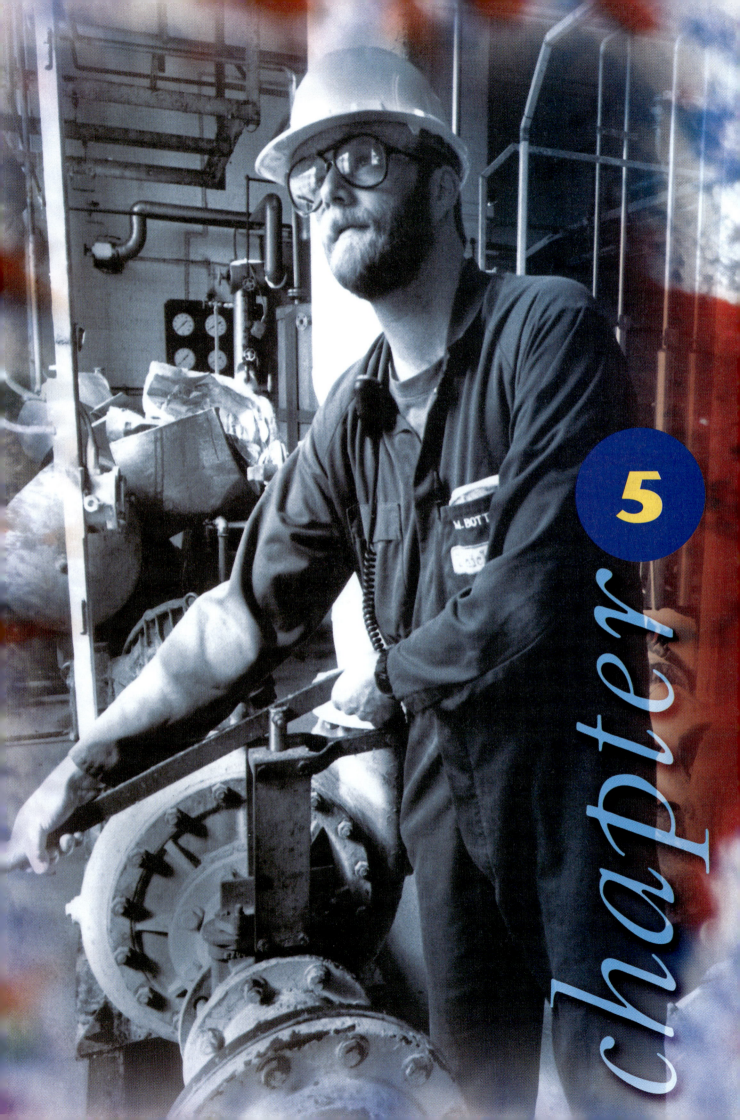

chapter

5

Key Terms

Aneurysm *(an-yoo-riz-m)*: A weakness in the wall of a blood vessel which may rupture.

Arteries: Large blood vessels that carry oxygen-rich blood from the heart to all parts of the body.

Blood volume: The total amount of blood circulating within the body.

Capillaries *(ca-pil-er-eez)*: Tiny blood vessels linking arteries and veins that transfer oxygen and other nutrients from the blood to all body cells and remove waste products.

Clotting: The process by which blood thickens at a wound site to seal an opening in a blood vessel and stop bleeding.

Direct pressure: The pressure applied on a wound to control bleeding.

External bleeding: Visible bleeding.

Haemophilia *(hee-mo-fil-ee-a)*: A disease more common in males caused by a lack of one or more clotting factors in the blood. Excessive bleeding internally and externally may follow minor trauma and may also occur spontaneously in the absence of trauma.

Haemorrhage *(hem-o-rage)*: A loss of a large amount of blood in a short period of time.

Internal bleeding: Bleeding inside the body.

Pressure bandage: A bandage applied firmly to create pressure on a wound to control bleeding.

Shock: The failure of the circulatory system to provide adequate oxygen-rich blood to all parts of the body.

Varicose veins: Veins that become swollen with pooled blood due to failure of the valves.

Veins: Blood vessels that carry blood low in oxygen from all parts of the body to the heart.

Bleeding is the escape of blood from arteries, veins or capillaries. A large amount of bleeding occurring in a short amount of time is called a haemorrhage. Bleeding is either internal or external. Internal bleeding is often difficult to detect in the early stages. External bleeding is usually obvious because it is visible.

To function well and keep all organs alive, the body must have enough blood circulating at sufficient pressure to reach all the body's tissues all the time. Uncontrolled bleeding, whether internal or external, is a life-threatening emergency (Figure 5-1). As you learned in the previous chapters, severe bleeding can result in death. You check for severe bleeding during the primary survey. However, you may not identify **internal bleeding** until you perform the secondary survey. In this chapter, you will learn how to recognise and care for serious internal and **external bleeding**. With external bleeding, the victim also needs wound care, which is described in Chapter 12.

BLOOD AND BLOOD VESSELS

Blood Components

Blood consists of liquid and solid components and comprises approximately 8 per cent of the body's total weight. The liquid part of the blood is called plasma. The solid components are the red and white blood cells and platelets.

Plasma makes up about half of the total **blood volume.** Composed mostly of water, plasma maintains the blood volume needed for normal function of the circulatory system. Plasma also contains nutrients essential for energy production, growth and cell maintenance, and carries waste products for elimination.

White blood cells are a key disease-fighting part of the immune system. They defend the body against invading micro-organisms. They also aid in producing antibodies, which help the body resist infection.

Red blood cells account for most of the solid components of the blood. They are produced in the marrow in the hollow centre of large bones such as the large bones of the arm (humerus) and thigh (femur). Red blood

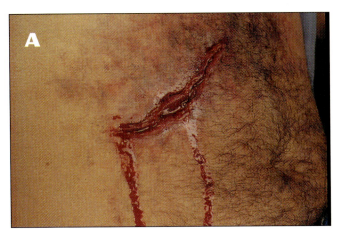
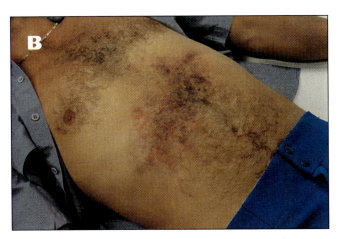

FIGURE 5-1A *External bleeding is more easily recognised than* **B** *internal bleeding.*

cells number nearly 260 million in each drop of blood. The red blood cells transport oxygen from the lungs to the body cells and carbon dioxide from the cells to the lungs. Red blood cells outnumber white blood cells by about 1000 to 1.

Platelets are disc-shaped structures in the blood. Platelets are an essential part of the blood's **clotting** mechanism because of their tendency to bind together; they help stop bleeding by forming blood clots at wound sites which form the framework for healing. Until blood clots form, bleeding must be controlled artificially.

Blood Functions

The blood has three major functions:

1. Transport of oxygen, nutrients and wastes.
2. Protection against disease by transport of antibodies to defend against germs, and assistance with clotting and healing in response to injury.
3. Maintenance of constant body temperature by circulating throughout the body.

Blood Vessels

Blood is channelled through blood vessels. There are three major types of blood vessels: **arteries**, **capillaries** and **veins** (Figure 5-2). Arteries carry oxygen-rich blood away from the heart. Arteries become smaller throughout the body until they connect to the capillaries. Capillaries are microscopic blood vessels linking arteries and veins. They transfer oxygen and other nutrients from the blood into the cells. Capillaries pick up waste products, such as carbon dioxide, from the cells and move them into the veins. The veins carry waste products from the cells to the kidneys, intestines and lungs, where waste products are eliminated.

The blood in the arteries is closer to the pumping action of the heart. Blood in the arteries therefore travels under greater pressure than blood in the capillaries or veins. Arterial blood flow pulses with the heartbeat; venous blood flows more evenly.

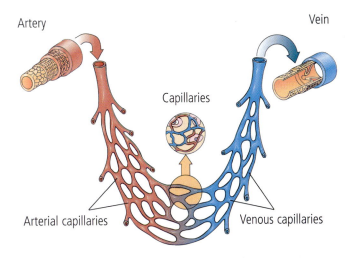

FIGURE 5-2 *Blood flows through the three major types of blood vessels: arteries, capillaries and veins.*

WHEN BLEEDING OCCURS

When bleeding occurs, the body begins a complex chain of events. The brain, heart and lungs immediately attempt to compensate for blood loss in order to maintain the flow of oxygen-rich blood to the body, particularly to the vital organs.

Other important reactions also occur on a microscopic level. Platelets collect at the wound site in an effort to stop blood loss through clotting. White blood cells prevent infection by attacking micro-organisms which commonly enter through breaks in the skin. The body manufactures extra red blood cells to help transport more oxygen to the cells.

Blood volume is also affected by bleeding. Normally, excess fluid is absorbed from the bloodstream by the kidneys, lungs, intestinal tract and skin. However, when bleeding occurs this excess fluid is re-absorbed into the bloodstream as plasma. This helps to maintain the critical balance of fluids needed by the body to keep blood volume constant.

Bleeding severe enough to critically reduce the blood volume is life-threatening and can be either internal or external.

The Beat Goes On

The Ice Age—Prehistoric Man

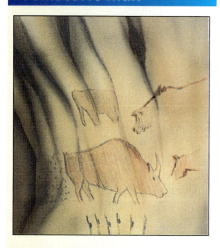

Primitive man draws a giant mammoth on a cave, with a red ochre marking resembling a heart in its chest.

500 B.C.—Greek Civilization

Ancient Greek physicians propound the theory of the humours, associating man's personality and health with four substances in the body—blood, black bile, yellow bile and phlegm. An imbalance can cause diseases or emotional problems. A curious practice called bloodletting develops in which physicians open a patient's vein and let him or her bleed to fix an imbalance in the humours.

900 to 1400—The Middle Ages

Bloodletting flourishes during the Middle Ages. Astrology's influence grows, leading doctors to use astrological charts to determine when and where to open a vein. Medical schools sprout up in England, France, Belgium and Italy.

3000 B.C.—The Fifth Dynasty

Egyptians believe that blood is created in the stomach and that vessels running from the heart are filled with blood, air, faeces and tears.

1628—The Renaissance Period

Dr William Harvey cuts into live frogs and snakes to observe the heart. Through his studies, Harvey determines that blood circulates through the heart, the lungs and the rest of the body.

Circa 200 A.D.—Late Roman Civilization

Galen, doctor of Roman Emperor Marcus Aurelius, theorises that blood is continuously formed in the liver and then moves in two systems: one that combines with the air and a second that forms from food to nourish the body.

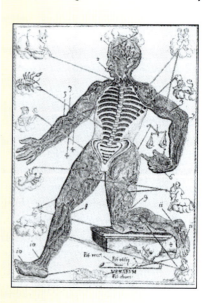

1661

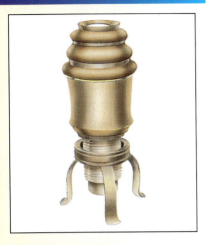

The invention of the microscope allows Italian-born physician Malpighi to see the tiny capillaries that link veins and arteries.

Early 1900's— The Twentieth Century

Dr Karl Landsteiner discovers that all human blood is not compatible and names the blood types. His work helps make blood transfusions commonplace.

1953

Dr John H. Gibbon invents a heart-lung machine to recirculate blood and provide oxygen during open-heart surgery, enabling more complex surgical techniques to develop.

1982

Dr William DeVries implants the first artificial heart in Barney Clark. The Seattle dentist survives 112 days, and the Jarvik-7 beats 12,912,499 times before Clark dies. In the 1980s, five artificial hearts are implanted. The longest survival period lasts 620 days. The body continues to treat the artificial heart as a "foreign body" and rejects it.

1665

The first blood transfusion mixes the blood of one dog with another. Transfusions range from successful to disastrous. One scientist proposes a transfusion between unhappily married people to try to reconcile the couple. After a man who receives sheep's blood dies, transfusion is outlawed in France.

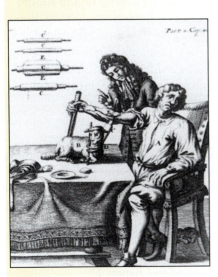

1967

The first heart transplant is attempted by Dr Christiaan Barnard in Cape Town, South Africa. Louis Washansky, a 54-year-old grocer, receives the heart of a woman hit by a speeding car. Washansky survives 18 days.

1944

When kidneys fail, poisons are released into the bloodstream that can cause vomiting, coma and eventually death. Dr Willem Kolff, a Dutch physician, develops one of the first artificial kidneys by sending the blood through a cellophane tubing that filters out the poisons.

The Future

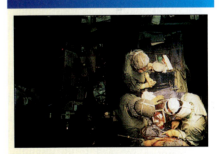

Through the ages, medical science has made extensive progress in saving lives. In Australia, almost one million donations of blood are collected each year from voluntary unpaid donors. This allows over 300,000 Australians a year to receive transfusions of blood or blood components. Between 1969 and 1993, almost 9000 Australians received kidney transplants, almost 600 received heart transplants, and over 600 received liver transplants. The early medical experiments of yesterday have become commonplace lifesaving procedures today.

How do the brain, heart and lungs attempt to compensate for blood loss?

Why will severe bleeding result in death if not controlled?

External Bleeding

External bleeding occurs when a blood vessel is opened externally, such as through a tear in the skin. You can usually see this type of bleeding. Most external bleeding you will encounter will be minor and usually stops by itself within 10 minutes when the blood clots. Sometimes, however, the damaged blood vessel is too large, or the blood is under too much pressure for effective clotting to occur. In these cases, bleeding can be life-threatening and you will need to recognise and control it promptly. You look for severe bleeding in the primary survey.

THE DISCOVERY OF TRAUMATIC ARTERIAL SPASM

About 200 years ago the English researcher John Hunter discovered and described how vasoconstriction can prevent a person from bleeding to death after an artery is severed or seriously injured. In his experiments with a boar and dog, he observed that the severed artery contracted so much in a short time that bleeding was reduced to an ooze. Clinical observations in World War I confirmed this in humans as well. Major arteries severed by bullets were sometimes seen to bleed little internally or externally. In World War II an airman whose foot was amputated by an aeroplane's propeller lost little blood. In another reported case, a motorcyclist's leg was amputated 5 cm below the knee in a crash, with blood loss of less than a quarter of a litre.

Signs of External Bleeding

The signs of life-threatening external bleeding include:

- Blood spurting from a wound.
- Blood that fails to clot after all measures have been taken to control bleeding.

Each type of blood vessel bleeds differently. Arterial bleeding is often rapid and profuse, and therefore it is life-threatening. As arterial blood is under more pressure it usually spurts from the wound, making it difficult for clots to form, so arterial bleeding is harder to control. Because of its high concentration of oxygen, arterial blood is a bright red colour.

Venous bleeding (bleeding from the veins) is easier to control than arterial bleeding. Veins are damaged more often because they are closer to the skin's surface. Venous blood is under less pressure than arterial blood and flows from the wound at a steady rate without spurting. Only damage to veins deep in the body, such as those in the trunk or thigh, produces profuse bleeding that is hard to control. Venous blood is dark red or maroon because it is low in oxygen.

Capillary bleeding, the most common type of bleeding, is usually slow because the vessels are small and the blood is under low pressure. It is often described as "oozing" from the wound. Clotting occurs easily with capillary bleeding. The blood is usually less red than arterial blood.

Why is arterial bleeding extremely dangerous?

Controlling External Bleeding

External bleeding is usually easy to control. Generally, the pressure created by placing a hand on the wound can control bleeding. This is known as applying **direct pressure**. Pressure placed on the wound restricts the blood flow through the wound and allows normal clotting to occur. Elevating the injured area also slows the flow of blood and encourages clotting. Pressure on a wound can be maintained by firmly applying a bulky pad and bandage to the injured area. A bandage applied to control bleeding is called a **pressure bandage.**

A tourniquet, a tight band placed around an arm or leg to help constrict blood flow to a wound, is rarely used because it too often does more harm than good. Initially a tourniquet may cause more bleeding below the band, as it prevents venous return. Eventually the tissues below the tourniquet are starved of blood and die from lack of nutrients and oxygen. The care of an amputation and major wounds is described in Chapter 12.

To control external bleeding, first expose the wound and check that there is no visible foreign body in the wound. Then follow these general steps:

1. Place direct pressure on the wound with a sterile dressing pad, or improvise with any clean cloth such as a towel or handkerchief. Using a pad or cloth will help keep the wound free from germs. Place a hand over the pad and apply firm pressure (Figure 5-3A). If you do not have a pad or cloth available, ask the victim to apply firm hand pressure. As a last resort, use your own hand.

2. If you do not suspect a broken bone, elevate the injured area above the level of the heart and let the victim rest in a comfortable position (Figure 5-3B).

3. Apply a pressure bandage to hold the pad or cloth in place. You may do this with a folded triangular bandage placed over the wound and tied over the site for extra pressure (Figure 5-3C), or with a roller bandage (Figure 5-3D).

4. If bleeding continues through or around the bandage, do not attempt to add more padding because the increased bulk will reduce the pressure on the wound. Remove the bandage and pad and reassess how they were applied. Replace the pad with a new one in the correct position.

5. Continue to monitor the victim's airway and breathing. Call an ambulance if necessary. Observe the victim closely for signs of shock (see Chapter 6) or any other indications of a deteriorating condition.

6. Periodically check the circulation beyond the bandage to make sure it is not too tight. Look for cold, pale skin, toes or fingers that do not return to normal colour after compressing the nail, or complaints of numbness or tingling (see Chapter 13).

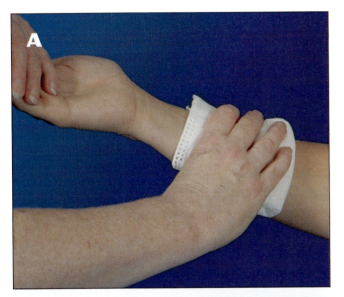
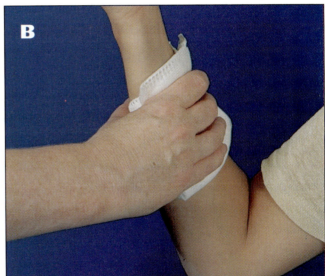
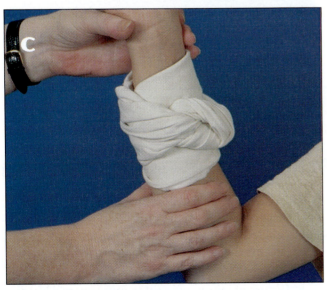
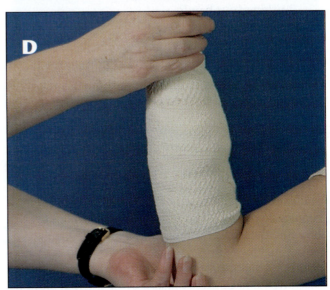

FIGURE 5-3 A *Apply direct pressure to the wound using a pad or clean cloth.* **B** *Elevate the injured area above the level of the heart if you do not suspect a fracture.* **C** *Apply a pressure bandage using either a folded triangular bandage, or;* **D** *a roller bandage.*

4 *Why should you remove a blood-soaked pad when bleeding is uncontrolled?*

Although most severe bleeding usually occurs from arteries, **varicose veins** can bleed heavily. Varicose veins are veins that have swollen due to a deterioration of the non-return valves in the veins. This allows the blood to pool at certain points rather than to flow back to the heart. Varicose veins can occur in any part of the body (for example, haemorrhoids) but are most commonly found in the legs due to the effects of gravity. A large volume of blood can be present in these veins and cause massive bleeding if the veins are injured or burst. If not stopped, this bleeding can lead to death. Use direct pressure to control bleeding from veins in the legs in the same way that you control other external bleeding. Elevation of the limb above the level of the heart dramatically reduces bleeding.

Preventing Disease Transmission

To reduce the risk of disease transmission when controlling bleeding, you should:

- Place an effective barrier between your skin and the victim's blood when you give first aid. Examples of such barriers are the victim's hand, latex gloves or even a clean, folded cloth.

- Wash your hands thoroughly with soap and water immediately after providing care, even if you wore gloves or used another barrier. Use a hand basin or tap, preferably not one in a food preparation area.

- Avoid eating, drinking and touching your mouth, nose or eyes while providing care or before washing your hands.

Internal Bleeding

Internal bleeding is the escape of blood from arteries, veins or capillaries into spaces in the body. Capillary bleeding, indicated by mild bruising, is beneath the skin and is not serious. However, deeper bleeding involves arteries and veins and may result in severe blood loss.

Severe internal bleeding usually occurs in injuries caused by a violent blunt force, such as in a car crash or a fall from a height. Internal organs such as the spleen and liver can be damaged by blows to the body even though there may be no external signs of injury or bleeding. Internal bleeding may also occur when an object such as a knife penetrates the skin and damages internal structures. Some medical conditions such as a bleeding stomach ulcer can also cause internal bleeding. In any serious injury, suspect internal bleeding.

Internal bleeding can be as serious as external bleeding. Although the blood is not lost from the body,

Table 5–1

POSSIBLE INTERNAL SOURCES OF BLEEDING THROUGH ORIFICES

Orifice	Possible cause	Type of bleeding
Ear	Injured eardrum	Steady bright red bleeding
	Skull fracture	Trickle of blood mixed with clear fluid
Mouth	Jaw fracture or mouth injury	Bright red blood spat out
	Stomach or intestines	Vomited dark brown blood (looks like coffee grounds)
	Lung or airway injury	Coughed up bright red or frothy blood
	Oesophagus	Vomited bright red blood
Nose	Injured nasal passages or fracture	Heavy flow of bright red blood
	Skull fracture	Trickle of blood mixed with clear fluid
Rectum	Piles (haemorrhoids)	Steady bright red bleeding
	Intestinal bleeding	Tarry black stool
Vagina	Menstrual bleeding	Steady moderate to heavy bleeding with cramps
	Miscarriage, abortion	Sudden heavy flow, shock developing
Urethra	Kidney bleeding	Dark blood-stained urine
	Bladder or urinary tract bleeding	Clotted blood or diluted blood in urine

it is lost from the circulatory system and vital organs are deprived of oxygen. Internal bleeding can also cause problems if it presses on vital structures, such as blood inside the skull putting pressure on the brain or bleeding inside the chest preventing the lungs from expanding properly.

History, Symptoms, Signs and Behaviour Indicating Internal Bleeding

The body's inability to adjust to severe internal bleeding will eventually produce signs that indicate shock. Shock is discussed in more detail in Chapter 6.

Internal bleeding is more difficult to recognise than external bleeding because the signs are less obvious and may take time to appear. Suspect internal bleeding if any of the following are present:

- History of injury sufficient to cause internal bleeding.

- Medical condition that can cause internal bleeding, such as an ulcer, **haemophilia** or **aneurysm.**

- Pain and tenderness in soft tissues around the area, possibly with hardness, swelling and distension.
- Discolouration of the skin in the injured area.
- Anxiety or restlessness.
- Rapid, weak pulse.
- Rapid breathing.
- Skin that feels cool or moist or looks pale or bluish.
- Nausea and vomiting.
- Excessive thirst.
- Deteriorating conscious state.
- Bleeding from body orifices (see Table 5-1).

Controlling Internal Bleeding

Controlling internal bleeding depends on the severity and site of the bleeding. If you suspect internal bleeding caused by serious injury, call for an ambulance immediately. There is little you can do to effectively control serious internal bleeding. Calling an ambulance is the best help you can provide. Ambulance personnel must transport the victim rapidly to the hospital. Usually, the victim needs immediate surgery to correct the problem.

While waiting for the ambulance to arrive, follow the general guidelines of care for any emergency. These are:

1. Prevent further injury.
2. Monitor the ABC.
3. Help the victim to rest in the most comfortable position.
4. Maintain normal body temperature.
5. Reassure the victim.
6. Provide care for other specific conditions.

5 *What is the likely result of moving a person who is bleeding internally?*

Summary

- Recognising and controlling life-threatening bleeding is critical in an emergency.
- Check for severe external bleeding during the primary survey immediately after checking breathing and circulation. Care for bleeding with pressure, elevation and rest, and monitor the victim for shock.

- Suspect internal bleeding when a serious injury has occurred. When the victim's history, symptoms, signs and behaviour suggest internal bleeding, call an ambulance immediately and provide care until ambulance officers arrive and take over.
- Controlling external bleeding also includes wound care, which is described in Chapter 12.

Answers to Application Questions

1. When bleeding occurs, the brain, heart and lungs strive to supply adequate oxygen to all body tissues. First, body tissues that are not receiving adequate oxygen notify the brain. Then the brain sends instructions to the heart to beat faster so that it can pump more blood and deliver the needed oxygen. Simultaneously, the brain instructs the lungs to breathe faster to bring in the needed oxygen.

2. Severe bleeding results in death because blood loss decreases blood volume and deprives body tissues of the oxygen they need for survival.

3. Arterial bleeding is dangerous because the blood is under greater pressure than in the veins or capillaries. The greater the blood loss, the faster the heart beats to meet the body's demands for oxygen. However, by increasing its rate, the heart also increases the rate of blood loss. Arterial bleeding results in a large amount of blood loss in a short time, rapidly reducing the supply of oxygen which body tissues need for survival. It is also dangerous because the pressure in the arteries causes the surging of blood, which impedes clotting.

4. If bleeding persists, this indicates inadequate pressure is being applied or pressure is being applied to the wrong area. Bleeding will not be controlled until you remove the bandage and pad, reassess the wound and replace the pad in the correct area. Replace a blood-soaked pad with a clean one. Retain all blood-soaked material for medical personnel to assess blood loss.

5. Any unnecessary movement will stimulate the circulation and is likely to increase internal bleeding. Surgery is usually required to control internal bleeding. While waiting for the ambulance, helping the victim to rest in a comfortable position may be life saving.

Study Questions

1. **Match each term with the correct definition.**

    a. Haemorrhage.
    b. Arteries.
    c. Capillaries.
    d. Veins.
    e. Internal bleeding.
    f. External bleeding.
    g. Direct pressure.
    h. Pressure bandage.

    ____ Vessels that transport oxygen and other nutrients to cells and remove waste products.
    ____ Using your hand to apply pressure on the wound.
    ____ The loss of a large amount of blood in a short period of time.
    ____ Visible bleeding.
    ____ The escape of blood from an artery, vein or capillary into spaces in the body.
    ____ Vessels that transport blood low in oxygen, containing waste products.
    ____ Vessels that transport oxygen-rich blood to the capillaries for distribution to cells.
    ____ Used to maintain pressure on the wound to control bleeding.

2. **List two functions of the blood.**

3. **List two signs of life-threatening external bleeding.**

4. **Describe how to control external bleeding.**

5. **Match each step of care for controlling external bleeding with its specific task.**

    a. Apply direct pressure.
    b. Elevate the injured part.
    c. Apply pressure bandage over a firm pad.
    d. Keep the person at rest and the injured part still.
    e. Check circulation beyond the bandage.

    ____ Uses principles of gravity to slow blood flow to the injured area to help control bleeding.
    ____ Ensures bandage is not restricting circulation to other areas.
    ____ Maintains pressure on the wound and helps prevent infection.
    ____ Places pressure on the wound to slow blood flow and aid clotting.
    ____ Reduces the flow of blood to the injured area.

6. *List five symptoms and signs, and the behaviour of a victim of internal bleeding.*

Use the following scenario to answer questions 7, 8 and 9.

Your father returns home from a day of fishing. He has caught half a dozen trout and decides to clean the fish for dinner. He takes out his knife and begins to clean the fish. He is in the middle of a story about "the one that got away" when the knife slips and he severely cuts his hand. Calling out, he grabs his hand to hold the wound together.

7. *Sequence the actions you would take to care for your father's wound.*

_____ Apply a pressure bandage to maintain the pressure on the wound.

_____ Assist him into a position of rest with his arm supported.

_____ Take any clean material within reach, place it on the wound and apply direct pressure with your hand over the pad.

_____ Help him to hold his injured hand above the level of his heart.

Despite the pressure placed on the wound, you notice blood beginning to soak through the bandage. Your father becomes anxious, starts breathing faster and looks pale.

8. *Sequence the next actions you would take.*

_____ Provide reassurance and lightly cover him with a blanket, without overheating.

_____ Remove the blood-soaked pad, reassess the wound and apply a fresh pad and bandage over the wound.

_____ Assist your father to lie down and raise his legs.

_____ Call an ambulance.

9. *Describe how someone close by could help in this emergency.*

10. *What should you do if you suspect serious internal bleeding?*

   a. Call an ambulance immediately.

   b. Apply pressure at the closest pressure point.

   c. Place an ice pack on the affected area.

   d. Wrap a pressure pad and bandage around the affected area.

11. *List three things you can do to reduce the risk of disease transmission when controlling bleeding.*

Answers are in Appendix A (page 360).

Shock

YOU have already learned how some injuries and conditions can cause breathing and the pulse to stop. Severe bleeding also is life-threatening. Normally the body can cope with the physical stresses of illness and injury. However, when the body can no longer cope, the victim may lapse into another life-threatening condition called shock.

This chapter outlines how to recognise the symptoms and signs of shock and how to care for a victim with this condition.

For Review

A basic understanding of how the respiratory and circulatory systems function and of the inter-relationship of body systems (Chapter 2) will help your understanding of the chapter.

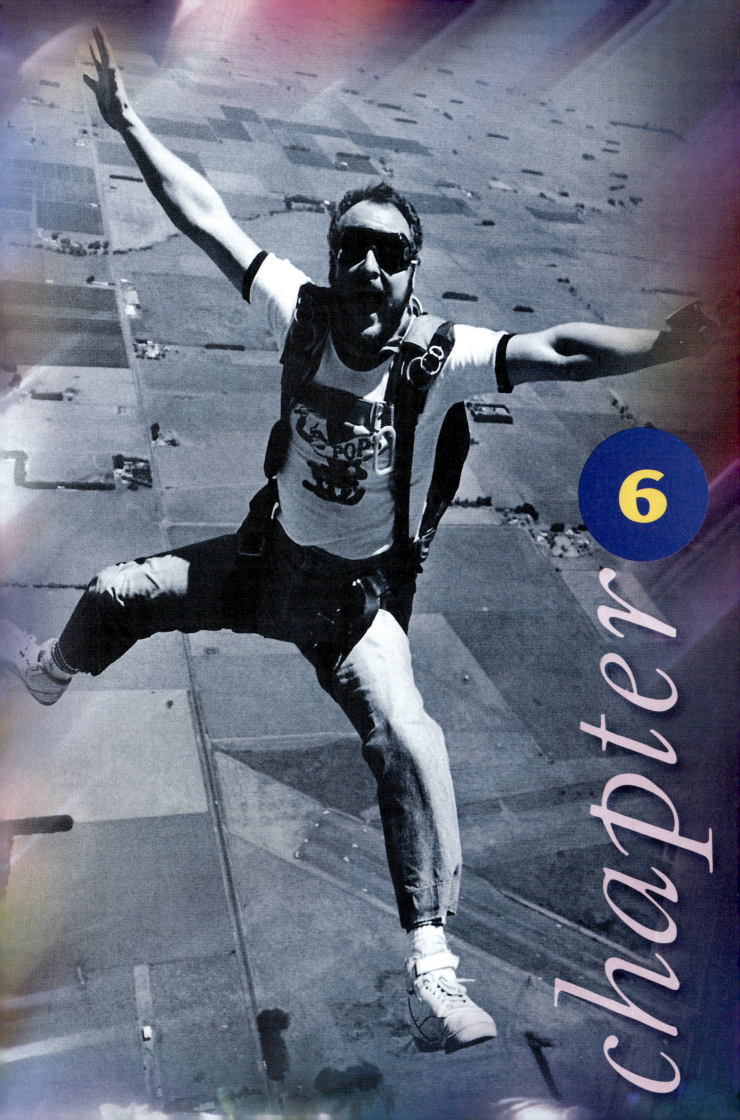

chapter

6

Key Terms

Blood volume: The total amount of blood circulating within the body.

Shock: The failure of the circulatory system to provide adequate oxygen-rich blood to all parts of the body.

Vital organs: Organs whose functions are essential to life, including the brain, heart and lungs.

10:55 PM. *On an isolated road, a large kangaroo leaps into the path of an oncoming car travelling at 100 kph. The driver, a 21 year old university student and athlete, cannot avoid the collision. In the crash, both of her legs are broken and are pinned in the wreckage.*

11:15 PM. *Another car finally approaches. Seeing the crashed car, the driver stops and comes forward to help. He finds the woman conscious but restless and in obvious pain. He says he will go to call an ambulance at the nearest house, a kilometre or two down the road. He assures her he will return.*

11:25 PM. *When the driver returns, he sees that the woman's condition has changed. She is now breathing faster, looks pale and appears drowsy. He takes hold of her hand in an effort to comfort her and feels that her skin is cold and moist. Her pulse is fast but so weak he can hardly feel it.*

11:30 PM. *The ambulance arrives 10 minutes after receiving the phone call. The man explains that the woman became drowsy and is no longer conscious. Her breathing has become very irregular. The ambulance crew goes to work immediately.*

11.40 PM. *Finally, the rescuers free her legs and remove her from the car. The man notices that she looks worse. He knows the hospital is still 10 minutes away.*

12.00 MIDNIGHT. *Despite the best efforts of everyone involved, the woman is pronounced dead a little over an hour after the crash. Her heart stopped beating en route to the hospital. Although the ambulance officers gave CPR and advanced cardiac life support measures, they were unable to save her. She was a victim of a progressively deteriorating condition called shock.*

When the body experiences injury or sudden illness, significant fear or pain, it responds in a number of ways. Survival depends on the body's ability to adapt to the physical stresses of illness or injury. When the body's compensation measures fail, the victim can progress into a life-threatening condition called **shock.** Shock complicates the effects of injury or sudden illness. In this chapter, you will learn to recognise and give care to minimise shock.

WHAT IS SHOCK

When **vital organs** do not receive enough oxygen-rich blood, they fail to function properly. This triggers a series of responses that lead to the condition known as shock. These responses are the body's attempt to maintain adequate blood flow to the vital organs, and thus prevent their failure.

WHAT CAUSES SHOCK?

When the body is healthy, three conditions are needed to maintain adequate blood flow:

- The heart must be working well.

- An adequate amount of oxygen-rich blood must be circulating in the body.

- The blood vessels must be intact and able to adjust blood flow.

When someone is injured or becomes suddenly ill, these normal body functions may be interrupted. In cases of minor injury or illness, this interruption is brief because the body is able to compensate quickly. However, with more severe injuries or illnesses, the body may be unable to adjust. When the body is unable to meet its demands for oxygen because blood fails to circulate adequately, shock occurs.

Causes of shock can include decreased blood volume, disturbances of heart rhythm and damage to the nervous system.

Decreased Blood Volume

For the heart to do its job properly, an adequate amount of blood must circulate within the body. The amount of blood circulating within the body is called the **blood volume.**

The body can compensate for some decrease in blood volume. Consider, for example, what happens when you donate blood. An adult can lose 500 ml of blood over 10 to 15 minutes without any real stress to the body. With severe injuries involving greater or more rapid blood loss, however, the body may not be able to adjust adequately.

Bleeding is not the only form of fluid loss that may result in shock. Extensive burns or other large fluid losses from the body, such as diarrhoea or vomiting, can also cause shock. Diarrhoea and vomiting can be particularly serious in children and the elderly.

Disturbances of Heart Rhythm

Any illness or injury which disrupts the heart's rhythm, such as a heart attack, may also lead to shock.

If the heart does not beat rhythmically, cardiac output and the circulation of blood will be affected. With some irregular heart rhythms, blood does not circulate at all.

Damage to the Nervous System

Normally, blood vessels decrease or increase the flow of blood to different areas of the body by constricting or dilating. This ability ensures that blood reaches the areas of the body that need it most, such as the vital organs.

Injuries or illnesses, especially those that affect the brain and spinal cord, can cause blood vessels to lose this ability to change size. Also, blood vessels can be affected if the nervous system is damaged by an infection, a drug or a poison.

1 *How can damage to the nervous system affect the ability of blood vessels to function?*

EFFECTS OF SHOCK ON THE BODY

When someone suffers a severe injury or sudden illness that affects the flow of blood, the heart beats faster and stronger at first to adjust to the increased demand for more oxygen. As the heart is beating faster, breathing must also speed up to meet the increased demands of the body for oxygen (Figure 6-1). You can detect these

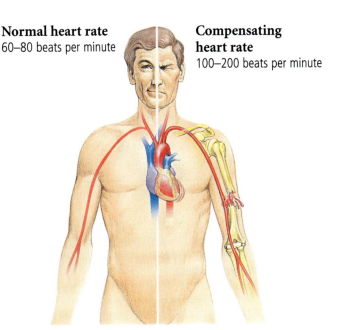

Normal heart rate
60–80 beats per minute

Compensating heart rate
100–200 beats per minute

FIGURE 6-1 *The heart beats faster to compensate for significant blood loss.*

Why does the body's need for oxygen increase with injury or illness?

Why is sweating a natural reaction to stress from injury or illness?

changes by feeling the pulse and counting the breathing rate when you check the vital signs during the secondary survey.

If the heart is damaged, it cannot pump blood properly. If blood vessels are damaged, the body cannot adjust blood flow. Regardless of the cause, when body cells receive inadequate oxygen, shock is triggered.

When shock occurs, the body attempts to prioritise its needs for blood by ensuring adequate flow to the vital organs, such as the heart, brain, lungs and kidneys. It does this by reducing the amount of blood circulating to the less important tissues of the arms, legs and skin. This is why the skin of a person in shock appears pale and feels cool. In later stages of shock, the skin, especially the lips and around the eyes, may appear blue from a prolonged lack of oxygen. Blood is also diverted from the stomach and digestive tract. The person may therefore feel nauseated if the stomach is empty or may vomit if the stomach is full from a recent meal.

Increased sweating is also a natural reaction to stress caused by injury or illness. This makes the skin feel moist.

SYMPTOMS AND SIGNS OF SHOCK

Although you may not always be able to determine the cause, remember that shock is a life-threatening condition. You should learn to recognise the symptoms and signs of shock in every sick and injured person (Figure 6-2).

Shock victims usually show many of the same symptoms and signs. A common symptom is restlessness or irritability. Often this is the first indicator that the body is experiencing a significant problem. Other recognisable symptoms and signs are:

- pale, cool, moist skin
- rapid breathing
- rapid and weak pulse
- excessive thirst
- nausea and/or vomiting
- altered conscious state.

As the victim's condition deteriorates, the symptoms and signs will become more pronounced.

SIGNS OF SHOCK

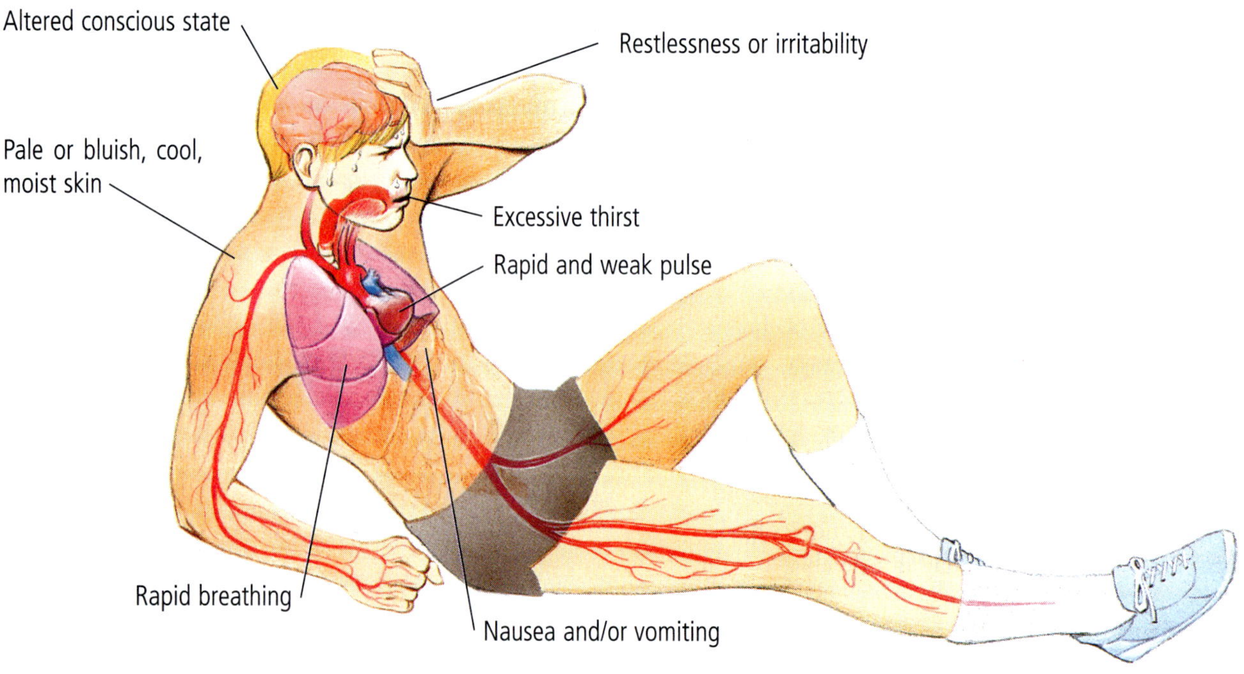

Altered conscious state

Restlessness or irritability

Pale or bluish, cool, moist skin

Excessive thirst

Rapid and weak pulse

Rapid breathing

Nausea and/or vomiting

FIGURE 6-2 *The symptoms and signs of shock may not be obvious immediately. Be alert for these in cases of injury or sudden illness. Provide care at once to help reduce the effects of shock.*

Knowing that shock is a progressive failure of body systems, explain how emotional stress might affect the onset and pace of shock.

4

Why could any significant injury or illness cause shock?

5

SHOCK: THE DOMINO EFFECT

- An injury causes severe bleeding.

- The heart attempts to compensate for the disruption of blood flow by beating faster. The victim first has a rapid pulse. More blood is lost. As blood volume drops, the pulse becomes weak or hard to find.

- The increased workload on the heart results in an increased oxygen demand. Therefore, breathing becomes faster.

- To maintain circulation of blood to the vital organs, blood vessels in the arms, legs and skin constrict. Therefore, the skin appears pale and feels cool. In response to the stress, the body perspires heavily and the skin feels moist.

- As a further boost to the circulation, blood is withdrawn from the stomach and digestive tract. Nausea results and vomiting may occur.

- Tissues of the arms and legs are now without oxygen and cells start to die. The brain now sends a signal to return blood to the arms and legs in an attempt to balance blood flow between these body parts and the vital organs.

- Vital organs are now without adequate oxygen. The heart tries to compensate by beating even faster. More blood is lost and the victim's condition worsens.

- Without oxygen, the vital organs fail to function properly. As the brain is affected, the person becomes restless and drowsy and eventually loses consciousness. As the heart is affected, it beats irregularly, resulting in an irregular pulse. The rhythm then becomes chaotic and the heart fails to pump blood. There is no longer a pulse. When the heart stops, breathing stops.

- The body's continuous attempt to compensate for severe blood loss eventually results in death.■

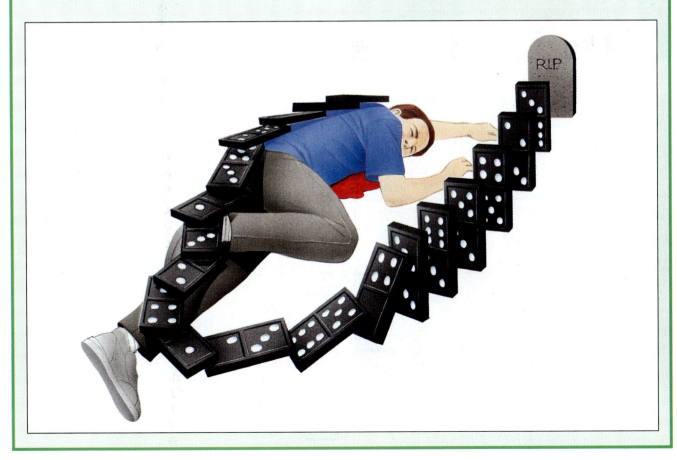

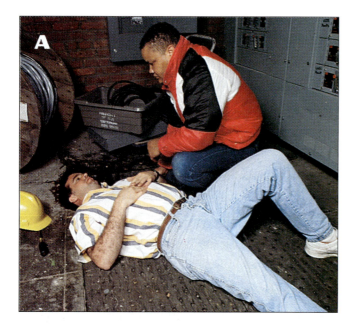

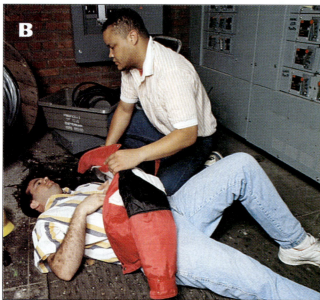

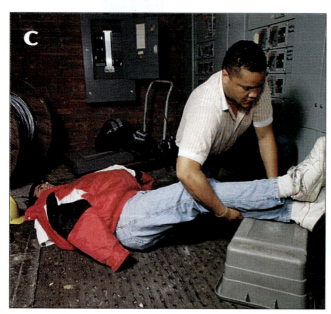

FIGURE 6-3 A *Monitor the ABC of a victim in shock.*
B *Maintain normal body temperature.* **C** *Elevate the victim's legs to keep blood circulating to the vital organs.*

CARE FOR SHOCK

The general care you give in any emergency will help reduce the effects of shock. Always follow the emergency action principles, and give the following specific care:

- Prevent further injury.

- Check the ABC and care for any airway, breathing or circulation problem you find by following the Basic Life Support flow chart on page 35 (Figure 6-3A).

- Control any external bleeding as soon as possible to minimise blood loss.

- Help the victim to rest comfortably. This is important because pain and fear can intensify the body's stress and accelerate the progression of shock.

- Help the victim to maintain normal body temperature (Figure 6-3B). If you need a blanket to help keep the victim warm, also place a blanket under the victim to avoid further heat loss (see Chapter 17).

- Reassure the victim.

- Provide care for specific conditions that are present.

- Continue checking the ABC and level of response.

- Elevate the legs slightly to assist the return of blood flow to vital organs, unless you suspect head, neck or back injuries, or possible broken bones in the hips or legs (Figure 6-3C). If you suspect a heart attack or stroke, or if you are unsure of the victim's condition, do not raise the legs.

- Do not give the victim anything to eat or drink, even though the person is likely to be thirsty. The victim's condition may be severe enough to require surgery, in which case it is important that the stomach be empty.

- Advise the victim not to smoke.

- Call an ambulance immediately. Shock cannot be managed effectively by first aid alone. A victim of shock may require advanced life support as soon as possible.

- If the victim's condition deteriorates, unconsciousness may occur, and the victim must be positioned on the side and a clear airway maintained.

Remember:

Thirst is a common feature of shock. However, any fluids given by mouth may cause vomiting or complications if surgery is needed.

Summary

- Do not wait for shock to develop before providing care to a victim of injury or sudden illness.

- Look for the symptoms and signs of shock in any victim who has experienced emotional or physical trauma, especially if there is blood loss or if the normal function of the heart is affected. Fear and pain also can cause shock and can make an existing condition worse.

- Always follow the emergency action principles to minimise the progressive stages of shock.

- Care for life-threatening conditions, such as breathing problems or severe external bleeding, before caring for lesser injuries.

- Remember that the key to managing shock effectively is to start giving care as soon as possible and calling for an ambulance.

Answers to Application Questions

1. Blood vessel function depends on the vessels receiving accurate instructions from the nervous system. Any time there is damage to the nervous system (brain, spinal cord or nerves), the transmission of impulses to the blood vessels may be impaired or completely cut off. Without adequate instructions, the ability of blood vessels to function effectively, specifically to change size, is greatly reduced.

2. The body's oxygen needs always increase with injury and illness, because the body uses more energy in its attempt to compensate for the effects of injury or illness while also performing all normal functions.

3. As activity within the body increases to compensate for injury or illness, body temperature rises. As you have read in Chapter 2, the body strives to maintain a constant temperature. Any rise in body temperature results in the body's attempt to cool itself down, as in sweating.

4. Think about the effect of emotional stress on the body under normal circumstances. How does your body respond when you are very angry, worried or afraid? Your heart rate may increase in response to the adrenalin released in your system. This is a protective mechanism which helps you move quickly away from danger. You may have trouble breathing, and you may sweat profusely. The degree of stress determines how severely the body is affected. Emotional stress can speed the onset of shock by placing additional demands on your body at a time when your body may be struggling to survive.

5. Shock occurs with any significant illness or injury when the body cannot compensate for the injury or illness and maintain normal body functions.

Study Questions

1. **Match each term with the correct definition.**

   a. Blood volume.

   b. Injury.

   c. Medical emergency.

   _____ Condition occurring when the body is subjected to external force.

   _____ Sudden illness resulting from problems occurring within the body.

   _____ Amount of blood circulating within the body.

2. **Reread the scenario at the beginning of the chapter and list four symptoms, signs and behaviour of shock you can identify there.**

3. **List two conditions that result in shock.**

4. **List at least five things you can do to care for shock.**

5. **Shock can occur as a result of:**

   a. inadequate blood volume

   b. severe diarrhoea

   c. fatigue

   d. over-exertion.

   e. a and b.

6. **When shock occurs, the body prioritises its needs for blood by sending blood first to:**

   a. the arms and legs

   b. the brain and heart

   c. the skin.

   d. a and c.

7. *The skin appears pale during shock as a result of:*

    a. constriction of blood vessels near the skin's surface

    b. the heart beating faster

    c. profuse sweating

8. *Early intervention is the key to managing shock effectively. Which of the following are included in the care for shock?*

    a. Maintaining normal body temperature.

    b. Monitoring airway, breathing and circulation.

    c. Helping the victim rest comfortably.

    d. b and c.

    e. a, b and c.

9. *Which body systems are affected by shock?*

    a. Circulatory and respiratory.

    b. All body systems.

    c. Circulatory, respiratory and nervous.

    d. Respiratory and nervous.

10. *Why is shock a life-threatening condition?*

11. *Why does elevating the victim's legs help manage shock?*

Answers are in Appendix A (page 361).

Breathing Emergencies

IN CHAPTER 4 you learned how to give expired air resuscitation (EAR) in situations of respiratory arrest—when the victim's breathing has stopped completely. However, in many other situations the victim still may be breathing but with difficulty. This condition is called respiratory distress and is an emergency requiring your immediate attention.

In addition to the general principles of first aid for all victims of respiratory distress, this chapter outlines how to give specific care depending on the cause of the breathing emergency.

For Review

A review of how the respiratory and circulatory systems function (Chapter 2), how to care for respiratory arrest (Chapter 4) and the steps of the primary survey (Chapter 3) will help your understanding of the chapter.

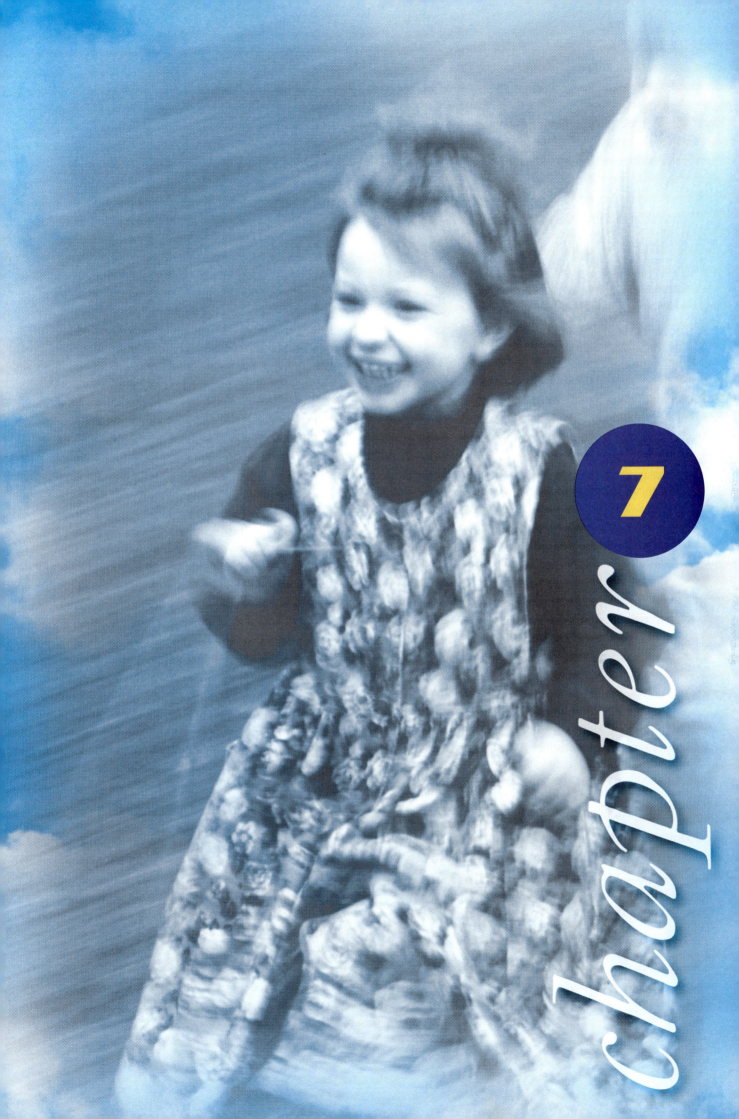

chapter

7

Key Terms

Airway obstruction: Partial or complete blockage of the airway which either prevents or makes it difficult for air to reach a person's lungs.

Asthma *(ass-ma)*: A condition in which the air passages become narrowed by muscle spasm, swelling of mucous membranes and increased mucus production.

Choking: Airway obstruction caused by a foreign body or swollen tissues.

Cyanosis *(sy-a-no-sis)*: A bluish discolouration of the skin, tongue and lining of the mouth.

Drowning: Death by suffocation when submerged in water or other liquid.

Exhale: To breathe air out of the lungs.

Hanging: The accidental or intentional suspension of the body's weight by something wrapped around the neck.

Hyperventilation *(hy-per-ven-til-ay-shon)*: A condition in which a person develops a carbon dioxide and oxygen imbalance in the body related to an altered pattern of breathing.

Inhale: To breathe air into the lungs.

Lungs: A pair of organs in the chest which provide the mechanism for taking oxygen in and removing carbon dioxide during breathing.

Pleural cavity: The space between the lungs and the chest wall.

Pneumothorax *(nyoo-mo-thor-aks)*: A collection of air or gas in the pleural space that causes the lung to collapse (pneumo = air, thorax = chest).

Respiratory distress: A condition in which breathing is difficult.

Spontaneous pneumothorax: A pneumothorax that occurs without any injury to the chest wall, caused by an internal rupture of lung tissue, following a violent bout of coughing, severe asthma attack, serious lung infection or rupture of a cyst on the surface of the lung.

Strangulation: The accidental or intentional squeezing of the neck and windpipe which obstructs a person's air supply.

Suffocation: The accidental or intentional cutting off of a person's air supply by an external object.

Tension pneumothorax: A type of pneumothorax that develops following a rupture of the chest wall or lung tissue when air collects in the pleural space and cannot get out.

Simon was a keen athlete and loved team sports most of all. He looked forward to his school sport practices each week, whatever the weather conditions.

One cold winter's day Simon started to play football and realised he was feeling very tired; just keeping up with the play was causing him to become increasingly short of breath, and he was coughing frequently. He found he had to stop every few minutes to catch his breath, but the cough kept interrupting every burst of activity to the point where he was unable to keep up with the game.

The physical education teacher realised that Simon was not well and told him to sit out the rest of the game. Simon tried to argue, but his attempts to talk brought on another coughing spasm and it felt as if his chest was filling with sticky mucus which he could not cough up. Feeling a little scared at his sudden breathing difficulties, Simon slowly walked off the oval to join some classmates on the sidelines.

When he sat down on a bench he found that his breathing was still getting worse, and he had to stand up and lean against a tree to get as much air as he could. Worried by Simon's distress, and recognising that Simon needed urgent medical help, the teacher sent another student to the school office to telephone for an ambulance. She stayed with Simon and tried to comfort and reassure him.

After initial medical treatment in hospital, Simon improved rapidly. Further tests confirmed the diagnosis and Simon was told he had exercise-induced asthma, which is common in young people, especially when exercising in the cold. The asthma specialist reassured Simon and told him that he would be able to return to his favourite sport provided that he followed his asthma management plan. In the future, Simon was to take "preventer" medication at regular times of the day, and "reliever" medication by puffer ten minutes before starting any physical exercise or sport.

After a few weeks of medication, Simon was as active in sports as he wanted to be and did not again experience that feeling of gasping for air. Because he understood the effects of asthma, he took the medication regularly and strictly followed the guidelines from his specialist.

All organs in the body need a continuous supply of oxygen to stay alive and to function efficiently. If the oxygen supply is interrupted, death or organ damage may result very quickly. In particular, the brain can be damaged after a very short time without oxygen.

A lack of oxygen to the body tissues can result when:

- there is too little oxygen in the air, as may occur where the air is full of smoke, in a tunnel, at high altitudes or when underwater diving

- there is an obstructed airway, when it is blocked by the tongue, foreign material or tissues swollen by allergic reaction or injury

- there is inefficient activity of the muscles of respiration caused by injuries to the chest wall or spinal cord, or by electric shock

- the breathing control centre in the brain is damaged by injury or affected by drugs or disease

- there is blood, water or other fluid in the air sacs of the lungs which interferes with the passage of oxygen from the lungs into the bloodstream

- the available oxygen cannot be used, as occurs with certain types of poisoning, such as carbon monoxide and cyanide

- the lungs are compressed by blood or air

In Chapter 4 you learned how to give expired air resuscitation (EAR) for victims who were not breathing. Those who are having difficulty breathing or whose breathing is so ineffective that the body is not getting the oxygen it needs also require emergency care. This chapter discusses these breathing emergencies and the first aid required.

RESPIRATORY DISTRESS

Respiratory distress may be caused by injury or illness, such as the following:

- An obstructed airway, such as choking.
- A respiratory illness such as pneumonia.
- A respiratory condition such as asthma or emphysema.
- Electric shock.
- Shock.
- Near-drowning.
- Heart attack or heart disease.
- Injury to the chest wall or lungs.
- Allergic reactions to foods, insect stings or other substances.
- Poisoning, such as inhaling or ingesting toxic substances.

Respiratory distress also may result from excitement, exercise or anxiety.

Table 7-1

SYMPTOMS AND SIGNS OF RESPIRATORY DISTRESS

Condition	Symptoms and signs
How victim feels	• Victim feels short of breath, dizzy or lightheaded. • Victim feels pain in the chest or tingling in hands and feet.
Abnormal breathing	• Breathing is slow or rapid. • Breaths are unusually deep or shallow. • Victim is gasping for breath or making wheezing, gurgling or high-pitched crowing noises.
Abnormal skin appearance	• Victim's skin may be unusually moist. • Victim's skin has a flushed, pale or bluish appearance. • Mucous membranes in the mouth are a bluish colour.

Symptoms and Signs of Respiratory Distress

Many symptoms and signs indicate respiratory distress. Victims may gasp for air or appear to breathe faster. The breathing rate may be slower than normal, as with a drug overdose. The breathing pattern may be laboured or unusually deep or shallow, or accompanied by unusual noises, such as wheezing or gurgling, or high-pitched sounds like crowing.

With laboured breathing, the breathing may appear to be "see-saw", with the failure of the chest to expand when the victim breathes in while the abdomen appears to move outwards. There is an in-drawing of the soft tissue above the collar bones and the sternum, between the ribs and at the lower chest. There is also a "flaring" of the winged part of the nostrils, especially in children.

The victim's skin appearance may indicate respiratory distress. At first, it may be unusually moist and appear flushed. Later, it may appear pale or bluish as the oxygen level in the blood falls. Remember, **cyanosis** is a late sign and is not always present.

Victims may say they feel dizzy or short of breath or say they can't breathe. They may feel lightheaded and they may feel pain in the chest or tingling in the hands and feet. Understandably, the victim may be anxious or fearful. Any one or more of these symptoms or signs are a clue that the victim may be in respiratory distress. Table 7-1 lists the symptoms and signs of respiratory distress.

Specific Causes of Respiratory Distress

Although respiratory distress is often caused by injury, several other conditions also can cause this problem.

These include asthma, hyperventilation, choking, near-drowning and electrical injuries. These conditions are discussed later in this chapter, together with the specific first aid required.

GENERAL PRINCIPLES OF FIRST AID FOR RESPIRATORY DISTRESS

Recognising the early symptoms and signs of respiratory distress and giving appropriate first aid are often the key to preventing an emergency. Respiratory distress may be the beginning of a life-threatening condition. For example, it can be the first sign of a more serious breathing emergency or even a heart attack. Respiratory distress can lead to respiratory arrest which, if not immediately cared for, will result in death.

Many of the symptoms and signs of different kinds of respiratory distress are similar. You do not need to know the specific cause to provide care effectively.

Remember to survey the scene to ensure your own safety before you approach the victim. Respiratory distress can be caused by toxic fumes which still may be present at the scene.

Complete your primary survey. If the victim is breathing, the heart must be beating. Check for any severe bleeding. A conscious person in respiratory distress is usually more comfortable in a sitting position (Figure 7-1). Provide enough air by opening a window, or ask bystanders to move back. Make sure someone has called the local emergency number for help, if you have not already done so.

If the victim is conscious, do a secondary survey. As you do this, remember that a person experiencing breathing difficulty may have trouble talking. Speak to any bystanders who may have relevant information which the victim can confirm by nodding. If possible, try to help reduce any anxiety which may contribute to the victim's breathing difficulty. If it is available, assist the victim to take prescribed medication for the condition.

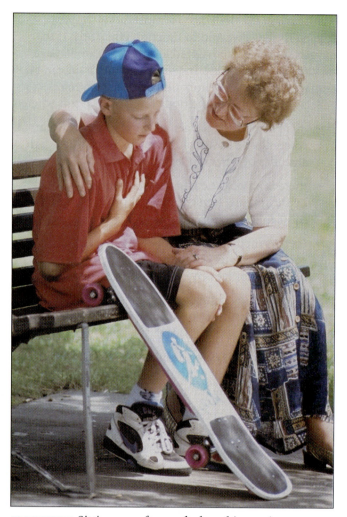

FIGURE 7-1 *Sitting can often make breathing easier.*

Continue to look and listen for any changes in the vital signs. Watch for additional signs of respiratory distress. Calm and reassure the victim. Help maintain normal body temperature by preventing chilling on a cool day or by providing shade on a hot day.

If the victim's breathing is rapid and there are signs of an injury or an underlying illness, call an ambulance because this person needs advanced care immediately.

The following sections describe specific conditions which cause respiratory distress and the first aid required.

FIRST AID FOR RESPIRATORY DISTRESS

- Conduct a primary survey.
- Call for an ambulance if necessary.
- Help the victim to rest comfortably and. quietly
- Carry out a secondary survey.
- Reassure the victim.
- Assist with relevant medication.
- Help the victim to maintain normal body temperature.
- Monitor the victim's vital signs. ▪

Remember:

You do not need to know the specific cause of a breathing emergency to provide first aid; follow the general principles of care previously described.

ASTHMA

Asthma is a condition in which the air passages to the lungs become narrowed by muscle spasm, swelling of the mucous membrane lining the lungs and increased mucus production in the lungs. The airways become narrowed and the victim has difficulty breathing. Air is trapped in the lungs because the victim cannot easily breathe out.

Asthma is particularly common in children, where it is the most common cause of school absenteeism and the most frequent cause of hospitalisation. In Australia, an average of 800 deaths per year result from asthma. Greater efforts are being made, via the National Asthma Campaign, to help parents, child care providers, teachers and coaches to recognise asthma and learn how to manage it.

Many different factors can trigger an asthma attack, including:

- Exposure to a sudden change in weather, especially cold or wet conditions.

- Exercise or physical activity (exercise-induced asthma, known as EIA), especially when there is no management plan for medication or pre-exercise warm-ups.

- Infections, especially respiratory infections.

- Allergic reaction to food, pollen or an insect sting.

- Emotional stress.

Ideally, someone who has asthma has developed a management plan with the doctor. A management plan which includes the use of "preventers" and "relievers" can help prevent attacks or reduce their severity if they do occur. "Preventers" such as Intal™ and corticosteroids such as Becotide™, Becloforte™ and Pulmicort™ help to prevent attacks when taken regularly to treat the underlying disease. "Relievers" are bronchodilator drugs such as Ventolin™, Respolin™ and Bricanyl™, which are taken before exercise or when an attack begins to relax muscles, reduce spasm and ease breathing. However, their action is short lived, and they do not prevent a subsequent attack of asthma.

Asthma medications are colour coded for easy recognition. The blue or grey coloured containers are "relievers"; cream, yellow, brown and red containers are used for the "preventers".

Many of these medications are taken through a "puffer", a small pressure canister which releases the medication into the mouth to be breathed in when the person depresses the device. Some medications are given through a "turbuhaler", from which a measured dose can be inhaled without the co-ordination problems or propellent usage of a puffer (Figure 7-2).

Sometimes a puffer is used with a spacer device which holds the medication for the user to inhale over several breaths (Figure 7-3). This is useful for children and for adults who have difficulty co-ordinating the

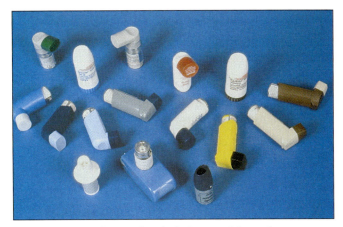

FIGURE 7-2 *Puffers and turbuhalers used for asthma medication.*

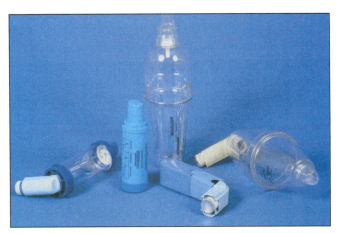

FIGURE 7-3 *Spacer devices used with asthma medication puffers to hold the medication and space it out over several breaths.*

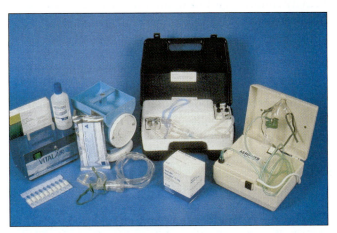

FIGURE 7-4 *A nebuliser converts medication into an aerosol mist spray for easy inhalation for some asthma sufferers.*

release of the medication from the puffer while breathing in. Spacers are often recommended for corticosteroids, which should not come into contact with tissues in the mouth. Very young or elderly asthma sufferers may use a nebuliser pump which converts the medication into an aerosol mist spray for easy inhalation (Figure 7-4).

Symptoms and Signs of an Asthma Attack

The onset of an attack can be recognised by one or more of the following symptoms and signs:

- Shortness of breath (especially when talking).
- Wheezing when exhaling; but remember, *not all asthma victims wheeze*.
- Dry or moist cough.
- Thirst due to loss of water vapour from the lungs.
- Increasing pulse rate.
- Drawing in of the spaces between the ribs and above the collar bones with the effort of breathing.
- Cyanosis.
- Collapse.

First Aid for Asthma Attack

If you know the person's management plan, follow its guidelines. Assist the victim to:

1. Take any prescribed medication promptly.
2. Rest from any physical activity, even if this appears at first to make the attack worse.
3. Sit with arms supported on a table or bench to make breathing easier.

Constantly observe the victim in case any deterioration occurs.

If there is definite improvement, normal activity can resume under close observation. Strenuous physical activity should be avoided unless a medical clearance has been given.

If there is no improvement after the initial steps have been taken, help the victim to take two more puffs of the "reliever" medication, and then either contact the person's doctor or call for an ambulance.

If there are signs of deterioration, call for an ambulance immediately. Signs of deterioration include:

- An inability to talk.
- Exhaustion.
- Cyanosis seen in the lips and tongue.
- Collapse.

Assist the victim to take up to four additional puffs of their "reliever" medication while waiting for trained help. If breathing stops, begin EAR promptly. Effort may be required to overcome the resistance to inflation.

Prevention of an Asthma Attack

People with asthma should have their lung function medically assessed. As part of their personal asthma management plan (Figure 7-5), many people will use a device called a peak flow meter which measures their lung function. A reduced reading indicates the need for increased "preventer" medication; improved readings indicate that the asthma is under control.

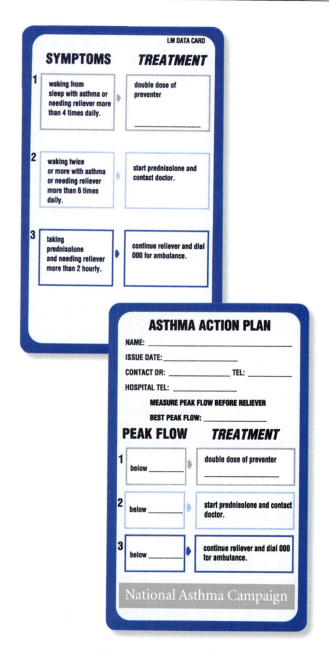

FIGURE 7-5 *An asthma management plan.*

Exercise-induced asthma (EIA) responds well to treatment if the person takes the prescribed medication appropriately. Generally the person with EIA is advised to take the prescribed medication 5 to 10 minutes before exercise and to use a structured warm-up routine before starting full physical activity.

Most asthma sufferers gain from good general health and fitness and can prevent or reduce asthma attacks with an effective management plan.

In an asthma attack, changes occur in the air passages and lungs. What are the effects of these changes on the victim?

HYPERVENTILATION

Hyperventilation is a condition in which a person develops an imbalance in the levels of oxygen and carbon dioxide in the body. The victim starts to breathe at a faster rate than is necessary. Hyperventilation may result from a variety of causes, including:

- Stress related to anxiety or fear.
- Head injury.
- Severe bleeding.
- Heart failure.
- Collapsed lung.
- Some poisons.
- Diabetic emergency.

Because the condition may be caused by a serious underlying medical disorder, the victim needs prompt medical assessment and treatment to avoid the possibility of serious complications. For example, a victim of a diabetic emergency may not have reduced carbon dioxide levels in the blood despite rapid and shallow breathing.

Symptoms and Signs of Hyperventilation

Someone who is hyperventilating has some or all of the following symptoms and signs:

- Shallow, rapid breathing.
- Feeling of suffocation.
- Fear and anxiety.
- Dizziness.
- Numbness or tingling of fingers and toes, often with claw-like spasm of the hand with the thumb pulled across the palm.
- Feeling of detachment from the body, as if no longer in control.

First Aid for Hyperventilation

To give first aid care for hyperventilation:

1. Remain calm and offer reassurance. Explain that the symptoms will disappear when breathing returns to normal.

2. Count each breath aloud and thus encourage a slower breathing rate. The victim who can co-operate and concentrate on taking slower breaths will improve quickly. Even when the victim seems to be fully recovered, a doctor should rule out any underlying medical problem.

> ## Remember:
>
> *A person with rapid and shallow breathing may have an underlying medical condition which requires immediate medical attention.*

2 *In a person who is hyperventilating as a result of emotional stress, what immediate change occurs in the carbon dioxide levels in the blood?*

NOTE: In the past, it was standard practice to ask the victim to breathe from a paper bag that was tightly sealed over the nose and mouth. The goal was to raise the level of carbon dioxide in the blood by having the person rebreathe the same air with less oxygen in it. This method is considered dangerous and is no longer recommended, even in cases of hyperventilation caused by stress, because of the dangers of lowering the oxygen level in the blood.

CHOKING

Choking occurs when the airway is totally or partially obstructed by swollen tissues or a foreign body, or when food or other material enters the windpipe instead of the gullet (Figure 7-6). Adults may be affected when they eat hurriedly or have reflexes affected by old age, alcohol or disease. Children are at particular risk because of their tendency to put small objects in their mouths. Peanuts are especially dangerous for children under the age of five.

Symptoms and Signs of Choking

A conscious choking victim may be unable to breathe at all in a case of total **airway obstruction,** or they may be moving only a small amount of air past a partial airway obstruction. The victim may display some or all of the following symptoms and signs:

- Inability to breathe, speak, cry or cough.
- Noisy breathing or wheezing.
- Clutching at the throat.

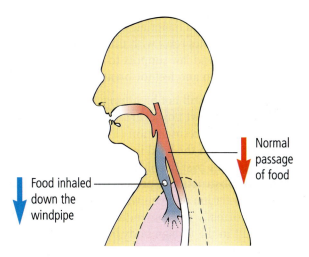

FIGURE 7-6 *Choking occurs if food or other material enters the windpipe instead of the gullet.*

- Red or congested face, with bulging neck veins.
- Anxiety, restlessness.
- Cyanosis.
- Collapse and unconsciousness.

First Aid for Choking

A victim with a partial airway obstruction **who is able to breathe, speak or cough** may be choking but does not need immediate first aid. Encourage the person to continue coughing in an attempt to expel the foreign object. *Do not slap the person on the back,* as this could force the object deeper into the airway. If the person continues to wheeze or breathe noisily but is getting some air, call for an ambulance immediately.

If a victim **cannot breathe or cough,** urgent care is required. Ensure that someone has called an ambulance and follow these first aid guidelines:

1. Quickly assist the victim to lie down.

2. With the victim lying down on one side, use the heel of your hand to give up to four sharp back blows between the shoulder blades (Figure 7-7).

3. Check to see if the foreign object has been expelled and the victim is able to breathe again.

4. If the victim is still unable to breathe, give up to four lateral chest thrusts in an attempt to expel the object. With the victim on one side, place one hand palm down against the armpit and the other hand beside it. Do not apply pressure below the ribs or over the abdomen. Give three or four quick thrusts to compress the chest and increase internal pressure to expel the object (Figure 7-8).

5. Check again to see if the foreign object has been expelled and the victim is able to breathe. The victim is likely to become unconscious quickly if the obstruction is not relieved.

6. Keep the unconscious victim lying on one side and try to clear the airway. Check the mouth for any visible foreign material, which may come loose when the muscles relax with unconsciousness. Use head tilt and jaw support to open the airway, and look, listen and feel for breathing.

7. If the victim is still not breathing, follow the Basic Life Support flow chart (see page 35) and give expired air resuscitation (EAR) as described in Chapter 4. With the head in the correct position, try to blow air past the obstruction into the lungs. When an obstruction is present, there will be resistance to inflation and you will need to blow harder than is normally recommended. Sometimes this will result in the foreign body being blown down into the lungs. This can be removed later during medical treatment.

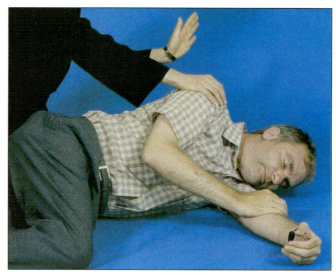

FIGURE 7-7 *Using the heel of your hand, give sharp back blows to dislodge a foreign object from the airway.*

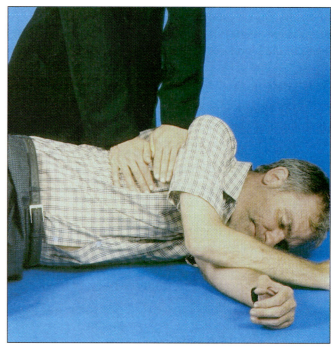

FIGURE 7-8 *If back blows are unsuccessful, use lateral chest thrusts to increase internal pressure to expel a foreign object from the airway.*

8. If air goes in and the chest rises, the victim is likely to breathe spontaneously and then should be turned onto the side in the recovery position.

9. If the obstruction is not cleared with EAR, repeat the back blows and chest thrusts as described in steps 2 to 4. Then try EAR again. If the obstruction is not cleared, continue to alternate back blows and lateral chest thrusts with EAR until the obstruction clears or the ambulance arrives.

Even when your efforts to clear the obstruction are successful and the victim is breathing normally again, medical attention is needed. The steps of first aid for choking are summarised in Figures 7-9 and 7-10 (on opposite page).

Suspected Choking Victim—Adult

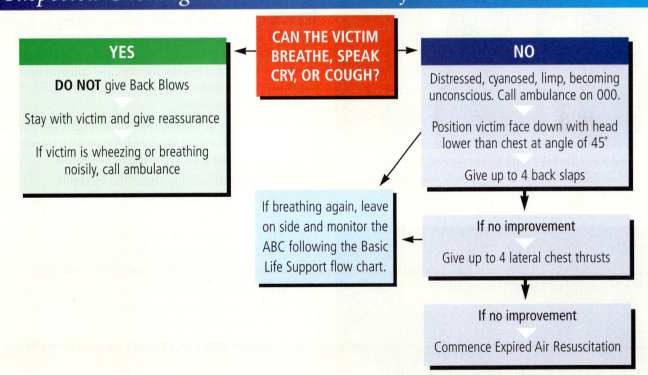

CAN THE VICTIM BREATHE, SPEAK CRY, OR COUGH?

YES

DO NOT give Back Blows

Stay with victim and give reassurance

If victim is wheezing or breathing noisily, call ambulance

NO

Distressed, cyanosed, limp, becoming unconscious. Call ambulance on 000.

Lie on side

Give up to 4 back blows

If no improvement

Give up to 4 lateral chest thrusts

If no improvement

Commence Expired Air Resuscitation

If breathing again, leave on side and monitor the ABC following the Basic Life Support flow chart.

FIGURE 7-9 *Summary of first aid for a choking adult.*

Suspected Choking Victim—Child or Infant

CAN THE VICTIM BREATHE, SPEAK CRY, OR COUGH?

YES

DO NOT give Back Blows

Stay with victim and give reassurance

If victim is wheezing or breathing noisily, call ambulance

NO

Distressed, cyanosed, limp, becoming unconscious. Call ambulance on 000.

Position victim face down with head lower than chest at angle of 45°

Give up to 4 back slaps

If no improvement

Give up to 4 lateral chest thrusts

If no improvement

Commence Expired Air Resuscitation

If breathing again, leave on side and monitor the ABC following the Basic Life Support flow chart.

FIGURE 7-10 *Summary of first aid for a choking child or infant.*

3 *How do items of food and small objects get stuck in your trachea when they should be in the oesophagus?*

4 *Why is choking a first aid emergency?*

First Aid for a Choking Infant or Child

For a choking infant or child, follow the general first aid procedure as for a choking adult described above. However, there are two differences to remember:

1. Instead of sharp back blows with the victim on the floor, you can put the infant or child on your lap face down, with the head lower than the chest, at an angle of 45°. Give up to four back slaps between the shoulder blades (Figure 7-11).

2. Give lateral chest thrusts with your hands positioned on both sides of the rib cage just below the armpits. Give three or four squeezing thrusts on both sides simultaneously (Figure 7-12). For a larger child, it may be safer to give chest thrusts with the child lying on the floor.

Although it is a dramatic event, choking is a rare cause of death in Australia.

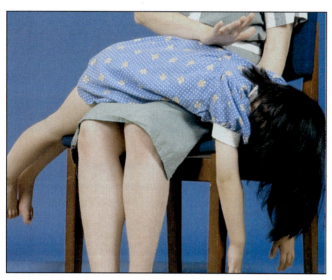

FIGURE 7-11 *Give back slaps rather than back blows to an infant or child to dislodge a foreign body from the airway.*

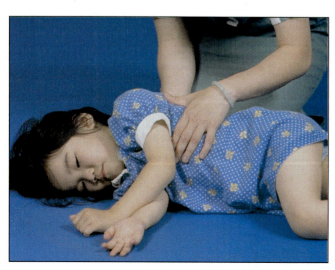

FIGURE 7-12 *If back slaps are unsuccessful, give lateral squeezing thrusts on both sides to dislodge a foreign body from the airway of an infant or a child.*

DROWNING

Drowning is death by suffocation when submerged in water. Most people who are close to drowning cannot or do not call for help. Their energy is spent just trying to keep their head above water. In near-drowning the victim survives submersion, although sometimes only temporarily. Near-drowning begins whenever small amounts of water are inhaled into the lungs, which happens when a person is gasping for air while struggling to stay afloat. Stimulation by the water causes spasm of the muscles of the larynx (voice box), which close the airway to prevent more water from entering the lungs. As a result, the lungs of most drowning or near-drowning victims are relatively dry, unless the victims have been submerged for prolonged periods of time. However, the spasm which blocks the airway to prevent water from entering the lungs also prevents air from going in. The victim suffocates and soon becomes unconscious. At some point after unconsciousness, the muscles relax, the victim spontaneously breathes and, if the victim is submerged, more water can enter the lungs. During immersion water is swallowed, increasing the risk of regurgitation of stomach contents during rescue and resuscitation.

First Aid for Drowning

Be sure someone has called for help, and then get to the victim as soon as possible without risking your own safety. If possible use something which floats, such as a life jacket, ring buoy, rescue tube, boat, raft or surfboard, to aid in the rescue. Remove the unconscious victim from the water as quickly as possible. Then follow these steps:

1. Once out of the water, you should turn the victim on one side and open the airway, which allows water or vomit to drain from the mouth.

2. Check for breathing, and if the victim is not breathing, start expired air resuscitation (see Chapter 4).

3. After five breaths, check for a carotid pulse. It may be difficult to detect a pulse in a cold near-drowning victim. Check for up to 1 minute.

4. If you cannot feel a pulse, start CPR. The body must be on a hard, firm, horizontal surface for compressions to be effective.

5. Continue EAR or CPR until medical help arrives.

Suspected Spinal Injury in Water

If a victim is found floating in shallow water, you should suspect a head or spine injury. Support the victim's head and neck and keep it aligned with the body. To turn an unconscious victim who is face down in the water, support the head, neck, chest and trunk and quickly turn the body as one unit. Remove the victim from the water as quickly as possible and follow steps 1 to 5 above.

Victims with high spinal injuries will show the following "telling" signs:

- No expansion of the chest. Expansion of the abdomen.
- Rapid dilatation of the stomach associated with vomiting.

A conscious victim can communicate the inability to move legs or arms or may complain of feelings of "pins and needles". If a conscious victim with a suspected spinal injury is in the water and is breathing, support that person's head, neck and trunk as one unit and, if there is no danger, wait for trained rescuers.

If you are physically unable to remove the unconscious victim from deep water, tow the victim to a shallow area. EAR can be commenced in shallow water if the victim is not breathing.

Trained rescuers may use a spinal injury board to remove the victim. Do not try to use such a board yourself unless you have current training and practice in its use, because it can cause further injury to the victim.

If no trained rescuers are readily available, you need to act promptly because prolonged immersion may cause deterioration in the victim's condition due to heat loss. In these circumstances, remove the victim from the water with minimum movement of the spine. Although most of the damage occurs at the time of impact, the injury can be made worse by forward movement or twisting of the neck.

Of all spinal injuries associated with aquatic sports, 85 per cent are flexion-compression injuries. The average age of victims is 22, and most of them are male. The most common site of injury is the level of the fifth and sixth cervical vertebrae; thus the victim can still breathe.

Handle all unconscious victims as gently as possible with minimal movement of the head and neck. Do not let your concern for a possible fracture interfere with your care for the airway.

> ## Remember:
> *Maintaining a clear and open airway takes priority over the management of a fracture, even a suspected fracture of the neck.*

HANGING, STRANGULATION, THROTTLING AND SUFFOCATION

Breathing emergencies may also result from **hanging**, **strangulation**, throttling or **suffocation** (Figure 7-13). Any of these will fully or partially cut off the victim's air supply. In each case, the victim may be conscious or unconscious. The person may start breathing again

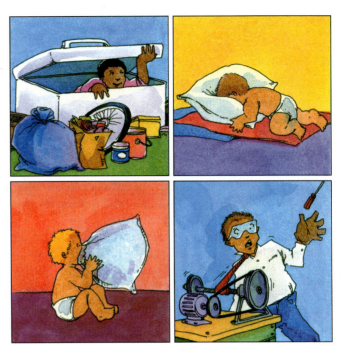

FIGURE 7-13 *Some causes of suffocation.*

spontaneously when the restricting factor is removed or the person may need expired air resuscitation. These are all breathing emergencies.

Symptoms and Signs of Hanging, Strangulation, Throttling and Suffocation

- Presence of suffocating or constricting material, or marks on the throat.
- Collapse and/or unconsciousness.
- Not breathing or difficulty breathing.
- Redness and congestion of face in the early stages.
- Cyanosis.
- Bulging neck veins.

First Aid for Hanging, Strangulation, Throttling and Suffocation

1. If the victim is hanging, support the body weight until the constricting material is removed.
2. Immediately remove any material which is suffocating the victim or constricting the neck or windpipe.
3. Help a conscious victim to rest, and give reassurance. A victim of hanging, strangulation or throttling should receive medical attention for possible injury, even if breathing seems normal.
4. Turn an unconscious victim onto the side and open the airway with head tilt and jaw support. Check for breathing. Make sure someone has called an ambulance.
5. If the victim is not breathing, begin expired air resuscitation (EAR).
6. Check for a pulse. If there is no pulse, begin CPR.

SAND TRAP

A 10-year-old frantically pleaded "don't let me die" as his rescuers raced to free him from a collapsed sand hole, saving his life with a snorkel.

Holidaying families mounted an amazing 25-minute rescue operation using boogie boards to hold back the sand and force a snorkel into the boy's mouth to allow him to breathe.

Daniel Konemann, of Raby in Sydney's south-west, was eventually dragged from the sand in deep shock after the drama on Tuesday.

He owed his life to the beachgoing families who won their battle against the collapsing sand under the co-ordination of a holidaying Victorian policeman. Their fight to save Daniel took place at the Murra-murang resort near Bateman's Bay on the NSW south coast.

The accident happened about 4:30 p.m. as the boy played on the beach around the hole he was digging.

"It was around six feet deep (about 2m) and like a mineshaft." Mr. Campbell [the resort proprietor] said.

"The first we knew was when his little sister started screaming."

Terrified sister, Rebecca, 11, was soon joined by mother Lyn Konemann and stepfather Jeff Greenall, who had been watching from nearby.

Staff from the resort, families on the beach and off-duty policeman David Foley immediately joined the rescue.

Mr. Campbell said the hole started caving in around the boy before sand built up and covered his head. …

"They put the snorkel in his mouth and brought over boogie boards to support the sides of the hole."

Mr. Campbell said the boy's head became completely buried as the sands continued to cave in. The snorkel provided his only airway for more than two minutes. …

After almost half an hour the boy was pulled from the sand in deep shock and taken to the hospital.

Daniel yesterday told of his horror as the weight of the sand closed in.

"Every time I breathed in and out the sand was crushing me and I thought I could probably die," Daniel said. "Luckily, Jeff got the snorkel and held me by the mouth while everyone was digging to get me out.

"They started to use boogie boards to stop the sand from caving back in and eventually got one of my arms out.

"I was very scared the whole time. I won't be digging any more holes like that again." …

The Advertiser, Adelaide, 7 January 1993.

INHALATION OF FUMES

Inhalation of toxic gases and fumes can cause a breathing emergency. Leaking gas or a fire can cause the oxygen level in the air to become dangerously low.

Inhalation of smoke can decrease the oxygen reaching the lungs and cause swelling and burning inside the airway. This may cause severe respiratory distress and increase the difficulty in maintaining normal oxygen supply to the brain. Carbon monoxide, from engine exhaust, is colourless and odourless; it affects the blood cells, preventing oxygen from reaching tissues even after the victim has been removed to a safe place (see Chapter 10).

Solvents include many commercial products such as paint thinners and removers, petroleum products and adhesives. Incorrect use of such products in a non-ventilated space can lead to inhalation at dangerous levels and death. Some people, including young people, intentionally inhale the fumes of such substances for their stimulant effects.

Symptoms and Signs of Inhalation of Fumes

Because different fumes can have different effects, the symptoms and signs vary. The victim may demonstrate only one or two of the following:

- Not breathing or difficulty breathing.
- Skin colour pale, cyanotic or turning cherry pink.
- Burns or stains around the mouth or nose.
- Symptoms and signs of shock (see Chapter 6).
- Confusion, disorientation, listlessness, intoxication.
- Collapse and/or unconsciousness.

First Aid for Inhalation of Fumes

Immediately call for the appropriate emergency help, such as the fire service and ambulance. If the area is made dangerous by smoke, fire or fumes, do not enter it. If it is safe to do so, ventilate the area immediately (for example, by opening the door of a garage) and try to remove the victim.

If fire is known or suspected to be present, feel the temperature of a door with the back of your hand before opening it—if it is hot, do not open it. When you do open a door, stand to one side first with your face turned away to guard against the explosive effects of air under pressure. If there is smoke in the room, stay low to the floor as you move to the victim. Drag the victim out by the feet.

Follow these guidelines for first aid for the victim:

1. Remove the victim to a safe place with fresh air.

2. Be sure someone has called for an ambulance.

3. Smother any smouldering clothing, or remove any substance causing continuing fumes.

4. Turn the unconscious victim into the recovery position. Clear and open the airway, and check for breathing. Give resuscitation as needed, following the Basic Life Support flow chart (see page 35).

5. If the victim is conscious, or unconscious and breathing spontaneously, conduct a secondary survey and provide first aid for other problems found, such as burns.

ELECTRICAL INJURIES

Contact with an electrical current can cause spasm of chest muscles and cessation of breathing and/or heartbeat, and may also cause burns. Typical electrical emergencies result from a faulty switch or appliance cord, children playing with or coming into contact with a cord or plug, contact between an electrical appliance and water, fallen power lines following a storm or accident, and lightning strike. Each year in Australia there are a number of deaths from lightning strikes which occur when a person is the tallest feature in the landscape, such as an open playing field, golf course or boat.

Symptoms and Signs of Electrical Injuries

The scene may provide indications of an electrical injury. Look for objects burned by lightning or for power lines, cords or appliances near the victim. Following are symptoms and signs of an electrical injury:

- Unconsciousness.
- Respiratory arrest.
- Cardiac arrest.
- Entry and exit burns on the victim where the electric current passed through the body.
- Symptoms and signs of shock (see Chapter 6).

First Aid for Electrical Injuries

Your first concern is to make sure the electrical current is not still a risk. *Do not touch the victim until you are certain there is no electrical current still present.* With a regular household appliance, switch off the main power or remove the plug if it is safe to touch the supply cord. With high-voltage currents, such as from a fallen power line or industrial equipment, stay at least 6 metres away

STRIKING DISTANCE

Lightning occurs when particles of water, ice and air moving inside storm clouds lose electrons. Eventually, the cloud becomes divided into layers of positive and negative particles. Most electrical currents run between the layers inside the cloud. However, occasionally, the negative charge flashes toward the ground, which has a positive charge. An electrical current snakes back and forth between the ground and the cloud many times in the seconds that we see a flash crackle down from the sky. Anything tall—a tower, a tree or a person—becomes a path for the electrical current.

Travelling at speeds up to 500 km per second, a lightning strike can hurl a person through the air, burn off clothing, stop the breathing and sometimes also stop the heart. The most severe lightning strikes carry up to 50 million volts of electricity—enough to keep 13,000 homes running. Lightning can "flash" over a person's body or, in its more dangerous path, it can travel through blood vessels and nerves to reach the ground.

Besides burns, lightning can also cause neurological damage, fractures and loss of hearing or eyesight. The victim may sometimes describe the episode as getting hit on the head or hearing an explosion, but may at times be confused or amnesic.

Use common sense around thunderstorms. If you see a storm approaching in the distance, do not wait until you are drenched to seek shelter. If a thunderstorm threatens, you are advised to shelter:

- inside a large building or home
- inside a car and roll up the windows

Avoid:

- swimming or boating as soon as you see or hear a storm (water conducts electricity)
- using the telephone, except in an emergency

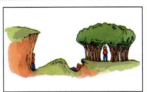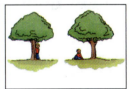

- telephone poles and tall trees if you are caught outside
- hilltops (try to crouch down in a ravine or valley)

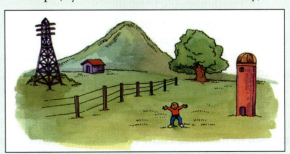

- farm equipment and small vehicles such as motorcycles, bicycles and golf carts
- wire fences, clothes lines, metal pipes and rails and other conductors

Source: *Modern First Aid* by A.S. Playfair.

from the power because the electricity can arc quite a distance, especially in wet conditions. Call the electricity supply authority and then wait for the arrival of trained staff or for assurance that the power has been turned off.

In the case of a fallen power line touching or near a car with a victim inside, do not try to reach the victim. Tell anyone inside to remain in the car until the area is safe. It is safe inside the vehicle, but trying to leave the car will expose a person to further danger.

When it is safe to approach the victim of an electrical injury, follow these guidelines:

1. Turn an unconscious victim onto the side. Open the airway and check for breathing, following the Basic Life Support flow chart (page 35). Make sure an ambulance has been called. Follow the ABC of the primary survey.

2. Be alert for the symptoms and signs of shock and give first aid to minimise shock (see Chapter 6).

3. Give care for any burns.

4. Continue to monitor the victim's condition until the ambulance arrives.

5 *Why is it essential to stay at least 6 metres away from a fallen high-voltage cable?*

SPONTANEOUS PNEUMOTHORAX

A **pneumothorax** occurs when air enters the **pleural cavity** (the space between the lungs and chest wall). Normally this space is at less than atmospheric pressure, ensuring that air will be pulled into the lungs when the chest wall expands and the diaphragm descends. If the chest wall is punctured, atmospheric air will be drawn into the pleural cavity causing the lung on that side to collapse. (See Chapter 12 for a discussion of penetrating chest and back wounds.)

This condition can occur without any injury to the chest wall when there is an internal rupture of lung tissue. This condition is then known as a **spontaneous pneumothorax** and can follow a violent bout of coughing, severe asthma attack, serious lung infection or rupture of a cyst on the surface of the lung. As the name suggests, it generally occurs without warning but can lead to life-threatening breathing problems unless prompt first aid is given.

Symptoms and Signs of Spontaneous Pneumothorax

Many victims have very few symptoms in the early stages, but others may show severe distress within minutes.

Therefore, the victim may have some or all of the following:

- Chest pain, often under the shoulder blade on the affected side and/or a sharp pain at the shoulder tip on each attempt to breathe in.
- Breathing difficulties, especially the inability to take a full or deep breath.
- Restricted or absent movement of the chest wall on the affected side.
- Cough.
- A rapid and weak pulse.
- Symptoms and signs of shock.

If a complication known as **tension pneumothorax** develops, the victim may collapse and even die from the effects of the increased pressure on the heart and unaffected lung. This is due to the continued entry of air into the pleural cavity which squeezes the remaining organs in the chest as pressure builds up inside.

First Aid for Pneumothorax

In a victim with breathing difficulty but no apparent chest wound you may not be able to recognise the problem as a pneumothorax. For any breathing problem for which there is no obvious cause, follow these guidelines:

1. Help a conscious victim into the position which is most comfortable for breathing, generally sitting up with support.

2. Reassure and calm the victim while completing a primary survey.

3. Send someone to call for an ambulance and monitor the vital signs while waiting for help to arrive.

4. Give emergency care as necessary, following the Basic Life Support flow chart (page 35).

If a tension pneumothorax develops and breathing stops, expired air resuscitation may keep the victim alive until the increased pressure in the chest can be relieved by medical care. If the circulation fails, cardiopulmonary resuscitation may be life-saving.

WINDING AND HICCUPS

Although rarely breathing emergencies, winding and hiccups can be problems which need first aid.

First Aid for Winding

A person can be winded by a blow to the solar plexus (on the back wall of the abdomen behind the stomach). A blow over the upper abdomen may cause breathing difficulty.

The symptoms and signs of being winded include:

- Breathing difficulty.
- Inability to speak.
- Victim bent over, possibly holding the upper abdomen.
- Abdominal pain, nausea or vomiting.

If someone has been winded, you should:

1. Help a conscious victim into a position which is most comfortable for breathing.

2. Reassure and calm the victim until the breathing difficulty passes.

3. Obtain medical attention if the symptoms persist.

4. Turn an unconscious victim onto the side and open the airway. Although respiratory arrest is unlikely, check for breathing and complete a primary survey.

First Aid for Hiccups

Hiccups, caused by involuntary contractions of the diaphragm, seldom last long and usually stop spontaneously. Tell the person to sit comfortably and quietly, and advise the victim to try breath-holding for short periods. Alternatively, take long, slow drinks of water from the far side of a cup or glass. This requires good concentration and co-ordination which can break the hiccupping cycle. If the hiccups continue for several hours, the person should seek medical attention.

Summary

In this chapter you have learned to recognise and care for breathing emergencies from a variety of causes.

In the primary survey you should check for the symptoms and signs of respiratory distress, including abnormal breathing, abnormal skin appearance and feelings of dizziness, shortness of breath and chest pain.

The general principles of first aid for respiratory distress include:

- Call for an ambulance.
- Help the victim to rest comfortably.
- Carry out a secondary survey to check for other problems.
- Reassure the victim.
- Help the victim to maintain a normal body temperature.
- Continue to monitor the victim's vital signs.

Provide additional specific first aid when you know the cause of the respiratory distress to be:

- Asthma.
- Hyperventilation.
- Choking.
- Near-drowning.
- Hanging, strangulation, throttling or suffocation.
- Inhalation of fumes.
- Electrical injury.
- Pneumothorax.
- Winding or hiccups.

Answers to Application Questions

1. During an asthma attack, air can become trapped in the lungs because the swollen bronchial passages will not allow a sufficient amount of air to pass through and be exhaled. Excessive mucus production from swollen mucous membranes causes further breathing difficulty. The effects on the victim include shortness of breath, increasing pulse, wheezing and coughing.

2. As a result of hyperventilation, blood carbon dioxide levels fall.

3. During breathing, the epiglottis opens, allowing air to enter the trachea and move into the lungs. When you eat, the epiglottis covers the opening of the trachea so that food and liquids cannot enter the lungs. Choking can occur when a person inadvertently breathes in and swallows at the same time. When this happens, the epiglottis receives mixed signals. It receives messages to protect the trachea from food and objects, but also to allow air to enter. The epiglottis cannot perform both functions at the same time. In these situations, the epiglottis may open, resulting in air, food and liquids entering the trachea.

4. Choking can result in respiratory arrest, cutting off the oxygen supply to the body. If care does not begin immediately, body tissues will begin to die, and body systems will fail. If the condition is not corrected promptly, body systems fail, resulting in death.

5. High-voltage electricity can arc significant distances. Arcing has been known to occur up to 6 metres. Do not try to rescue the victim until the electricity supply authorities have declared the area to be safe.

Study Questions

1. **Match each term with the correct definition.**

   a. Airway obstruction.

   b. Asthma.

   c. Breathing emergency.

   d. Hyperventilation.

   e. Choking.

   f. Bronchodilator.

   g. Cyanosis.

   h. Respiratory distress.

   _____ Medication to treat asthma attack.

   _____ Condition of imbalance in oxygen and carbon dioxide in the body related to breathing too fast.

   _____ Blockage of the airway which prevents air from reaching the victim's lungs.

   _____ Bluish colour of skin and mucous membranes indicating a breathing emergency.

   _____ Condition in which breathing becomes difficult.

   _____ Condition in which air passages are narrowed by muscle spasm, swelling of mucous membranes and increased mucus production.

   _____ Blockage of the airway caused by a foreign body.

   _____ Emergency in which breathing is so impaired that life is threatened.

2. **List four symptoms and signs of respiratory distress.**

3. **List three causes of choking.**

4. **What are the symptoms and signs of an asthma attack?**

5. **Asthma, hyperventilation and inhalation of fumes:**

   a. may result in respiratory distress

   b. require EAR

   c. are always life threatening.

   d. a and c.

   e. a, b and c.

6. **You should call an ambulance for a person suffering an asthma attack:**

   a. as soon as the attack begins

   b. if the attack is worsening or not responding to prescribed medication

   c. only if the casualty asks you to.

7. *Are the following statements true or false?*

a. Cyanosis is a sign of respiratory distress.   T / F

b. You should give expired air resuscitation to a conscious casualty   T / F
    who is choking.

c. A person who is hyperventilating should breathe in and out of a paper bag.   T / F

d   An allergic reaction can cause respiratory distress.   T / F

e. All asthma victims wheeze.   T / F

f. Respiratory distress can lead to respiratory arrest.   T / F

g. A person with asthma should have a personal asthma management plan.   T / F

h. Hyperventilation will resolve itself and does not need medical assessment.   T / F

i. Carbon monoxide is visible in the air.   T / F

j. You should stand under a tree if caught outside in an electrical storm.   T / F

8. *After giving back blows and lateral chest thrusts to an unconscious choking victim who is still not breathing, you should:*

a. try EAR

b. keep repeating back blows and chest thrusts

c. start CPR.

d. a, b and c.

9. *While eating dinner, a friend suddenly starts to cough and make high-pitched noises. You should:*

a. give back slaps

b. give lateral chest thrusts immediately

c. encourage your friend to continue coughing to try to dislodge the object.

d. help your friend to lie down

10. *The care for drowning includes:*

a. pumping the abdomen to clear out swallowed water

b. EAR if needed

c. not bothering to check for a pulse but starting CPR immediately.

d. All of the above.

11. *The care for electrical injuries includes:*

a. caring for any burns present

b. steps to minimise shock

c. monitoring the ABC.

d. All of the above.

Answers are in Appendix A (page 361).

First Aid for the Adult Victim of Choking

Determine if the person is choking
- Ask "Are you choking?"

If the person is still able to breathe, speak, cry or cough ...
- Encourage the person to continue coughing.
- Reassure the person.
- Continue to monitor the situation.
- If there is wheezing or noisy breathing, call an ambulance.
- Do not use back blows, because this may make the situation worse.

If the person is unable to breathe, speak, cry or cough ...

Give up to 4 back blows
- Help the person lie on the floor on the side.
- Give up to 4 back blows between the shoulder blades with the heel of your hand.

If the victim is still unable to breathe, speak, cry or cough ...

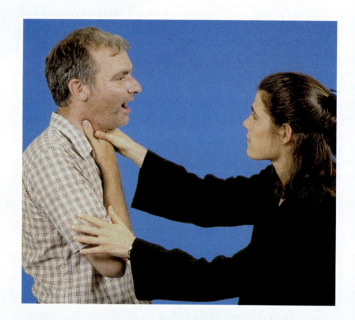

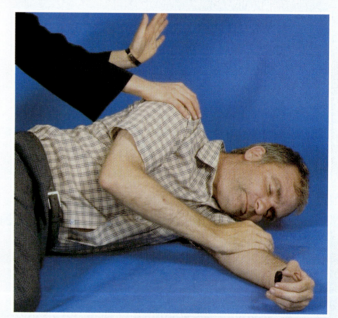

Give up to 4 chest thrusts
- Leave the victim on the side.
- Place the palm of one hand on the side of the ribs against the armpit, and place the other hand beside it.
- Give up to 4 quick downward thrusts.
- It is likely that the person will become unconscious quickly if the obstruction is not relieved.

If the victim becomes unconscious, keep the victim on the side and ...

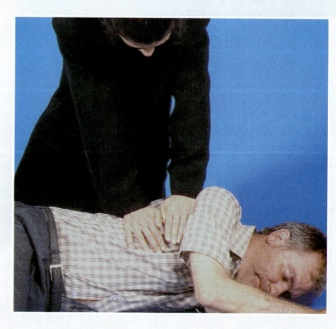

PRACTICE GUIDE

Check the airway

- Check mouth and throat for any visible foreign matter which can be removed with your fingers.
- Tilt head and support jaw.

Check breathing

- Maintain head tilt and jaw support.
- Look, listen and feel for any signs of breathing, such as wheezing or laboured breaths.

If the victim is breathing ...

- Leave the victim on the side and monitor the ABC.
- Await arrival of ambulance personnel.

If the victim is not breathing ...

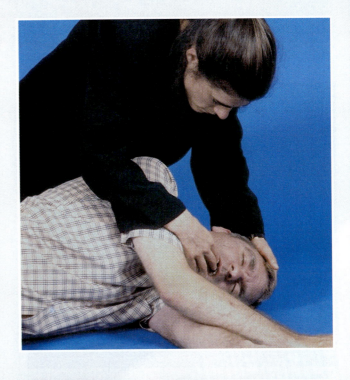

Turn the victim on the back and begin EAR.

Ensure head is correctly positioned with head tilt and jaw support.

- Give 5 full breaths.
- Watch the chest rise to ensure air is going in.
- If obstruction is present, there will be resistance to inflation and the chest will not rise. Continue EAR to try to blow air past the obstruction or spasm in the airway.

If you are successful and the chest rises ...

- Check for a pulse.

If the victim has a pulse but is not breathing, continue EAR until breathing recommences.

If the victim does not have a pulse, begin CPR.

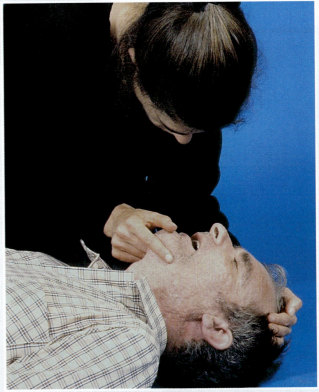

Review progress

If the chest does not rise with inflation attempts ...

- Roll the person onto the side and give up to 4 back blows and up to 4 chest thrusts as before.
- Check the airway and breathing.

If victim is still not breathing ...

- Roll victim onto back and continue resuscitation attempts.

- Continue to alternate EAR with back blows and chest thrusts until:

—obstruction is dislodged.

—victim starts to breathe.

—trained personnel take over.

Note: *Sometimes EAR will result in the foreign body being blown down into the lung. This can be removed later during medical treatment.*

First Aid for an Infant or Child Victim of Choking

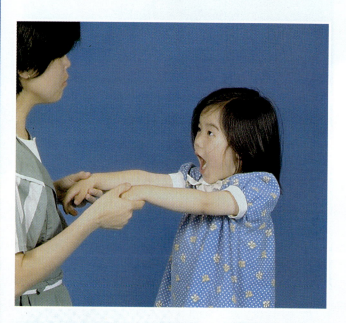

Determine if the infant or child is choking

- Consider whether the child is breathing, crying, speaking or coughing.

If the infant or child is still able to breathe, speak, cry or cough ...

- Allow or encourage the infant or child to continue coughing.
- Continue to monitor the situation.
- If there is wheezing or noisy breathing, call an ambulance.
- Do not use back blows, because this may make the situation worse.

If the infant or child is unable to breathe, speak, cry or cough ...

Give up to 4 back blows

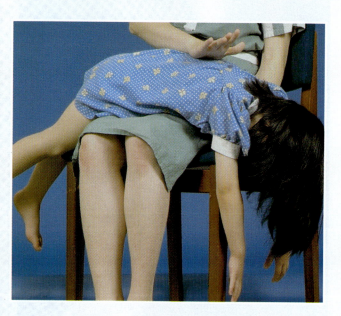

- Position the infant or child face down across your lap with head low.
- Give up to 4 back blows between the shoulder blades with the heel of your hand.

If the infant or child is still conscious but still unable to breathe, speak, cry or cough ...

Give up to 4 chest thrusts

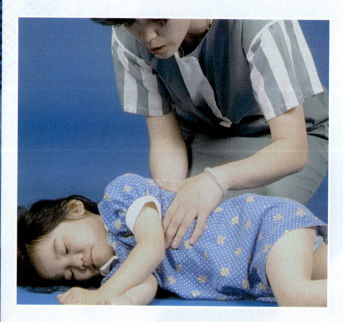

- Place your hands on both sides of the ribs against the armpit.
- Give 3 or 4 quick squeezing thrusts simultaneously on both sides.
- It is likely that the infant or child will become unconscious quickly if the obstruction is not relieved.

If the infant or child becomes unconscious, turn him or her on the side and ...

Check airway

- Check mouth and throat for any visible foreign matter that can be removed with your fingers.
- Support the jaw with the head in neutral position or slightly tilted.

Check breathing

- Maintain head position and jaw support.
- Look, listen and feel for any signs of breathing, such as wheezing or laboured breaths.

If the infant or child is breathing ...

- Leave the infant or child on the side and monitor the ABC.
- Await arrival of ambulance personnel.

If the infant or child is not breathing ...

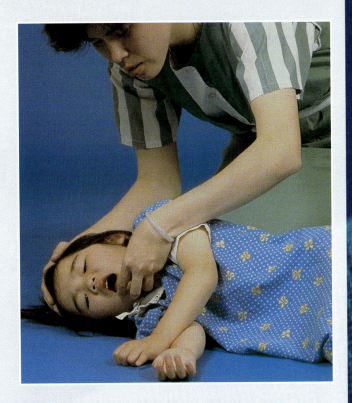

Turn the victim on the back and begin EAR

- Ensure the head is correctly positioned and jaw supported.
- Give 5 breaths or puffs.
- Watch the chest rise to ensure air goes in.
- If obstruction is present, there will be resistance to inflation and the chest will not rise. Continue EAR to try to blow air past the obstruction or spasm in the airway.

If you are successful and chest rises ...

- Check for a pulse

If the infant or child has a pulse but is not breathing, continue EAR until breathing recommences.

If the infant or child does not have a pulse, begin CPR.

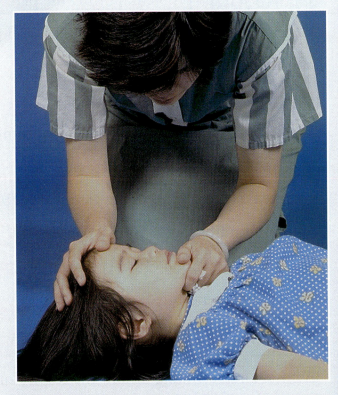

Review progress

If the chest does not rise with inflation attempts ...

- Position the infant or child face down on your lap with the head low.
- Give up to 4 back blows and up to 4 squeezing chest thrusts as before.
- Check the airway and breathing.

If the infant or child is still not breathing ...

- Turn the infant or child onto back and continue resuscitation attempts.
- Continue to alternate EAR with back blows and chest squeezing thrusts until:
    —obstruction is dislodged.
    —the infant or child starts to breathe.
    —trained personnel take over.

Note: *Sometimes EAR will result in the foreign body being blown down into the lung. This can be removed later during medical treatment.*

PRACTICE GUIDE

Cardiac Emergencies

CHAPTER 4 outlined how to give CPR to victims in cardiac arrest—when the heart has stopped completely. However, in other situations, the victim may still have a pulse but have a heart problem, putting the person at risk of a cardiac arrest. Heart attack and congestive heart failure are two common cardiac emergencies requiring first aid. It is important that you learn the symptoms and signs of these emergencies, and the correct first aid to give to the victim. As well, you can modify your own risk factors and reduce the likelihood of heart disease or a cardiac emergency.

For Review

A basic understanding of how the respiratory and circulatory systems function (Chapter 2), how to care for cardiac arrest (Chapter 4) and knowledge of the steps of the primary survey (Chapter 3) will help your understanding of the chapter.

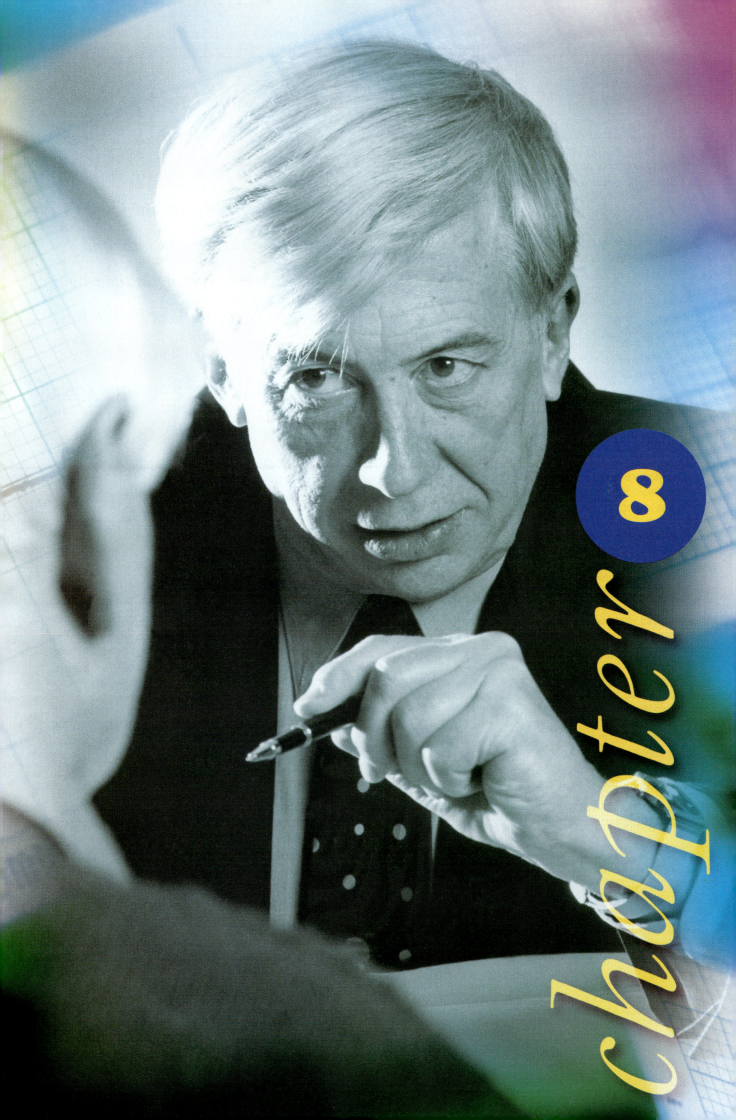

chapter **8**

Key Terms

Angina *(an-jy-na)*: A condition which occurs when the coronary arteries become seriously narrowed by disease and the supply of oxygenated blood to the heart becomes insufficient for the increased oxygen needed during activity. It is characterised by pain or pressure in the chest which is relieved by rest and/or medication.

Anticoagulant *(anti-co-ag-yu-lant)*: A substance or drug that stops or reduces the coagulation, or clotting, of the blood; used to prevent blood clots within the body.

Atherosclerosis *(ath-e-ro-scle-ro-sis)* : Condition in which blood vessels are narrowed by the build-up of cholesterol and other deposits.

Cardiovascular *(car-dee-o-vask-yoo-lar)* **disease**: Disease of the heart and blood vessels.

Cholesterol: A fatty substance made by the body and found in certain foods. Too much cholesterol in the blood can cause fatty deposits on artery walls which may restrict or block blood flow.

Congestive heart failure: A condition in which the heart is weak and functions poorly because of chronic heart disease or old age.

Coronary *(co-ron-ry)* **arteries**: Arteries which supply the heart muscle with oxygen-rich blood.

Coronary thrombosis *(throm-bo-sis)*: A clot which blocks a coronary artery.

Embolus *(em-bo-lus)*: Air or fatty deposit which travels in the circulatory system, eventually lodging in and blocking a small blood vessel.

Ischaemia *(is-kee-mee-a)*: A decreased supply of oxygen-rich blood to a body organ or part, often marked by pain and organ failure.

Myocardial *(my-o-car-dee-al)* **infarction** *(in-fark-shon)*: Damage which occurs to the heart muscle when blood supply in the coronary arteries is blocked; called heart attack.

Risk factors: Conditions or behaviours which increase the chance that a person will develop a disease.

The long-awaited break had arrived at last! Elizabeth put aside her stressful office job and John sent the children off to grandmother. It was the Queen's Birthday weekend, and John and Elizabeth were relaxing in their holiday flat at the beach on Port Phillip Bay. After a relaxing day walking along the beach, watching the waves and seagulls, they went to bed early.

At about two in the morning, Elizabeth woke to John's desperate words: "This pain in my chest—I'm scared!" She put on the light and saw his face was grey and he was sweating profusely. He seemed to be having trouble breathing. He said the pain felt like a vice squeezing his chest.

Elizabeth quickly called 000, and within 10 minutes the ambulance arrived. John was suffering a heart attack. The ambulance officers stabilised him in about 30 minutes and transported him to the nearby hospital.

John recovered well with medical treatment. Elizabeth often wondered what would have happened if she had not wakened to make the call that night.

In the primary survey, you identify and care for immediate threats to a victim's life. Your first aid priorities are the victim's airway, breathing and circulation (the ABC). In Chapter 4, you learned how to give CPR for a victim whose heart has stopped beating. In this chapter, you will learn how to recognise and provide care for other sudden illnesses involving the heart, such as a heart attack.

This chapter also identifies the important **risk factors** for **cardiovascular disease,** and provides an opportunity to promote good cardiovascular health in addition to learning CPR. People too often focus only on what to do after a cardiac arrest occurs. It is possible to modify your behaviour in order to prevent cardiovascular disease.

HEART ATTACK

Like all living tissue, the cells of the heart need a continuous supply of oxygen. The **coronary arteries** supply the heart muscle with oxygen-rich blood (Figure 8-1A). If heart muscle tissue is deprived of blood, it becomes damaged. If enough tissue is affected, the heart cannot pump effectively. When heart tissue dies it is called a heart attack, or **myocardial infarction**.

A heart attack damages heart muscle and interrupts the heart's electrical system. This may result in an irregular heartbeat and prevent blood from circulating effectively.

It is possible for the heartbeat to become slow, rapid or irregular as a result of heart disease. Sometimes these changes in rhythm can be serious and even cause cardiac arrest.

If the change in rhythm is serious enough, an artificial pacemaker may be fitted. This operates through a small wire which runs into the heart muscle and is connected to a battery implanted under the skin.

A person with an artificial pacemaker will still need CPR if cardiac arrest occurs as this indicates that the pacemaker is not working.

Common Causes of Heart Attack

Heart attack is usually the result of cardiovascular disease. Cardiovascular disease—disease of the heart and blood vessels—is the leading cause of death for adults in Australia. Many Australians suffer some form of cardiovascular disease. In 1992, cardiovascular disease caused 54,912 deaths. Of these, 31,482 were due to heart attack.*

Cardiovascular disease develops slowly. Fatty deposits of **cholesterol** and other material may gradually build up on the inner walls of the coronary arteries. This condition, called **atherosclerosis,** causes progressive narrowing of these vessels and is called coronary artery disease. When coronary arteries narrow, a clot may develop due to the slowing of blood at the site. This causes a heart attack (Figure 8-1B). Also, an **embolus,** a small piece of fatty tissue, may break off and travel to another vessel where it blocks the flow. Atherosclerosis will also involve arteries in other parts of the body such as the brain, which can lead to a stroke (see Chapter 9).

Atherosclerosis develops gradually, and it can go undetected for many years. Even with significantly

*National Heart Foundation of Australia, *Heart Facts 1992,* p. 4.

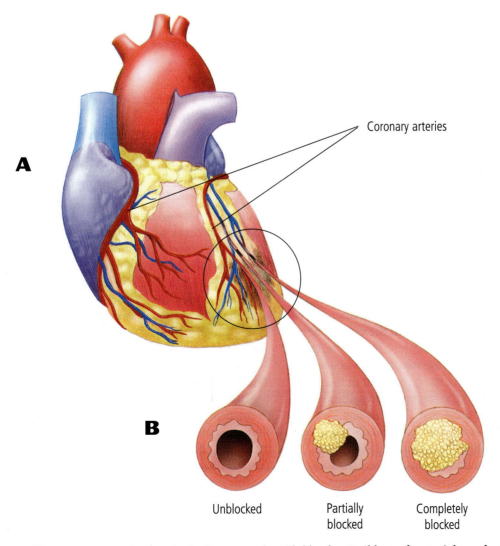

Coronary arteries

A

B

Unblocked

Partially blocked

Completely blocked

FIGURE 8-1 A *The coronary arteries supply the heart muscle with blood.* **B** *Build-up of materials on the inner walls of these arteries reduces blood flow to the heart muscle and may cause a heart attack.*

THE HEART AS A PUMP

Too often we take our hearts for granted. As a mechanical pump, the heart is extremely reliable. The heart beats about 70 times each minute, or more than 100,000 times a day. During the average lifetime, the heart will beat nearly three billion times. The heart pumps about 8 litres of blood per minute, or more than 10,000 litres per day. The heart pumps blood through about 100,000 km of blood vessels. ■

reduced blood flow to the heart muscle, there may be no symptoms or signs of heart trouble. Most people with atherosclerosis are unaware of it but, as the narrowing progresses, some people experience early warning signs when the heart does not receive enough blood, especially during exercise or exertion (sometimes called angina). Others may suffer a heart attack or even cardiac arrest without any previous warning. Fortunately, this process can be slowed or stopped by lifestyle changes, such as forming healthy eating habits. Later in this chapter you will learn what you can do to keep your heart healthy.

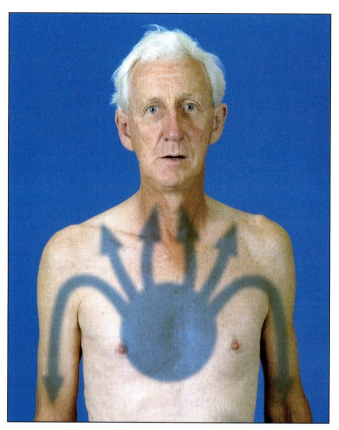

FIGURE 8-2 *Heart attack pain is most often felt in the centre of the chest, behind the sternum. It may spread to the shoulder, arm, neck or jaw.*

1 *How does atherosclerosis result in a heart attack?*

Symptoms and Signs of a Heart Attack

The most prominent symptom of a heart attack is persistent chest pain or discomfort. However, it is not always easy to distinguish between the pain of a heart attack and chest pain caused by indigestion, muscle spasm or other conditions.

The pain of a heart attack can range from discomfort to an unbearable crushing sensation in the chest. The victim may describe it as an uncomfortable pressure, squeezing, tightness, aching, constricting or a heavy sensation in the chest. Often, the pain is felt in the centre of the chest behind the sternum (breastbone). It may spread to the shoulder, arm, neck or jaw (Figure 8-2). The pain is constant and usually not relieved by resting, changing position or taking oral medication. Any chest pain which is severe, lasts longer than 10 minutes or is accompanied by other heart attack signs should receive emergency medical care immediately.

Although a heart attack is often dramatic, victims can have relatively mild symptoms, often mistaken for

indigestion. Some heart attack victims feel no chest pain or discomfort.

People with coronary artery disease may experience chest pain or pressure which comes and goes at different times. This type of pain is called **angina.** Angina develops when the coronary arteries are narrow and the heart needs more oxygen, especially during physical activity or emotional stress. This lack of oxygen can cause a constricting chest pain which may spread to the neck, jaw and arms. Pain associated with angina usually lasts less than 10 minutes. A person who suffers from angina will have prescribed medication to help relieve the pain. Reducing the heart's demand for oxygen, such as by stopping physical activity, and taking prescribed medication, often relieves angina symptoms.

Another sign of a heart attack is breathing difficulty. The victim may be breathing faster than normal because the body is trying to get much-needed oxygen to the heart. The victim's pulse may be faster or slower than normal, or irregular. The victim's skin may be pale or bluish, particularly around the nose and mouth. The face may be moist from perspiration. Some heart attack victims sweat profusely. These signs result from the stress experienced by the body when the heart does not work effectively.

Any heart attack may lead to cardiac arrest, so it is important to recognise and act on these symptoms and signs. Prompt action may prevent cardiac arrest. A heart attack victim whose heart is still beating has a far better chance of survival than a victim whose heart has stopped. Most people who die from a heart attack do so within 1 to 2 hours after the first signs. Many could have been saved if the victim or someone on the scene had been aware of the signs of a heart attack and acted promptly. As most heart attacks result from clotting within the coronary arteries (sometimes called **coronary thrombosis**), early treatment with medication which dissolves clots, has proven to be helpful in minimising damage to the heart.

Many heart attack victims delay seeking care. Nearly half of all heart attack victims wait 2 or more hours before going to the hospital. Victims often do not realise they are having a heart attack, or they may dismiss the symptoms as being that of indigestion or muscle soreness.

Remember:

The key symptom of a heart attack is persistent chest pain. If the chest pain or discomfort is severe or does not go away within 10 minutes, call an ambulance immediately and begin care for a heart attack.

Caring for a Heart Attack

The most important first aid measure is to recognise that any of the symptoms and signs listed in Table 8-1 may be those of a heart attack. Therefore, you must take immediate action if any of these appear. A heart attack victim may deny the seriousness of the symptoms being experienced. Do not let this influence you. If you think that someone might be having a heart attack, you must act. First, advise the victim to stop all activity and rest comfortably. Many heart attack victims find it easier to breathe while sitting upright (Figure 8-3).

Continue with your secondary survey. If the victim is experiencing persistent chest pain, ask for the following information:

- When did the pain start?
- What brought it on?
- Does anything lessen it?
- What does it feel like?
- Where does it hurt?

Table 8-1

SYMPTOMS AND SIGNS OF A HEART ATTACK

Condition	Symptoms and signs
Persistent chest pain or discomfort	Persistent pain or pressure in the chest which is not relieved by resting, changing position or oral medication. Pain may range from discomfort to an unbearable crushing sensation, with pain spreading to the throat or jaw, or down one or both arms.
Breathing difficulty	Breathing is noisy. Victim feels short of breath. Breathing is faster than normal.
Changes in pulse rate	Pulse may be faster or slower than normal, or may be irregular.
Skin appearance	Skin may be pale or bluish. Face may be moist, or victim may sweat profusely.

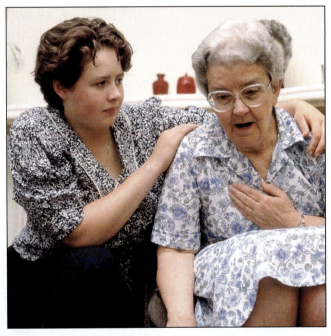

FIGURE 8-3 *The heart attack victim should rest in a position which helps breathing.*

2 *Why do some heart attack victims suffer cardiac arrest?*

Check if the victim has a history of heart disease. Some people with heart disease have prescribed medications for chest pain. You can help by getting the medication for the victim. A common medication prescribed for angina is glyceryl trinitrate, taken as a small tablet or puffer spray which is absorbed under the tongue, or on a continuous basis through a patch placed on the chest wall. Once absorbed into the body, this medication enlarges the blood vessels to make it easier for blood to reach heart muscle tissue. The pain is relieved because oxygen delivery to the heart is increased and the heart does not have to work so hard.

If you still think that the victim may be having a heart attack, or if you are unsure about the victim's condition, ask a bystander to call an ambulance for help. If you are alone, make the call yourself. Surviving a heart attack often depends on how soon the victim receives advanced medical care. **Unless you are in a remote area, do not try to drive the victim to the hospital yourself,** because cardiac arrest can occur at any time. Call the emergency number immediately, before the condition worsens and the heart stops beating.

Keep a calm and reassuring manner when caring for a heart attack victim. Comforting the victim helps reduce anxiety and eases some of the discomfort. Watch the victim closely until ambulance personnel arrive. Continue to monitor the vital signs, and watch for any changes in appearance or behaviour. Be prepared to give CPR because the heart attack may deteriorate into cardiac arrest.

The box below summarises the first aid care for a heart attack.

3 *Why do heart attack victims often deny that they are having a heart attack?*

Aspirin

Aspirin has been shown to be a powerful **anticoagulant** medication in addition to its anti-inflammatory and pain-relieving properties. Many authorities now recommend that half an aspirin should be given as soon as possible to a victim with chest pain related to a heart attack because the aspirin may reduce the formation and extent of a blood clot in the blocked coronary artery. However, other authorities have expressed caution until more research has been completed.

At present, it is recommended in Australia that aspirin should not be given by first aiders or family members in this situation because there is a risk of causing further complications, especially when the chest pain is not due to a heart attack. Aspirin may be given by ambulance personnel when transporting the victim of a suspected heart attack, so that any delay in administering it will be short. Unfortunately, although a valuable medication, aspirin can cause complications such as internal bleeding if given in excess or inappropriately.

CARE FOR A HEART ATTACK

- Recognise the symptoms and signs of a heart attack.

- Convince the victim to stop activity and rest.

- Help the victim to rest comfortably.

- Try to obtain information about the victim's condition.

- Comfort the victim.

- Call the local emergency number for help.

- Assist with any prescribed medication.

- Monitor vital signs.

- Be prepared to give CPR if victim's heart stops beating. ▪

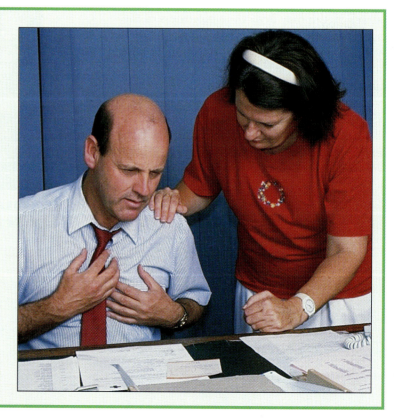

CONGESTIVE HEART FAILURE

Congestive heart failure is a term used to describe a condition in which the heart cannot pump normally. It does not mean that the heart is about to stop or fail completely.

Heart failure usually develops due to chronic heart disease or old age. Excess fluid in the lungs causes breathing difficulty, and elsewhere in the body it results in swelling, particularly of the legs and ankles.

Symptoms and Signs of Congestive Heart Failure

Heart failure has many symptoms and signs, including:

- General tiredness and breathlessness during exercise or strong emotion.
- Coughing and wheezing, sometimes with gurgling breathing.
- Swollen feet, ankles, legs and abdomen.
- A feeling of general ill health.

In people with advanced illness, the symptoms and signs worsen. In particular, breathlessness may occur with little activity or even at rest, and may become so bad that the person cannot lie down.

Caring for Congestive Heart Failure

Treatment for congestive heart failure can improve general health and help the person live longer. People with this condition may be prescribed regular medication and are usually advised to exercise in moderation and avoid salty foods and alcohol.

A person with heart failure may be quite well most of the time, but can suffer sudden deterioration if another illness occurs or medication is not taken.

In those instances, heart failure can become a serious emergency. You should monitor the person carefully and call an ambulance if necessary. Follow these general guidelines for care:

1. Help the victim to rest comfortably in a sitting position. Loosen any tight clothing especially at neck and waist (Figure 8-4).

2. Reassure and calm the victim.

3. Monitor breathing and pulse often. If the person's condition seems to get worse, call for an ambulance. Write down the breathing and pulse rates for the ambulance officers or doctor.

4. Be prepared to roll the victim onto the side if unconsciousness occurs. Maintain the airway and follow the Basic Life Support flow chart (see page 35).

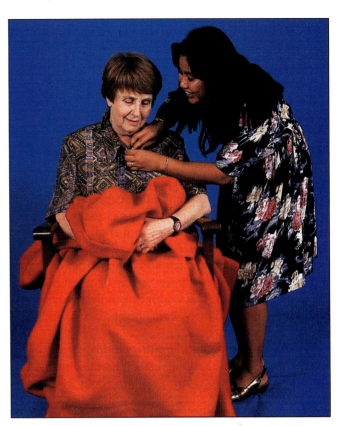

FIGURE 8-4 *Help a victim with congestive heart failure to sit comfortably.*

PREVENTING CARDIOVASCULAR DISEASE

Although a heart attack may seem to strike suddenly, the lifestyle of many Australians may be gradually endangering their hearts. Eventually this can result in cardiovascular disease. Potentially harmful behaviour frequently begins early in life. For example, many children develop tastes for "junk" foods high in fat or cholesterol with little or no nutritional value. Sometimes, children are not encouraged to exercise.

Several studies have shown that coronary artery disease actually begins in the teenage years, when most smoking begins. Teenagers are more likely to begin smoking if their parents smoke. Smoking also contributes to other diseases, as well as cardiovascular disease.

Risk Factors for Heart Disease

Scientists have identified numerous risk factors which increase the chances of a person developing heart disease. Some risk factors for heart disease cannot be changed, but many can be controlled. Men are at higher risk of heart disease than women, and a family history of heart disease also increases your risk.

Smoking, diets high in fats, high blood pressure, obesity and lack of routine exercise are all linked to increased incidence of heart disease. When one risk factor, such as high blood pressure, is combined with others, such as obesity or cigarette smoking, the possibility of a heart attack or stroke is greatly increased.

Controlling Risk Factors

Controlling risk factors involves adjusting your lifestyle to minimise the chance of future cardiovascular disease (Figure 8-5). The three major risk factors you can control are cigarette smoking, high blood pressure and high blood cholesterol levels.

Cigarette smokers have more than twice the chance of having a heart attack than non-smokers and two to four times the chance of cardiac arrest.

Uncontrolled high blood pressure can damage blood vessels in the heart and other organs. High blood pressure may be controlled by losing excess weight and changing your diet. If this is not enough, medications may be prescribed.

Diets high in saturated fats and cholesterol increase the risk of heart disease, however, some cholesterol in the body is essential. The amount of cholesterol in the blood is determined by how much your body produces and by the food you eat.

More important to an unhealthy blood cholesterol level is saturated fat. Saturated fats raise the blood cholesterol level by interfering with the body's ability to remove cholesterol from the blood.

Rather than trying to eliminate saturated fats and cholesterol from your diet, limit your intake. Moderation is the key. Read labels carefully: a "cholesterol-free" product may be high in unwanted saturated fat.

Two additional ways to help prevent heart disease are to control your weight and exercise regularly.

For further information on a healthy lifestyle, see Chapter 20.

4 *Which cardiovascular disease risk factors can be controlled by the individual?*

Results of Managing Risk Factors

Managing your risk factors for cardiovascular disease really works. During the past 25 years, deaths from cardiovascular disease have decreased by 64 per cent in Australia. As a result, as many as 25,000 lives may have been saved. Also, deaths from stroke have declined 71 per cent for men and 74 per cent for women.*

Deaths from these causes have probably declined as a result of improved detection and treatment, as well as lifestyle changes. People who become more aware of their risk factors for heart disease can take action to control them and improve their chances of living a long and healthy life. The time to reduce your risks for cardiovascular disease is now.

*National Heart Foundation of Australia, *Heart Facts* 1992, pp. 10-11, 15.

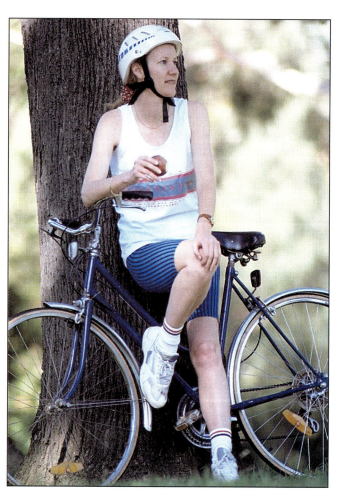

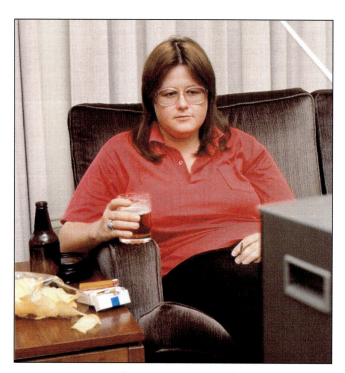

FIGURE 8-5 *Do not let risk factors control you by smoking, eating badly, doing no exercise and being overweight; instead, you control them by not smoking, eating a low-cholesterol diet, exercising regularly and maintaining normal weight.*

Summary

- Cardiac emergencies, including heart attack and congestive heart failure, are life-threatening and may lead to cardiac arrest.

- It is important that you recognise the symptoms and signs of cardiac emergencies and act promptly. If you are in any doubt about the severity of a problem which causes the symptoms and signs of a cardiac emergency, call an ambulance immediately.

- Cardiovascular disease can often be prevented by modifying your lifestyle to eliminate risk factors such as smoking, dietary fat, obesity and lack of exercise.

Answers to Application Questions

1. The narrowing of coronary arteries from atherosclerosis severely restricts or completely cuts off the delivery of oxygen-rich blood to the heart. When heart muscle does not receive enough oxygen, the resulting tissue damage limits the heart's ability to pump effectively. This is what is known as a heart attack.

2. A heart attack becomes cardiac arrest when so much of the heart muscle is damaged that the heart is unable to contract regularly and subsequently stops beating. There is no way to predict the extent of the damage sustained by the heart during a heart attack or to predict when a heart attack might become cardiac arrest. Therefore, it is very important to recognise and acknowledge symptoms and signs of a heart attack and to seek professional help quickly.

3. Victims deny they are having a heart attack for a variety of reasons. No one wants to have a heart attack. In fact, most people are so afraid of having a heart attack that they deny symptoms. Others do not want their families and loved ones to worry about them. They may be embarrassed about being ill or by the commotion a hospital visit causes. Shock and poor oxygenation can also cause confusion and an inability to assess the situation.

4. An individual is able to modify 3 major risk factors and reduce the risks of cardiovascular disease. The controllable risk factors are smoking, high blood pressure and high blood cholesterol. If a person stops smoking, controls high blood pressure by losing weight and reduces the amount of saturated fats in their daily diet, cardiovascular disease may be avoided.

Study Questions

1. *Match each term with the correct definition.*

    a. Congestive heart failure.

    b. Cholesterol.

    c. Coronary arteries.

    d. Heart.

    e. Heart attack.

    f. Cardiovascular disease.

    g. Risk factors.

    h. Angina.

    _____ A muscular organ which pumps blood throughout the body.

    _____ A fatty substance which builds up on the inner walls of arteries.

    _____ The leading cause of death for adults in Australia.

    _____ Temporary chest pain caused by a lack of oxygen to the heart.

    _____ Blood vessels which supply the heart with oxygen-rich blood.

    _____ Conditions or behaviours which increase the chance of developing disease.

    _____ A sudden illness involving damage to heart muscle tissue caused by insufficient oxygen-rich blood reaching the cells.

    _____ A gradually developing weakness of the heart which affects its ability to pump blood.

2. *List three risk factors for heart disease which are controllable.*

3. *The most prominent symptom of a heart attack is:*

    a. profuse sweating

    b. pale skin

    c. persistent chest pain

    d. difficulty in breathing.

4. *Chest pain associated with heart attack is:*

    a. an uncomfortable pressure

    b. persistent pain which may spread to the shoulder, arm, neck or jaw

    c. usually relieved by changing positions

    d. a and b

    e. a, b and c

5. *If a person with chest pain has a known history of heart disease, you should:*

   a. give them a prescribed dose of their treatment immediately
   b. drive the victim to the hospital in your car immediately
   c. ring your doctor for advice before giving medication
   d. send for an ambulance immediately

6. *During a heart attack:*

   a. the heart may function inadequately
   b. some heart muscle is damaged by lack of oxygen
   c. the heart may stop
   d. a, b.and c

7. *To care effectively for a person having a heart attack, you should:*

   a. position the victim for CPR
   b. call an ambulance immediately
   c. begin EAR
   d. all of the above

8. *To care for a conscious victim you suspect has congestive heart failure, the first thing you should do is:*

   a. turn the person onto the side and maintain an open airway
   b. assist the person to rest sitting up
   c. assist the person with prescribed medication
   d. start CPR immediately
   e. b and c

9. *CPR is needed:*

   a. when the victim is not breathing
   b. when the victim's heart stops beating
   c. for every heart attack victim
   d. when the heart attack victim loses consciousness

10. *Your elderly neighbour phones you and says she is not feeling well. When you get there, she appears short of breath and you notice that her lips are bluish in colour. She says that she is seeing a doctor regularly for a heart condition and has recently had a cold. You should first:*

   a. help her to rest comfortably in a seated position, reassure her and monitor her closely
   b. get her a cup of tea and tell her to ring the doctor in the morning
   c. lie her down and phone her husband at work
   d. take her for a walk outside for some fresh air.

Answers are in Appendix A (page 361).

Altered Conscious States

N CHAPTER 3 you were shown how to begin the primary survey of a victim by assessing them for responsiveness. This step is crucial because unconsciousness can be a sign of a life-threatening emergency. Unconsciousness, or an altered state of consciousness, signals that something is wrong in the body. It can result from many different injuries and illnesses. Whatever the cause, it requires immediate care.

This chapter outlines how to recognise changes in the conscious state and the care to give the victim.

For Review

A review of when to call an ambulance (Chapter 3) and familiarity with the body systems (Chapter 2) will help your understanding of the chapter.

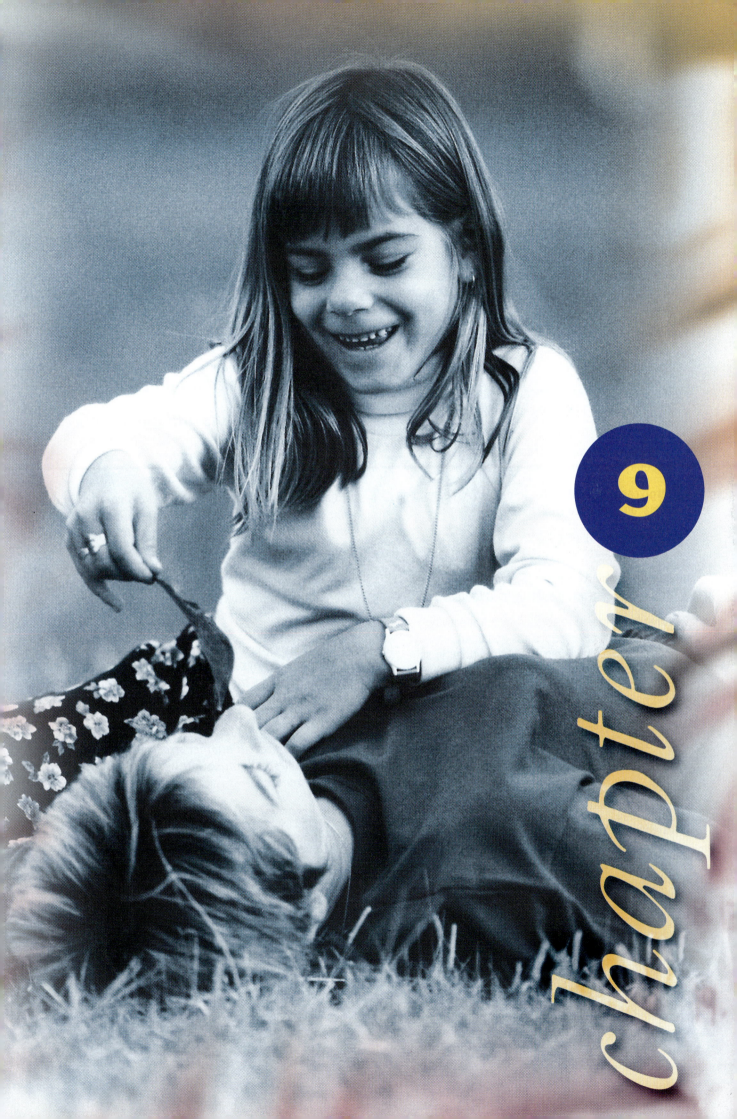

9

chapter

Key Terms

Brain: The centre of the nervous system that controls all body functions.

Cerebral compression: A condition of increased pressure inside the skull which compresses brain tissue and disrupts functioning.

Concussion: A temporary impairment of brain function, usually without permanent damage to the brain.

Diabetes *(dy-a-bee-teez)*: Diabetes mellitus is a condition in which the body does not produce enough insulin.

Embolism *(em-bo-liz-m)*: A piece of foreign material or tissue which travels through the bloodstream and blocks a blood vessel.

Epilepsy *(ep-i-lep-see)*: A chronic condition characterised by seizures, which usually can be controlled by medication.

Fainting: A loss of consciousness resulting from a temporary reduction of blood flow to the brain.

Hyperglycaemia *(hy-per-gly-see-mee-a)*: A greater than normal amount of sugar in the bloodstream.

Hypoglycaemia *(hy-po-gly-see-mee-a)*: A less than normal amount of sugar in the bloodstream.

Insulin *(in-su-lin)*: A hormone that enables the body to use sugar for energy; frequently used to treat diabetes.

Seizure: A disorder in the brain's electrical activity, marked by loss of consciousness and often uncontrollable muscle movement; may occur in an infant or child as a result of a sudden high temperature (often called a convulsion).

Stroke: A disruption of blood flow to a part of the brain which causes permanent damage, usually caused by a blood clot or bleeding vessel; also called a cerebrovascular accident (CVA).

Thrombus: A blood clot attached to the wall of a vein or artery which can block blood flow.

Transient ischaemic *(is-kee-mic)* **attack (TIA):** A temporary disruption of blood flow to the brain; sometimes called a mini-stroke.

It was lunchtime. Ross, a 60-year-old book editor, was having lunch with a colleague in the company cafeteria when suddenly he lost his sense of balance and his vision dimmed. His colleague immediately called Tom, a trained first aider in the office, who recognised the symptoms as a possible stroke. Tom called an ambulance and gave care until the ambulance officers arrived 10 minutes later.

On the brief trip to the hospital Ross vomited and blacked out. At the hospital doctors performed an immediate CAT scan which identified a major artery in the brain blocked by a clot. Ross's family was informed that he had suffered a stroke and might have severe permanent disability. However, they were told that there were promising results from a drug which was being tested for reversal of the damage resulting from a stroke. The family gave permission for the treatment, and Ross was given the drug intravenously.

After only 3 days Ross was walking again, and he was discharged in less than 2 weeks with no disabilities. Thanks to the prompt actions of the first aider, the ambulance officers and the medical staff, Ross has been able to return to an active life. To stay as healthy as possible and prevent another stroke, he has reduced his fat and cholesterol intake, lost weight and started regular exercise.

Any alteration in conscious state is a sign that something serious and possibly life-threatening is wrong with the victim. This chapter describes how to assess a victim's conscious state and how to care generally for the unconscious victim. It also describes the most common kinds of head injuries and medical conditions which can cause unconsciousness, such as diabetes, stroke and seizures, and the first aid to provide for each condition.

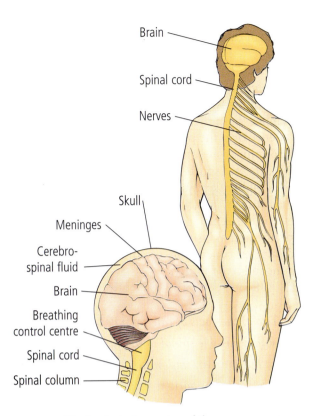

FIGURE 9-1 *The brain is the centre of the nervous system and controls all body functions.*

CONSCIOUSNESS AND THE NERVOUS SYSTEM

As you learned in Chapter 2, the brain is the centre of the nervous system and controls all body functions. The brain regulates the respiratory and circulatory systems, as it does all body systems, and thus controls breathing and the heart beat (Figure 9-1).

Any injury significant enough to cause unconsciousness or altered consciousness could cause injury to the brain itself and therefore should be considered serious. The brain can move within the skull, and therefore it can be injured by violent motion or pressure as well as by direct trauma to the head. Brain cells which die because of injury or illness are not replaced, because brain cells do not regenerate. Body functions controlled by the area of the brain that is damaged may be permanently affected or lost. An altered conscious state may be the first sign of such injury, and the victim may need emergency care immediately to prevent further damage.

Many medical conditions can cause unconsciousness or an altered conscious state. The medical problem may not originate in the brain although it may first reveal itself through its impact on the conscious state. For example, **diabetes,** a metabolic disease which results in hormonal imbalances, can cause an emergency in which the blood sugar level drops too low in the body. In this situation the brain cannot function as it should, the conscious state is affected, and the person may become unconscious. Similar to the unconsciousness caused by a head injury, this form of unconsciousness also indicates a need for immediate medical attention.

Determining Conscious State

To determine a person's conscious state, use the "shake and shout" method described in Chapter 3. Gently shake the victim's shoulders and loudly ask for the person's name. Because the victim may be unable to speak, give a simple command such as "Squeeze my hand. Now let it go." Never assess the conscious state by testing the victim's ability to feel pain, because this can cause distress to a person who is unable to speak or communicate.

> ### Remember:
> *A person who does not respond to "shake and shout" is unconscious.*

There are three levels of responsiveness:

- **Fully conscious:** The person can respond normally to questions and requests.
- **Semi-conscious:** The person is partly responsive and may answer questions in a way that shows confusion, disorientation or altered thinking.
- **Unconscious:** The person does not respond at all to the shouted command or to touch.

GENERAL CARE OF THE UNCONSCIOUS VICTIM

If the victim is unresponsive, turn the person onto the side, keeping the head and neck supported. Care for the airway, breathing and circulation following the Basic Life Support flow chart (see page 35). Call for an ambulance, and while waiting for help follow these additional guidelines:

1. If the unconscious victim is breathing and has a pulse, control any bleeding and put a dressing on a serious wound (see Chapter 5). Support any body areas where there is obvious injury.

2. Loosen any tight clothing at the neck, waist and chest. Look for a Medic Alert bracelet or pendant, or medical ID card (see Figure 1-7 in Chapter 1).

3. With the victim still on the side, perform a quick secondary survey for any other injuries and give appropriate care.

4. Help maintain body temperature by covering the person who is exposed to cold or damp or by shading the victim from the sun and by giving protection from heat. In addition, protection may be needed under the victim in extremely hot or cold conditions.

5. Continue to monitor the victim's conscious state, breathing and circulation.

6. Do not try to give fluids or food to an unconscious victim, and do not leave the person alone.

If possible, write down anything you observe about the victim's conscious state, whether it is improving or deteriorating. Record any changes in the victim while unconscious. Give this information to the ambulance officers when they arrive.

If you know or suspect a specific cause of the person's unconsciousness, you may need to give additional first aid. This care is described in the following sections on head injuries and illness which may cause an altered conscious state.

If the victim regains consciousness before the ambulance arrives, a medical assessment is still required. Whatever caused the unconscious state may continue as a medical problem and may again lead to a life-threatening condition.

CAUSES OF UNCONSCIOUSNESS

Unconsciousness may result from many different injuries and illnesses. Common causes include the following:

- Head injuries.
- Diabetes.
- Stroke.
- Seizures such as epilepsy.
- Fainting.

You should provide specific first aid for each of these conditions and illnesses, as described in the following sections.

HEAD INJURIES

The brain can be damaged or affected by any blow to the head or other area of the body which affects the head, such as a whiplash injury or falling heavily on the feet. It is often difficult to tell initially whether a head injury is minor or serious; however, a first aider should watch for any change in the victim's conscious state as this is the first indicator of a more serious problem.

Head injuries are not always obvious—an injury to the head which causes a scalp wound, bruising or bleeding may also cause a skull fracture (see Figure 12-11 in Chapter 12). The victim needs a medical examination immediately. A victim with a head injury may also have a spinal injury and so should be moved carefully. Remember that providing an open airway *always* takes precedence over the possibility of a spinal injury.

Head injuries are most commonly caused by car crashes, contact sports and occupational work that involves high-risk physical activity. Head injuries may also result from falls, which are more common among elderly or ill people.

Specific first aid is needed for the most common head injuries: concussion, cerebral compression, skull fracture and scalp injury.

1 *Two of the goals of care for a head injury victim with a possible spinal injury are to maintain an open airway and minimise movement. Is one more important than the other? Why?*

Concussion

Any significant force to the head may cause **concussion,** which results in a temporary impairment of brain function. The damage can occur on the opposite side of the brain from the site of the injury due to collision of brain tissue with the inside of the skull (Figure 9-2). It usually does not result in permanent physical damage to brain tissue, although extensive bruising or bleeding can occur. Concussion is sometimes called "brain shaking", and it can occur without apparent loss of consciousness.

The symptoms and signs of concussion may include:

- Brief or more extended periods of unconsciousness.

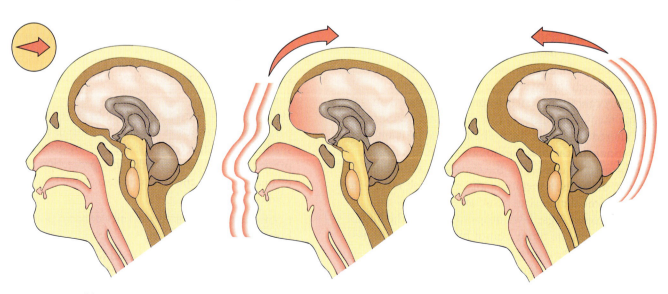

FIGURE 9-2 *A blow to one side of the head can cause injury to the opposite side of the brain.*

- a report of "seeing stars" or double vision
- confusion or temporary loss of short-term memory, e.g. of events just prior to the injury
- headache
- nausea and vomiting
- numbness, tingling or weakness in the arms and legs
- lack of eye-hand co-ordination or stumbling

Anyone suspected of having concussion should be observed closely and examined by a doctor because of the possibility of an associated, more serious injury. When taking immediate care of someone with concussion:

1. Assess the victim's conscious state by checking response to touch and spoken commands.

2. If unconscious, position the victim on the side and care for the airway, breathing and circulation following the Basic Life Support flow chart (see page 35).

3. If conscious, continue to observe the victim closely and note any improvement or deterioration. The victim should still see a doctor because obvious symptoms or signs may not appear for many hours.

4. Conduct a secondary survey and care for other conditions such as a scalp wound.

If you are unsure about the victim's condition, or if the casualty was unconscious for any period of time, arrange transport to a doctor or hospital.

Cerebral Compression

Cerebral compression is a condition which occurs when pressure within the skull increases. This may be caused by trauma to the head which damages brain tissue or by a blood clot forming within the skull.

Serious bleeding inside the skull compresses the brain and can lead to death. The pressure caused by bleeding or the swelling of injured brain tissue compresses the brain and may cut off oxygen to parts of the brain (Figure 9-3). Compression over the brain centres which control breathing and the heart rate can lead to breathing or cardiac emergencies.

The following symptoms and signs of cerebral compression may develop quickly or gradually, depending on the severity of the injury:

- Diminishing conscious state.
- Noisy or irregular breathing.
- Slow but full and bounding pulse.
- Weakness on one side of the body.
- Unequal pupils.
- Flushed face.
- Fever.

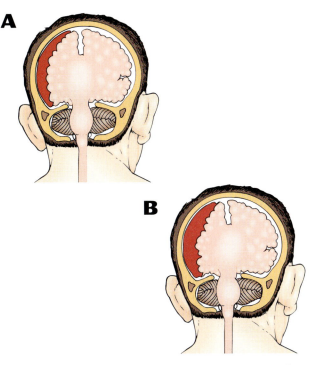

FIGURE 9-3 *Bleeding inside the skull creates pressure that compresses the brain and may cut off oxygen to parts of the brain.* **A** *Slight bleeding.* **B** *Severe compression.*

Follow these guidelines for care of a victim with possible cerebral compression:

1. Call an ambulance even if the victim is conscious, because urgent medical assessment is required.

2. If unconscious, position the victim on the side and care for the airway, breathing and circulation, following the Basic Life Support flow chart (see page 35).

3. If conscious, help the person to rest comfortably while waiting for the ambulance. Continually monitor the ABC and prepare to turn the victim on the side if the conscious state deteriorates.

4. Conduct a secondary survey and care for other conditions such as a scalp wound or skull fracture.

Skull Fracture

A blow to the head or a fall onto the head can cause a fracture of the skull, which in turn can damage the brain. Even if such a fracture does not at first seem serious, the fracture may cause cerebral compression. Consider all head injuries to be serious. Even if there is no apparent wound, the brain is easily damaged.

The symptoms and signs of a skull fracture may include:

- signs of head injury such as bruising or lacerations
- change in conscious state
- unequal pupils
- bloodshot or black-eye
- leakage of blood or fluid from the ear or nose

Follow these guidelines to care for a victim with a possible skull fracture:

1. Call an ambulance, even if the victim is conscious.

2. If unconscious, position the victim on the side and care for the airway, breathing and circulation, following the Basic Life Support flow chart (see page 35).

3. If conscious, help the victim into a half sitting position, and support the head and shoulders. Continually monitor the ABC and prepare to turn the victim onto the side if the conscious state deteriorates.

4. If there is discharge from the ear, tilt the victim's head toward that ear. Cover the ear with a dressing but do not try to plug the ear canal because this may increase pressure on the brain or introduce infection.

5. Give care to minimise shock (Chapter 6).

Scalp Injury

Scalp bleeding can be minor or severe. The bleeding is usually controlled with direct pressure. Be careful to press gently at first because the skull may be fractured. If you feel a depression, a spongy area or bone fragments, do not put direct pressure on the wound. Attempt to control bleeding with pressure on the area around the wound (Figure 9-4). Examine the injured area carefully because the victim's hair may hide part of the wound. If you are unsure about the extent of a scalp injury, call for an ambulance.

For a laceration of the scalp which does not involve obvious injury to underlying structures, give the wound care described in Chapter 12.

Preventing Head and Spine Injuries

Injuries to the head may also involve injuries to the spine. These injuries are a major cause of death and disability. However, many such injuries can be prevented by using safety practices in all areas of your life. It is important to reduce risks to yourself and to others around you.

Safety practices which can help prevent injuries to the head and spine include:

- wearing safety belts
- where appropriate, wearing approved helmets, eyewear, faceguards and mouthguards
- preventing falls
- taking safety precautions in sport and recreational activities
- avoiding inappropriate use of drugs
- inspecting work and recreational equipment periodically
- thinking and talking about safety

Wearing Safety Belts

Always wear a safety belt when travelling in a car, and be sure all passengers wear one. Airbags, available in some cars, provide additional protection but do not replace the use of safety belts. All small children riding in a car must be in an approved safety seat correct for the child's age and weight. A baby weighing under 9 kg should travel in an infant restraint facing the rear of the vehicle to protect the infant's head and neck (Figure 9-5).

Wearing Helmets and Eyewear

Helmets can prevent many needless injuries to the head and spine. They are designed for different purposes, with varying degrees of protection, depending on their

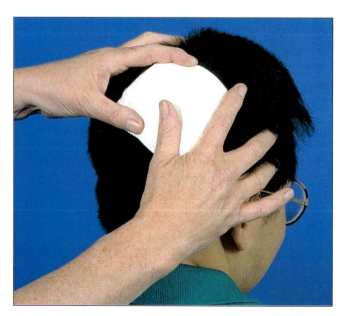

FIGURE 9-4 *To avoid putting direct pressure on a deep scalp wound, apply pressure with your hands to the area around the wound.*

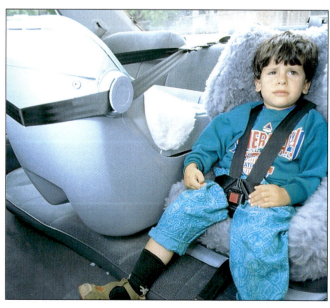

FIGURE 9-5 *Children and infants in cars must ride in Australian Standard approved safety seats.*

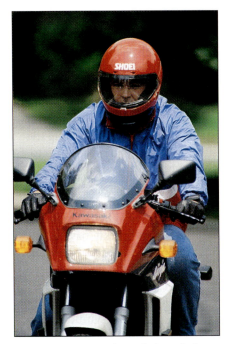
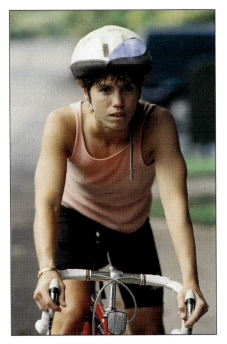
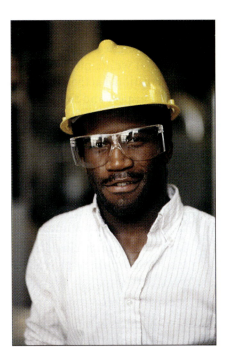

FIGURE 9-6 *Wearing a helmet helps protect against head and spine injuries.*

intended use (Figure 9-6). For example, the industrial work helmet called a "hard hat" provides adequate protection against falling debris but does not offer the proper protection for riding a motorcycle.

Any open form of transportation, such as a motorcycle, a moped, a dune buggy and even a bicycle exposes the head and spine to injury. Wearing a helmet can help reduce such injuries. The ideal motorcycle helmet, sometimes called a "full-face helmet", protects the lower face and jaw and has a large, clear or tinted face shield. Bicycle riders should wear an Australian Standards-approved helmet appropriate for the type of riding. In all cases, the helmet should be the correct size and fit comfortably and securely. In some States and Territories, the wearing of bike helmets is compulsory.

Preventing Falls

Most falls occur around the home, with young children and the elderly being the most frequent victims. You can take precautions to prevent falls. Uncarpeted floors should be of a nonslip type. Stairs should have nonslip treads and handrails. Rugs should be secured to the floor with double-sided tape. Clean up any spills promptly. The bathroom should be safe for all those using it. If necessary, install handrails by the bath, shower and toilet (Figure 9-7).

Taking Safety Precautions in Sport and Recreational Activities

Participants in sport or recreational activities should know their own physical limitations. Proper protective equipment is necessary for any activity in which serious injury may occur. In all sports involving physical contact, participants should wear mouthguards. It is most important that everyone should know and follow the rules, which not only make the activity fair but also

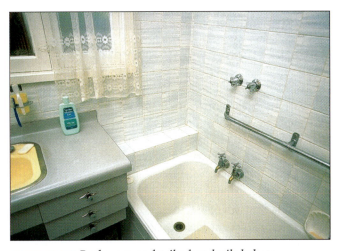

FIGURE 9-7 *Bathroom and toilet handrails help to prevent falls.*

help prevent injuries. The coach or a more experienced participant may impose additional rules for the safety of newcomers. Never participate in a new activity until you know the rules and risks involved.

Avoiding Inappropriate Use of Drugs

Alcohol and other drugs used inappropriately cause or contribute to many serious motor vehicle collisions and water-related injuries which result in head and spine injuries. Drugs impair judgment and reflexes, causing your body to respond abnormally (see Chapter 19). Drugs can give the user a feeling of false confidence. Under the influence of drugs, a person might not brake the car quickly enough or might dive into shallow water. Prescription and common pharmacy medications may also have side effects, such as drowsiness, which may make driving or operating machinery dangerous. Always follow your doctor's instructions and the directions on medication labels.

Thinking and Talking About Safety

People too often neglect thinking about safety in their daily lives; yet we are most vulnerable to injury at work, during recreational activities or while travelling. Take the time to inspect and think about your daily environment. Evaluate your habits. Answer the following questions:

- Are there things you could do in your home or work-place to help prevent injuries to yourself or others?

- Are you taking unnecessary risks in any activities?

- Do you follow rules intended for your safety?

- Do you frequently check the tyres on your car, truck, motorbike or bicycle?

- Do you ever attempt any activity without being in the right physical condition to do so safely?

Talk with others about preventing injuries at work, at home and during recreation. Children need guidance to help prevent injuries that could permanently affect their lives. Talk to them about safety on bikes, in the playground and at home. Their future may depend on your experience and advice.

ILLNESSES AFFECTING THE CONSCIOUS STATE

Alterations in the conscious state related to certain illnesses can occur suddenly. Often there are no warning signs to alert you that something is happening. At other times, the victim may feel ill or say that something "feels wrong".

The symptoms and signs of illness that affect the conscious state may include:

- a feeling of light-headedness, dizziness or weakness
- nausea or vomiting
- breathing changes
- pulse changes
- change in skin colour

In general, the fact that a person looks and feels ill means there is a problem.

Many different conditions, such as diabetes, **stroke, epilepsy,** poisoning and shock, can cause a change in conscious state. In an emergency, you do not need to know the exact cause to provide appropriate care for the victim, but you must know how to recognise a change in conscious state. Knowing and following the emergency action principles are all you need to do to care for a victim in whom you recognise an altered conscious state.

Faced with an unknown illness, you may not be sure whether to call for emergency medical help. Sometimes, as with simple **fainting,** the illness quickly passes. In this case, an ambulance may not be needed. However, if the problem is not resolved quickly and easily, or if you have any doubts about its severity, always call 000 or your local emergency number. It is better to err on the side of caution. Chapter 3 describes the symptoms and signs which indicate when to call for an ambulance.

The following sections provide information about some sudden illnesses you may encounter which result in an altered conscious state: diabetic emergencies, fainting, stroke, seizure, epilepsy and others. As you read, you will see that the care for all of these illnesses follows the same general guidelines:

1. Prevent further injury.

2. Monitor the ABC.

3. Call an ambulance when necessary.

4. Help the victim to rest comfortably.

5. Minimise shock by maintaining normal body temperature.

6. Provide reassurance.

7. Provide any specific care necessary.

Diabetic Emergencies

In order to function normally, body cells need sugar for energy. Through the digestive process, the body breaks

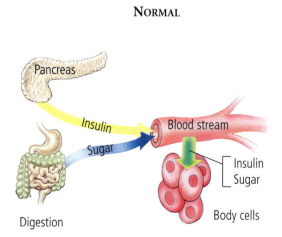

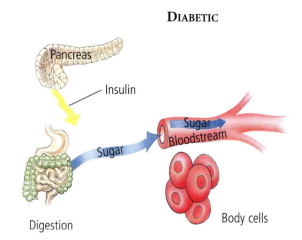

FIGURE 9-8 *The hormone insulin is needed to take sugar from the blood into the body cells.*

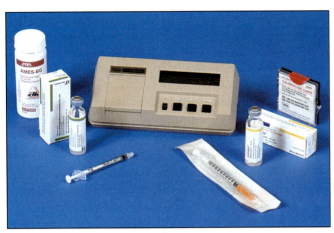

FIGURE 9-9 *Insulin-dependent people with diabetes inject insulin to regulate the amount of sugar in their body. A blood glucose meter is used to monitor blood glucose levels.*

down food into sugars, which are absorbed into the bloodstream. However, sugar cannot pass freely from the blood into the body cells. **Insulin,** a hormone produced in the pancreas, is necessary to take sugar into the cells. Without a proper balance of sugar and insulin, the cells will starve and the body will not function properly (Figure 9-8).

The condition in which the body does not produce enough insulin is called diabetes mellitus or sugar diabetes. There are about 500,000 Australians diagnosed as sufferers of diabetes.

There are two major types of diabetes. Type I, insulin-dependent diabetes, occurs when the body produces little or no insulin. Because this type of diabetes tends to begin in childhood, it is often called juvenile-onset diabetes. Most insulin-dependent people with diabetes have to inject insulin into their bodies daily.

Type II, non-insulin-dependent diabetes, occurs when the body produces insulin but not in sufficient quantity for the body's needs. This condition is called

mature-onset diabetes and most often occurs in older adults.

Anyone with diabetes must carefully monitor both their diet and exercise. Most also monitor their blood glucose very simply with the use of a blood glucose meter. Insulin-dependent people with diabetes must also regulate their use of insulin (Figure 9-9). When a person with diabetes fails to control these factors, either of two problems can occur—too much or too little sugar in the body. This imbalance causes illness.

When the insulin level in the body is too low, the sugar level in the blood is high. This condition is called **hyperglycaemia** (Figure 9-10A). Sugar is present in the blood but cannot be transported from the blood into the cells without insulin. When this occurs, body cells become starved of sugar. The body tries to get enough energy by using other stored food and energy sources such as fats. However, converting fats to energy produces waste products and increases the acidity level in the blood, causing a condition called acidosis. As this occurs, the person becomes ill. If it continues, the hyperglycaemic condition deteriorates into its most serious form, diabetic coma.

On the other hand, when the insulin level in the body is too high, the person has a low sugar level. This condition is known as **hypoglycaemia** (Figure 9-10B). The sugar level can become too low if the person with diabetes:

- takes too much insulin
- fails to eat adequately
- over-exercises and burns off sugar faster than normal
- becomes ill, especially with diarrhoea or vomiting
- experiences great emotional stress

In this situation, the small amount of sugar is used up rapidly, and there is not enough for the brain to function properly.

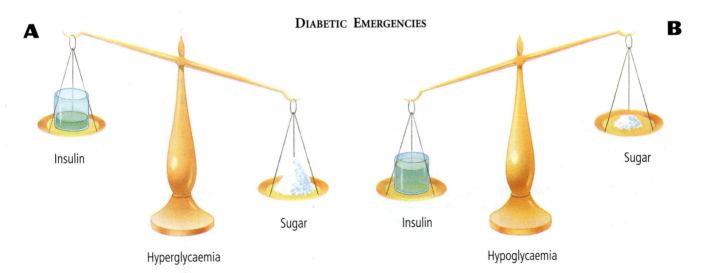

DIABETIC EMERGENCIES

A

Insulin

Sugar

Hyperglycaemia

B

Sugar

Insulin

Hypoglycaemia

FIGURE 9-10 A *Hyperglycaemia occurs when there is insufficient insulin in the body, causing a high level of sugar in the blood.* **B** *Hypoglycaemia occurs when the insulin level in the body is high, causing a low level of sugar in the blood.*

Symptoms and Signs of Diabetic Emergencies

The symptoms and signs of hyperglycaemia and hypoglycaemia differ somewhat. In particular, hyperglycaemia has a slow onset, and hypoglycaemia has a rapid onset and deterioration. The major symptoms and signs are, however, similar:

- Changes in the level of consciousness, including dizziness, drowsiness and confusion, sometimes mistaken for drunkenness.
- Rapid breathing.
- Rapid pulse.
- The victim feeling and looking ill.

It is not important for you to differentiate between hyperglycaemia and hypoglycaemia because the basic emergency care for both conditions is the same.

Care for Diabetic Emergencies

1. Conduct a primary survey and care for any life-threatening conditions.

2. If the victim is conscious, carry out a secondary survey looking for any visible abnormality, and look for a Medic Alert tag.

3. If the conscious victim can take food or fluids, give sugar as soon as possible (Figure 9-11). Most lollies, fruit juices and non-diet soft drinks have enough sugar to be effective. Common table sugar, either dry or dissolved in a glass of water, also works well to restore the victim to normal. If the person's problem is low sugar (hypoglycaemia), the sugar you give will help quickly. If the person already has too much sugar (hyperglycaemia), the excess sugar will do no further harm. Often a person with diabetes knows what is wrong and

will ask for something with sugar in it, or may be carrying a readily available source of sugar for such occasions. Call an ambulance if the person does not feel better within a few minutes of taking the sugar. A small meal, such as a sandwich, should be eaten by the fully conscious person to further assist in raising and maintaining the blood sugar. The person should still see a doctor for further assessment.

4. If the person becomes unconscious, call an ambulance and do not give anything by mouth. Instead, provide the general care for an unconscious victim as described previously. Monitor the ABC and maintain normal body temperature.

Stroke

A stroke, also called a cerebrovascular accident (CVA), is a disruption of blood flow to part of the brain, which is serious enough to damage brain tissue (Figure 9-12).

Most commonly, a stroke is caused by a blood clot, called a **thrombus** or **embolism,** that forms or lodges in the arteries that supply blood to the brain. Another common cause is bleeding from a ruptured artery in the brain. A head injury, high blood pressure, a weak area in an artery wall (aneurysm) or fat deposits lining

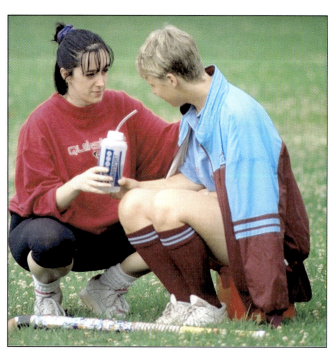

FIGURE 9-11 *If the victim of a diabetic emergency is conscious, give food or fluids containing sugar.*

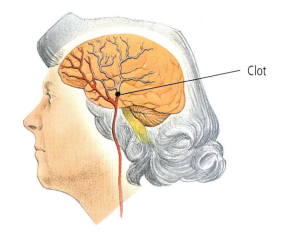

Clot

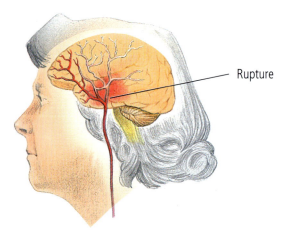

Rupture

FIGURE 9-12 *A stroke can be caused by a blood clot or bleeding from a ruptured artery in the brain.*

an artery (atherosclerosis) may cause stroke. Less commonly, a tumour or swelling from a head injury may compress an artery and cause a stroke.

A **transient ischaemic attack** (TIA) is a temporary episode which is like a stroke. TIAs are sometimes called "mini-strokes". Like a stroke, a TIA is caused by reduced blood flow to part of the brain. Unlike a stroke, the symptoms and signs of a TIA disappear within a few minutes or hours, although the person is not out of danger. Someone who experiences a TIA has a nearly 10 times greater chance of having a stroke in the future. Because you cannot tell a stroke from a TIA, you need only remember that any stroke-like symptoms and signs require immediate medical attention.

2 *Why does stroke result in damage to brain tissue?*

Symptoms and Signs of a Stroke

- The victim suddenly looking or feeling ill or behaving abnormally.
- Sudden weakness and numbness of the face, arm or leg, usually only on one side of the body.
- Difficulty talking or understanding speech.
- Blurred or dimmed vision.
- Unequal pupils.
- Sudden, severe headache.
- Dizziness, confusion or changes in mood.
- Ringing in the ears.
- Loss of bowel or bladder control.
- Possible unconsciousness.

Care for a Stroke

1. If the victim is unconscious, follow the steps of the Basic Life Support flow chart (see page 35). Position the victim on the side, make sure the airway is clear and open, and care for any life-threatening conditions which may occur. Call an ambulance immediately.

2. Stay with the victim and continue to monitor the conscious state, airway, breathing and circulation.

3. If the victim is conscious, carry out a secondary survey. If you see the symptoms and signs of a stroke, call for an ambulance.

4. Because a stroke can make the victim fearful and anxious, offer comfort and reassurance. Often the person does not understand what has happened.

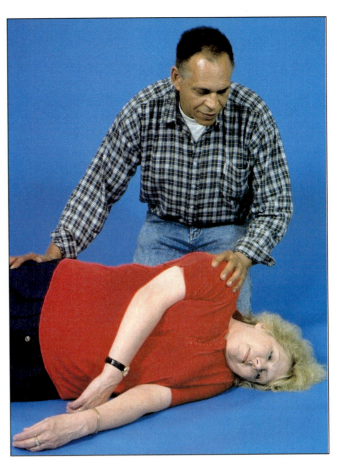

FIGURE 9-13 *Position a stroke victim on the side to help fluids or vomit drain from the victim's mouth.*

5. Help the victim to rest in a comfortable position, usually with head and shoulders supported.

6. Do not give the victim anything to eat or drink.

7. If the victim is drooling or having difficulty swallowing, place the person on the affected side to help drain any fluids or vomit from the mouth (Figure 9-13).

Ten years ago, a stroke almost always caused irreversible brain damage. Today this is not necessarily true. New drugs and medical procedures can limit or, in some cases, reduce the damage caused by stroke. Therefore you should quickly call an ambulance in order to get the best care for the victim as soon as possible.

3 *If you suspect that a conscious person has had a stroke, you should not give the person anything to eat or drink. Why?*

Preventing a Stroke

The risk factors for stroke and TIA are similar to those for heart disease. Some risk factors are beyond your control, such as age, gender or family history of stroke, TIA, diabetes or heart disease.

THE BRAIN MAKES A COMEBACK

Neuroscientists have been mystified for years by the capricious effects of strokes. For many stroke survivors talking becomes a tangle of words, a word like "piddlypop" spilling out in place of "hello". One man spoke normally unless he was asked to name fruits and vegetables. Each stroke survivor seemed to have a unique, perplexing set of problems, and doctors found recovery equally unpredictable.

Research into brain function after a stroke has shed new light on the way the brain works. Many strokes are caused when blood flow to the brain is cut off by a blood clot or haemorrhage. The oxygen-deprived brain cells rupture and die. Neuroscientists once believed that the cells died from lack of oxygen. However, their conclusion did not explain why stroke survivors sometimes got worse over a period of several hours.

The oxygen-deprived brain cells actually start an avalanche of death when they rupture. The ruptured cells release huge quantities of the amino acid glutamate that gushes into surviving brain cells and destroys them. Normally, small amounts of glutamate act as transmitters between the cells, but large amounts are extremely damaging.

Researchers are developing several drugs to try to block the amino acid avalanche after a stroke, including the use of drugs which have been used following a heart attack. Streptokinase is used to dissolve clots in the bloodstream and shows good potential use for stroke victims whose symptoms are produced by a blood clot in the brain. In the future the safe and effective use of such drugs may become more common. Unfortunately, a stroke resulting from a burst blood vessel will be made worse by streptokinase, which is why a CAT scan is performed before the drug is administered.

Strokes still present many mysteries, but with thousands of Australians surviving strokes, doctors are hopeful that the drugs will eventually eliminate the long-term effects. ■

You can, however, control other risk factors. One of the most important is hypertension, or high blood pressure. Hypertension increases your risk of stroke approximately seven times. High blood pressure puts pressure on arteries and makes them more likely to burst. Often, you can control high blood pressure by losing weight, changing your diet, exercising regularly and managing stress.

Cigarette smoking is another major risk factor for a stroke. It increases blood pressure and makes blood more likely to clot.

Diets high in saturated fats and cholesterol increase your chance of a stroke by increasing the possibility of fatty materials building up on the walls of blood vessels. Keep your intake of these foods at a moderate level.

Regular exercise increases blood circulation, which develops more channels for blood flow. These provide alternate routes for blood if the primary channels become blocked.

Epilepsy and Other Seizures

When the normal functions of the brain are disrupted by injury, disease, fever or infection, the electrical activity of the brain becomes irregular. This irregularity can cause a loss of body control known as a **seizure.**

Seizures can occur in a number of conditions. A victim of a head injury, poisoning or other condition severely impairing the supply of blood or oxygen to the brain may have a seizure. Seizures in children under the age of 6 years may result from a high fever caused by any illness.

Seizures are also caused by a chronic condition known as epilepsy. About 2 per cent of the Australian population has been diagnosed as having epilepsy. Epilepsy is usually controlled with medication, although some people with epilepsy have seizures from time to time. Others who go a long time without a seizure may think the condition has gone away and stop taking their medication. These people may then have a seizure again.

Symptoms and Signs of a Seizure

Before a seizure occurs, the person may experience an aura. An aura is an unusual sensation or feeling such as a visual hallucination; a strange sound, taste, or smell; or an urgent need to get to safety. The person may have time to tell bystanders and sit down before the seizure occurs if the aura is recognised.

Seizures range from mild blackouts, which others may mistake for daydreaming, to sudden, uncontrolled muscular contractions (convulsions) lasting several minutes. Infants and young children are at risk of seizures brought on by high fever.

Care for a Seizure

Although it may be frightening to see someone unexpectedly having a seizure, you can easily help care for the person. Remember that the person cannot control the seizure and the violent muscular contractions which may occur. Follow these guidelines:

1. Do not try to stop the seizure. Do not hold or restrain the person because this could cause musculoskeletal injuries.

2. Protect the victim from injury. Move away nearby objects, such as furniture, that might cause injury. Protect the person's head by placing thin padding, such as folded clothing, beneath it.

3. Manage the airway. Position the victim on one side as soon as possible when the seizure diminishes, so that any fluid such as saliva, blood or vomit will drain from the mouth.

4. Do not try to place anything between the person's teeth. People having seizures rarely bite their tongues or cheeks with enough force to cause any significant bleeding. However, some blood may be present, so positioning the person on the side as soon as possible will help any blood drain out of the mouth.

5. After the seizure, the victim will be drowsy and disorientated and should be kept on one side until fully conscious. Carry out a secondary survey to check for any injury during the seizure.

6. Be reassuring and comforting. If the seizure occurred in public, the victim may be embarrassed and self-conscious. Ask bystanders not to crowd around the person, who will be tired and want to rest. Occasionally the person may be incontinent, so you should provide some covering for the clothing if possible.

7. Stay with the person until they are fully conscious and aware of the surroundings.

8. If the victim is known to have periodic seizures, you do not need to call an ambulance. The person will usually recover from a seizure in a few minutes.

9. Call for an ambulance if:
   - the seizure lasts more than a few minutes
   - the victim has repeated seizures
   - the victim appears to be injured
   - the victim is pregnant
   - the victim is known to have diabetes
   - the victim is an infant or child
   - the person does not have a history of previous seizures
   - the seizure takes place in water
   - the victim fails to regain consciousness after the seizure
   - you are uncertain about the cause of the seizure

Convulsions Associated with a High Temperature

Convulsions associated with a high temperature can occur in infants and children, most often between the ages of 6 months and 3 years. They are caused by a high fever from any illness, such as infections, most of which are viral. Although frightening, these seizures are seldom dangerous. They generally stop occurring by 6 years of age and do not cause long-term problems. The symptoms and signs may include the following:
- Unwell appearance.
- High fever.

RESETTING THE THERMOSTAT

In the human brain there is a heat regulating centre which operates at a certain set point to maintain body temperature (normally 36.5 to 37.5°C). This set point can become raised due to the effects of an illness and, in a child, a sudden rise in temperature can cause a convulsion.

It is an instinctive response to try to cool down a child who is hot, whatever the cause. However, cooling a child too vigorously can be counter-productive and may cause the child's temperature to rise further.

Consider the analogy of central heating in a house. If the thermostat is set on high, the heater works until that temperature is reached. If someone leaves a door open, the heater works hard to try to keep the temperature at the set level, and stops only if the thermostat is lowered.

The thermostat in the brain works similarly. No matter how much external cooling is applied, the body will work hard to keep the body temperature at the set level until the thermostat is lowered. Sponging a child with cool water or fanning the skin acts like an open door, and the body will work hard to keep the temperature at the set level.

Paracetamol acts to "turn down the thermostat" by lowering the set point in the brain, thus allowing the body to cool down. Once the thermostat has been reset to a lower level, about an hour after paracetamol has been given, the child can then be sponged if the skin still feels hot. This helps the body temperature to come down. Remember, never let the child shiver, as shivering is one of the body's ways of raising the temperature.

Note: This principle of not trying to lower the temperature quickly applies only to children with fever. As you will learn in Chapter 11, an adult or older child suffering from a life-threatening heat illness such as heat stroke needs the body temperature brought down quickly. ■

- Hot, flushed, sweating skin.
- Eyes rolling up or squinting.
- Stiffness of the body with arched spine.
- Twitching of the face or jerking of the limbs.
- Congestion of the face and neck.
- Saliva frothing from the mouth.

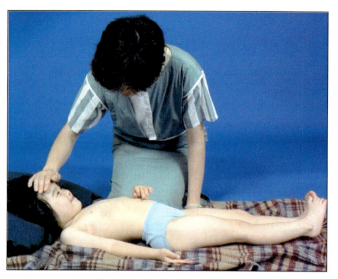

FIGURE 9-14 *Reduce fever by undressing the child to minimal clothing and giving paracetamol as directed.*

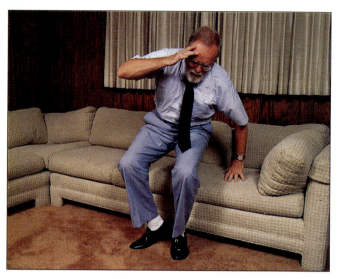

FIGURE 9-15 *A sudden change in position can sometimes trigger fainting.*

To provide care, follow the same guidelines as for seizures in adults. Position the child on the side, care for the airway and protect the child from injury. In addition:

1. Undress the child to minimal clothing to help bring down body temperature (Figure 9-14).

2. Do not let the child become chilled.

3. You do not need to rush the child to a hospital as the convulsions will stop as soon as the body temperature is lowered. Once the convulsions have stopped, call the doctor regarding treatment of the illness causing the high fever. You may be advised to give paracetamol to help bring the temperature down. Call for an ambulance if the convulsions do not stop when the temperature is lowered.

 4 *Will a child be obviously unwell before a convulsion associated with a fever?*

Fainting

One of the most common sudden illnesses is fainting. Fainting is a partial or complete loss of consciousness. It is caused by a temporary reduction of blood flow to the brain, such as when blood pools in the legs and lower body, reducing blood flow to the head. When the brain is suddenly deprived of its normal blood flow, it momentarily shuts down and the person faints.

Fainting can be triggered by an emotional shock such as the sight of blood. It may be caused by pain, by specific medical conditions such as heart disease, by standing for long periods of time, or by over-exertion.

Some people, such as pregnant women or the elderly, are more likely to faint when suddenly changing positions, such as moving from sitting or lying to standing up (Figure 9-15). Fainting may occur any time there is a change inside the body which momentarily reduces the blood flow to the brain.

Symptoms and Signs of Fainting

Fainting may occur with or without warning. The following symptoms and signs may occur:

* Feeling light-headed or dizzy.

* The signs of shock, such as pale, cool, moist skin.

* Nausea.

* Numbness or tingling in the fingers and toes.

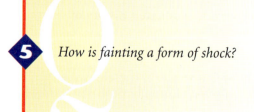 **5** *How is fainting a form of shock?*

Care for Fainting

Usually, fainting resolves itself. When the victim collapses, normal circulation to the brain resumes. The victim usually regains consciousness within a minute.

Fainting itself does not usually harm the victim, but injury may occur from falling. Follow these guidelines for care:

1. If you can reach the person who is starting to collapse, assist the person to the ground or other flat surface.

2. If the victim is responding, leave the person lying flat. Check the ABC. If unconscious, place the

victim on the side and follow the Basic Life Support flow chart (see page 35).

3. If possible, raise the legs 20 to 30 cm (Figure 9-16).

4. Loosen any restrictive clothing at waist or neck, such as a belt, tie or collar.

5. Do not give the victim anything to eat or drink.

Usually the victim of fainting recovers quickly with no lasting effects. However, because you cannot determine whether the fainting is linked to a more serious condition, the victim should seek medical attention.

6 *Why do people who have fainted regain consciousness after collapsing to the ground?*

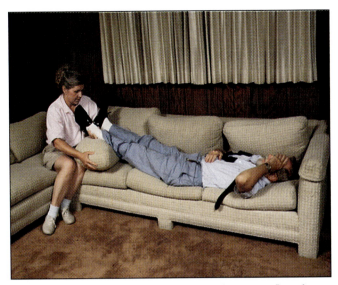

FIGURE 9-16 *To care for fainting, place the victim flat, elevate the feet and loosen any restrictive clothing such as a belt, tie or collar.*

Summary

- Determine the victim's conscious state by the "shake and shout" method.

- Care for the unconscious victim includes positioning on the side, monitoring the ABC, and additional care for any bleeding, wounds or other conditions.

- For head injuries causing an altered conscious state, first give the general care for an unconscious victim and then provide additional first aid for concussion, cerebral compression or skull fracture.

- Head injuries can be prevented by using safety equipment, safeguarding against falls, following sports safety precautions and avoiding the use of unnecessary drugs.

- For a diabetic emergency, care includes giving sugar to a conscious victim, or caring for an unconscious victim by following the general guidelines.

- Care for a stroke victim includes helping a conscious victim to rest without taking any food or drink, or caring for an unconscious victim by following the general guidelines.

- The risk of a stroke can be reduced by controlling blood pressure, losing weight, increasing exercise and by not smoking.

- Care of a victim having a seizure includes protecting the person from injury, positioning the victim to maintain the airway and care after the seizure.

- First aid for an infant or child having a convulsion caused by fever includes steps to quickly lower body temperature.

- Care for a person who faints includes protecting the person during the collapse, positioning the person while unconscious and monitoring the ABC.

Answers to Application Questions

1. Both are important, but maintaining an open airway is more important. A person who is not breathing will quickly die, at which point other injuries cease to be important. It is highly unlikely that you would cause further damage by carefully turning the victim onto one side and clearing and opening the airway.

2. Stroke causes damage to brain tissues by disrupting blood flow and, therefore, delivery of oxygen to the brain. Without oxygen, cells die—the brain is no exception.

3. You cannot tell the extent of damage suffered by the victim of a suspected stroke or TIA. Damage that limits the victim's ability to eat and drink may have occurred.

4. No. About 30 per cent of convulsions due to fever occur when the parent or guardian is unaware that the child has a fever. The convulsions often occur with the sudden rise in the child's temperature, before anyone notices a problem. It is thought to be the rise in temperature which causes the convulsion, rather than the level the temperature reaches.

5. Fainting is a form of shock because it involves the failure of the circulatory system to adequately circulate blood to all parts of the body.

6. When people collapse after fainting, the body no longer works against gravity to pump blood to the brain. When the body is flat, blood that has pooled in the legs and trunk can more readily return to the heart. Normal blood flow to the brain resumes and consciousness returns.

Study Questions

1. *Match each term with the correct definition.*

    a. Diabetes.
    b. Epilepsy.
    c. Fainting.
    d. Hyperglycaemia.
    e. Hypoglycaemia.
    f. Insulin.
    g. Seizure.
    h. Stroke.

    _____ A hormone that enables the body to use sugar.
    _____ A temporary reduction of blood to the brain, resulting in loss of consciousness.
    _____ A disruption of blood flow to the brain that causes brain tissue damage.
    _____ An interruption of the brain's electrical activity, causing loss of consciousness and body control.
    _____ A condition in which there is too little sugar in the bloodstream.
    _____ A condition in which the body cannot produce or adequately use insulin.
    _____ A condition in which there is too much sugar in the bloodstream.
    _____ A chronic condition characterised by seizures and usually controlled by medication.

2. *List the steps of general care for the unconscious victim.*

3. *Which of the following is not a level of consciousness?*
    a. Unconscious.
    b. Conscious.
    c. Hysteria.
    d. Semi-conscious.

4. *List at least five ways to prevent head and spine injuries.*

5. *Pressure on the brain caused by bleeding inside the skull can cause:*
    a. damage to brain tissue
    b. breathing problems
    c. cardiac problems.
    d. All of the above.
    e. None of the above.

6. *If you think the victim may have a skull fracture, you should:*
    a. put direct pressure on the wound to stop bleeding
    b. squeeze the nostrils shut to stop any fluid leaking out
    c. give CPR immediately
    d. position the victim sitting halfway up with head supported.

7. *List at least three instances in which you should call an ambulance for a seizure victim.*

8. *If you were caring for someone who looked pale, was unconscious and was breathing irregularly, what would you do?*
   a. Call an ambulance.
   b. Maintain body temperature and monitor the ABC.
   c. Give sugar to the victim.
   d. Tell the victim to call the doctor.
   e. a and b.

9. *Your father has diabetes. He also suffered a stroke a year ago. You find him lying on the floor unconscious. What should you do?*
   a. Phone his doctor for urgent advice.
   b. Lift up his head and try to give him a sugary drink.
   c. Place him on the side, monitor his ABC and call for an ambulance.
   d. Inject him with insulin yourself and then call an ambulance.

10. *In caring for the victim of a seizure, you should:*
   a. move any objects that might cause injury
   b. try to hold the person still
   c. place a spoon between the person's teeth
   d. splash the person with water
   e. try to keep the person upright.

11. *To manage the airway of a seizure victim:*
   a. Place an object between the victim's teeth
   b. Position the victim on the side as soon as possible
   c. Place a thick object, such as a rolled blanket, under the victim's head
   d. Move the victim into a sitting position.
   e. a and b.

12. *At the office, your boss complains that he has had a severe headache for several hours. His speech suddenly becomes slurred. He loses his balance and falls to the floor. What would you do?*
   a. Give him two Aspirin tablets.
   b. Help him find and take his high blood pressure medication.
   c. Suggest he go home.
   d. Call for an ambulance.
   e. Tell him to rest for a while.

Answers are in Appendix A (page 361).

Poisoning, Bites and Stings

POISONING takes the lives of many Australians every year. Many substances in our environment are poisonous, and you can accidentally come into contact with them in many different ways. Poisons can enter the body by being ingested, inhaled, absorbed or injected. Poisons may have severe effects, and knowing what first aid to give in cases of poisoning can help save a life.

This chapter outlines how to recognise poisoning and what care to give.

For Review

A review of the information on the lymphatic system (Chapter 2) and breathing emergencies (Chapter 7) will help your understanding of the chapter.

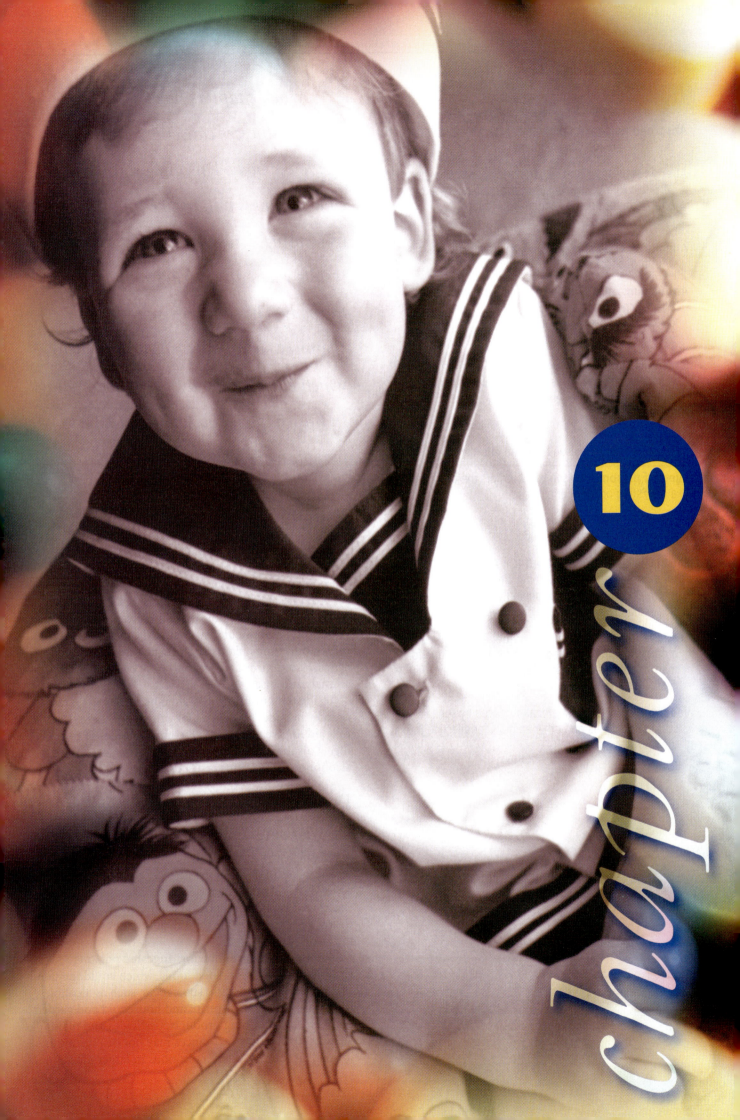

chapter

10

Key Terms

Absorbed poison: A poison that enters the body through the skin or mucous membranes.

Allergy: A disorder in which the body becomes over-sensitive to a particular substance; different allergies affect different tissues and may have local or general effects.

Anaphylaxis *(a-naf-il-ak-sis)*: A severe allergic reaction; a form of shock.

Antivenom: An antiserum containing antibodies against specific poisons in the venom of snakes, spiders or scorpions; used in treatment of bites or stings (formerly known as antivenene).

Envenomation *(en-ven-om-ay-shon)*: The injection of venom by a snake, spider or other animal to kill or immobilise its prey or enemy.

Ingested poison: A poison that is swallowed.

Inhaled poison: A poison breathed into the lungs.

Injected poison: A poison which enters the body through a bite, sting or hypodermic needle.

Poison: Any substance that causes injury, illness or death when introduced into the body.

Poisons Information Centre (PIC): A specialised reference centre in each capital city which provides information in cases of poisoning or suspected poisoning emergencies.

Pressure immobilisation technique: Application of a pressure bandage, used as a first aid technique for many bites and stings; it delays venom entering the circulation through the lymphatic system.

Venom: The poisonous material produced by snakes, scorpions, spiders and other animals for injecting into their prey or enemies.

Previous chapters have described sudden illnesses caused by conditions inside the body. Poisoning can also be a sudden illness but, unlike conditions such as fainting, stroke or epilepsy, poisoning results when an external substance enters the body. The substance may be a chemical, or it may be a germ or virus which enters the body via a bite or sting. In this chapter, you will learn how to recognise and care for poisoning.

Accidental poisonings in Australia have declined in recent years as a result of public education, child-resistant packaging of medicines and household products, and the work of Poisons Information Centres. Yet such poisonings remain a concern, and people still die or suffer injury and disability from such incidents.

Deaths occur from poisoning by solvents and house-hold products, agricultural chemicals, motor vehicle fumes, poisonous plants and other causes. Poisoning can also result from the injection of venom from some animals and insects.

Accidental poisoning can often be prevented. This chapter includes guidelines for prevention as well as the first aid to give victims of all common types of poisonings. Poisoning related to the abuse or misuse of drugs, alcohol or medications is discussed in Chapter 19.

POISONING

How Poisons Enter the Body

A **poison** is any substance which causes injury or illness when introduced into the body. Some poisons can cause death. Poisons include solids, liquids and fumes (gases and vapours). A poison can enter the body in four ways: ingestion, inhalation, absorption and injection (Figure 10-1).

Ingestion means swallowing. **Ingested poisons** include some contaminated foods, which could include mushrooms and shellfish; substances, such as alcohol; medications, such as aspirin; and household and garden items, such as cleaning products, pesticides and plants (Figure 10-2). Many substances may not be poisonous in small amounts but are poisonous in larger amounts.

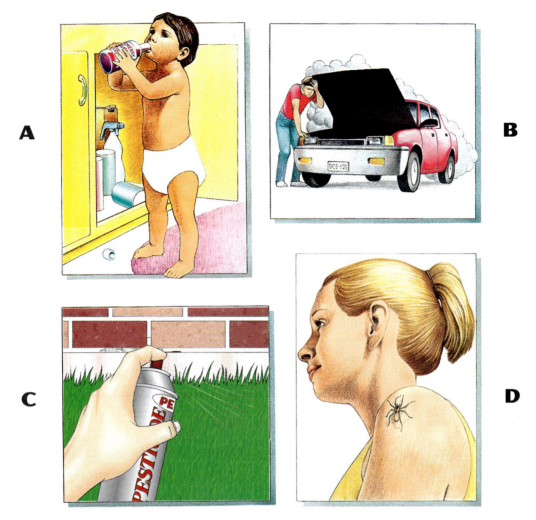

FIGURE 10-1 *A poison can enter the body by:* **A** *ingestion,* **B** *inhalation,* **C** *absorption and* **D** *injection.*

Poisoning by inhalation occurs when a person breathes in toxic fumes. **Inhaled poisons** include:

- Gases, such as carbon monoxide, from an engine or other combustion.

- Gases, such as carbon dioxide, which can occur naturally from decomposition.

- Gases, such as nitrous oxide, used for medical reasons.

- Gases, such as chlorine, found in commercial swimming pools.

- Fumes from household products, such as glues, paints and petrol.

- Fumes from drugs, such as cocaine.

- Other odourless fumes.

An **absorbed poison** enters the body after it comes into contact with the skin, mucous membranes and other body surfaces. Absorbed poisons come from chemicals and some plants such as stinging nettles and the rhus tree, as well as from fertilisers and pesticides used in lawn and plant care and many other substances.

Injected poisons enter the body through the bites or stings of insects, spiders, ticks, animals and snakes, or in the form of drugs or medications injected with a hypodermic needle and other sharp objects.

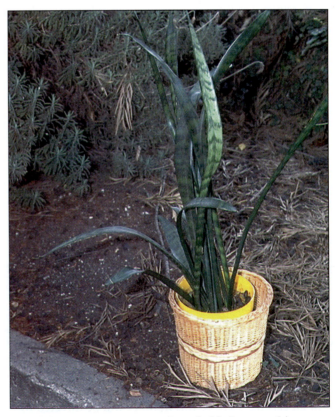

FIGURE 10-2 *Many common household plants, such as mother-in-law's tongue, are poisonous.*

Symptoms and Signs of Poisoning

The most important thing is to *recognise that a poisoning may have occurred.* As with other serious emergencies, such as a heart attack, shock or a head and spine injury, evaluate the scene, the condition of the victim and any information from the victim or bystanders. If you then have even a slight suspicion that the victim has been poisoned, seek medical assistance immediately.

As you approach the victim, survey the scene. Be aware of any unusual odours, flames, smoke, open or spilled containers, an open medicine cabinet, an overturned or damaged plant or other symptoms or signs of possible poisoning. Remember that the substance may be an odourless gas.

When you reach the victim, do a primary survey, then a secondary survey if the victim has no life-threatening conditions. The victim of poisoning generally looks ill and displays symptoms and signs common to other sudden illnesses. The symptoms and signs of poisoning can include nausea, vomiting, diarrhoea, chest or abdominal pain, breathing difficulty, sweating, altered conscious state and seizures.

Other signs of poisoning can be burn injuries around the lips or tongue, or on the skin. You may also suspect a poisoning based on any information you have from or about the victim. Look also for any drug paraphernalia or empty containers (see also Chapter 19).

If you suspect a poisoning, try to get answers to the following questions:

- What type of poison was taken?
- How much was taken?
- When was it taken?

This information will help you provide the most appropriate care.

Poisons Information Centres

A poisoning is sometimes a unique problem for the first aider as well as for the responding ambulance personnel. The severity of the poisoning depends on the type and amount of the substance, how it entered the body and the victim's size, weight and age. Some poisons act fast and have characteristic signs. Others act slowly and cannot be easily identified. Sometimes you will be able to identify the specific poison, sometimes not.

To help people deal with poisonings, a network of **Poisons Information Centres** (PICs) exists throughout Australia, located in the emergency departments of large hospitals. Medical professionals in these centres have access to a central computer holding information about virtually all poisonous substances. They will tell you how to help the poison victim. You should have the PIC number by your phone. During early 1995, a single national phone number—13 11 26—is being phased in for all centres. Calls to this number will be directed to the local PIC, and after hours to the nearest staffed centre.

If the scene is safe and the victim is conscious, call 13 11 26 first. The PIC will tell you what care to give and whether ambulance personnel are needed.

If the victim is unconscious, or if you do not know the PIC number, call your local emergency number.

1 *Why should you call the Poisons Information Centre for advice immediately when you suspect someone has been poisoned?*

FIRST AID FOR POISONING

Follow these general principles for any poisoning emergency:

1. Survey the scene to make sure it is safe to approach and to gather clues about what happened.
2. If necessary, remove the victim from the source of the poison if it is safe to do so.
3. Do a primary survey to assess the victim's airway, breathing and circulation.
4. Care for any life-threatening conditions.
5. If the victim is conscious, do a secondary survey to gather additional information.
6. Look for any containers and take them to the telephone.
7. Call your PIC or emergency number.
8. Follow the directions of the PIC or the emergency operator.

Do not give the victim anything to drink or eat unless advised to do so by medical professionals. If the poison is unknown and the victim vomits, save some of the vomit, which the hospital may analyse to identify the poison.

Ingested Poisons

Besides following the general principles for any poisoning, you may also need to provide additional care for specific types of ingested poisons. Generally these fall into two distinct categories: corrosive or non-corrosive poisons.

Non-Corrosive Poisons

The Poisons Information Centre may instruct you to induce vomiting if:

- the poison is not corrosive or petrol-based
- the victim is conscious
- the poison was ingested in the last 30 minutes

CASE STUDY

A hungry 22-year-old man, bushwalking with friends, ate some small mushrooms with pale stems when the party stopped for a rest. Within 8 hours he suffered stomach pain followed by vomiting and diarrhoea. By the time help was obtained, his conscious state had deteriorated, and he was transported to the nearest medical facility. After 2 days he became jaundiced and comatose and finally died. The autopsy revealed poisoning from the death cap mushroom. ■

For many years syrup of ipecac has been used to induce vomiting for poisonings in or around the home. However, syrup of ipecac must be used with caution because it can react badly with some poisons, and can have a 20-minute time delay or longer before it acts. In some centres, syrup of ipecac is still recommended for remote areas where there may be some delay before the victim obtains medical aid. *Do not give syrup of ipecac unless instructed to do so by the Poisons Information Centre or another medical adviser as it can have adverse effects.*

Follow the advice of the PIC or other medical professionals before diluting poisons taken in capsule or tablet form in case it is not the best treatment.

Hospitals and medical services may use activated charcoal to assist in absorbing ingested poisons, thereby reducing their effects by prevention of absorption. However, activated charcoal is not recommended as a part of first aid treatment.

There are some instances when vomiting *should not* be induced. These include when the victim:

- is unconscious
- is having a seizure
- is pregnant
- has no gag reflex
- is known to have heart disease
- has ingested a corrosive substance (an acid or alkali), a petroleum product (such as kerosene or petrol) or a substance which causes vomiting or convulsions or other nervous system stimulation

Corrosive Poisons

Corrosive chemicals such as acids or alkalies damage or destroy tissues. Vomiting these corrosives could burn the oesophagus, throat and mouth. Diluting the corrosive substances by giving the victim small amounts of milk or water to drink decreases the potential for tissue damage. The fumes from petroleum products such as kerosene or petrol may also damage delicate lung tissue if vomiting occurs. Always contact the Poisons Information Centre for further advice.

Remember:

What burns going down will burn again coming up.

Inhaled Poisons

Toxic fumes come from a variety of sources. They may have an odour or be odour free. Carbon dioxide, for example, is an inhaled poison which comes from many sources such as decomposing organic matter; methane may be found at the bottom of wells or in mines and sewers. Fumes from certain industrial and home spray chemicals are also toxic if inhaled.

Another inhaled poison is carbon monoxide (CO). It is present in car exhaust and can be produced by defective cooking equipment and fires. A pale or bluish skin colour that indicates a lack of oxygen may indicate carbon monoxide poisoning. For years, people were taught that carbon monoxide poisoning was indicated by a cherry-red colour of the skin and lips. This, however, is a poor *initial indicator* of carbon monoxide poisoning. The red colour occurs later, usually just before or after death. Do not use skin colour as an indicator of the seriousness of the poisoning.

All victims of inhaled poison need oxygen as soon as possible. First and foremost, however, remember the emergency action principles. Survey the scene to determine if it is safe for you to help. If you can remove the person from the source of the poison without endangering your own life, then do so. Sometimes all you need to do is help a conscious victim into fresh air and then call an ambulance. Remove an unconscious victim from the contaminated environment, maintain an open airway and call an ambulance. If the person is not breathing, give expired air resuscitation (EAR) and call an ambulance. There is no risk to the first aider giving EAR to a victim of carbon monoxide poisoning when it is performed where there is fresh air.

CASE STUDY

An 8-year-old girl travelling in an old car was found unconscious and not breathing on the back seat. Her 18-year-old sister, seated in the front seat, had checked her about 15 minutes earlier and believed she was sleeping. EAR was performed while the driver sped to a hospital, but on arrival the girl was in cardiac arrest. Advanced life support measures were unsuccessful and she had repeated cardiac arrests during treatment. Eleven hours after the incident occurred, she was pronounced dead. The autopsy confirmed that death was due to poisoning by carbon monoxide from engine fumes and inadequate ventilation. ■

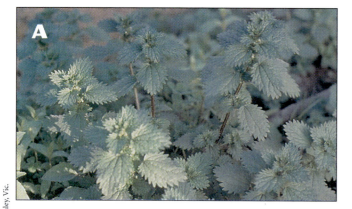

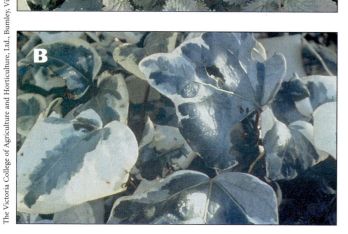

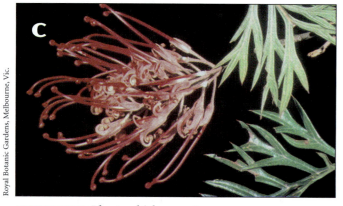

The Victoria College of Agriculture and Horticulture, Ltd., Burnley, Vic.

Royal Botanic Gardens, Melbourne, Vic.

FIGURE 10-3 *Plants which are poisonous on contact.*
A *Stinging nettle.* **B** *English ivy* **C** *Grevillea 'Robyn Gordon'.*

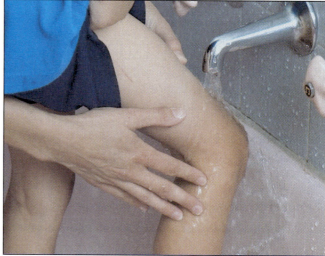

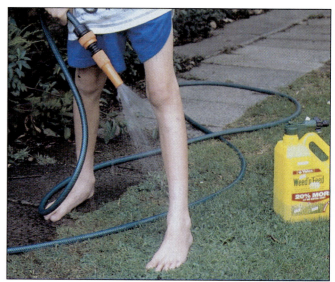

FIGURE 10-4 *Whenever chemical poisons come into contact with the skin or eyes, flush the affected area continuously with large amounts of water.*

Absorbed Poisons

People often have contact with poisonous substances which can be absorbed through the skin. Poisons absorbed through the skin include dry and wet chemicals, such as those used in yard and garden maintenance, industrial chemicals and plants (Figure 10-3).

To care for the person who has been in contact with a poison, follow these steps:

1. Immediately wash the affected area thoroughly with copious amounts of water (Figure 10-4).

2. Call the Poisons Information Centre or emergency number for advice.

3. Continue to flush the area until ambulance personnel arrive.

4. If running water is not available, brush off dry chemicals, such as lime. Take care that no one at the scene is affected.

Some dry chemicals such as dishwasher crystals are made more toxic by contact with water. But if continuous running water is available, it will flush the chemical from the skin before it can cause too much damage. Running water reduces the threat to you and quickly helps remove the substance from the victim.

Never apply lotions or other medications to the skin without contacting a Poisons Information Centre or a doctor first since they may cause further damage. If the condition becomes worse and large areas of the body or the face are affected, the person should see a doctor immediately.

Injected Poisons

Insect and animal stings and bites are among the most common sources of injected poisons. Due to lack of space, it is not possible to consider all possible types of stings and bites that could result in poisoning. The following sections describe the care for common bites and stings of snakes, marine animals, spiders and other venomous creatures. These bites and stings can be serious when they involve **envenomation**, the natural process of the creature's injection of **venom** to kill or immobilise its prey or enemy.

Pressure Immobilisation Technique

The most common method of treating many bites and stings is the **pressure immobilisation technique.** Originally introduced for snake bites, this method is also used for some other kinds of bites and stings. It is particularly important for those who have allergic reactions to injected venoms.

This method is effective because the pressure of the bandage over the bite area slows the rate at which venom enters the circulation. The toxic effects of the poison are therefore reduced, and some venom also becomes inactive when it is trapped in body tissues.

This method should not be used for bites and stings of red-back spiders, bees, wasps, ants, ticks, and venomous fish spine stings unless the victim has a known **allergy** *to the venom.*

The Practice Guide beginning on page 178 gives the detailed steps for applying a pressure immobilisation bandage. Following are key points of this technique:

1. Apply firm pressure over the bite site, using your hand if necessary.

2. Apply a crepe roller bandage to maintain pressure over the area of the bite.

3. For a bite on the leg or arm, use a second crepe roller bandage starting at the toes or fingertips and working upwards to cover as much of the limb as you can. Apply the bandage as tightly as you would for a sprained ankle but not so tightly as to cut off circulation below the bandage.

4. Immobilise the affected limb with a splint to reduce muscle movement. Help the victim to rest if possible and do not let the victim stand or walk. Bring transport to the victim, unless this will cause a delay of 2 hours or more.

5. Do not remove the bandages until the victim has reached medical care and then only if you are instructed to do so.

6. If the bandage is applied too tightly, circulation may be cut off below it. Signs of impaired circulation are discolouration of the fingers or toes below the bandage or the victim complains of sensations of coldness or numbness. If any of these symptoms or signs occur, loosen the bandage sufficiently to let blood flow return.

2 *If the pressure immobilisation technique works by limiting the spread of venom through the body, why is it not used in some types of bites and stings?*

Most bites occur on a lower limb, usually around the ankle. For bites on the head or trunk, do not try to use the pressure immobilisation technique but help the victim to rest completely until medical assistance is obtained.

Snake Bites

Australia is home to many of the most poisonous snakes in the world (see box on pages 164–165). The venoms of different poisonous snakes have different effects on various parts of the body, including the heart, blood and body tissues. The most serious common effect is paralysis of the breathing muscles which can lead to death. Only an expert can identify all snakes and know for certain whether a bite is from a poisonous snake. All snake bites should be treated as potentially lethal and immediate medical attention should be sought. Colour identification of a snake is most unreliable because many species change colour as the snake matures. It can be helpful if the snake is killed and brought for identification, but you should NEVER endanger yourself to do so. Many major hospitals have a "Venom Detection Kit" which assists in the precise identification of venom left at the bite site on the victim's skin (Figure 10-5).

Symptoms and signs of poisonous snake bites may appear either quickly or over the course of many hours. They include:

- paired or single fang marks in the skin
- nausea, vomiting
- headache
- altered conscious state
- double vision or blurred vision
- problems with speaking and/or swallowing
- weakness in extremities and/or paralysis
- respiratory distress or cardiac arrest
- clotting defects

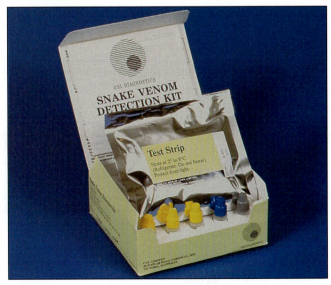

FIGURE 10-5 *A venom detection kit is used in major hospitals to identify venom following a snake bite.*

THE MOST VENOMOUS

- Australian copperhead (*Austrelaps superbus*)
- Beaked sea snake (*Enhydrina schistosa*)
- Black mamba (*Dendroaspis polylepis*)*
- Blue-bellied black snake (*Pseudechis guttatus*)
- Brown snake (*Pseudonaja textilis*)
- Chappell Island tiger snake (*Notechis ater serventyi*)
- Collett's snake (*Pseudechis colletti*)
- Death adder (*Acanthophis antarcticus*)
- Dugite (*Pseudonaja affinis*)
- Eastern diamond-back rattlesnake (*Crotalus adamananteus*)*
- Gwardar (*Pseudonaja nuchalis*)
- Indian cobra (*Naja naja*)*
- King brown, or Mulga snake (*Pseudechis australis*)
- King cobra (*Ophiophagus hannah*)*

- Papuan black snake (*Pseudechis papuanus*)
- Reevesby Island tiger snake (*Notechis ater niger*)
- Red-bellied black snake (*Pseudechis porphyriacus*)
- Rough-scaled snake (*Tropidechis carinatus*)
- Small-eyed snake (*Cryptophis nigrescens*)
- Spotted snake (*Demansia olivacea*)
- Taipan (*Oxyuranus scutellatus*)
- Tiger snake (*Notechis scutatus*)
- Western Australian tiger snake (*Notechis ater occidentalis*)
- Western Taipan, or small-scaled snake (*Oxyuranus microleidotus*)
- Yellow-banded snake (*Hoplocephalus stephensii*)

*Not native to Australia. ∎

Eastern Brown Snake   ### Highlands Copperhead

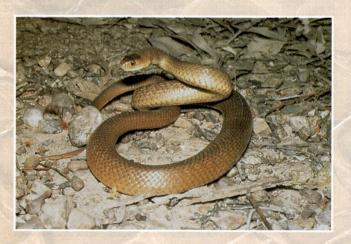

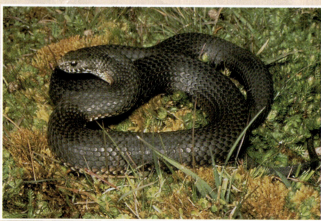

SNAKES IN THE WORLD

Red-Bellied Black Snake

Tiger Snake

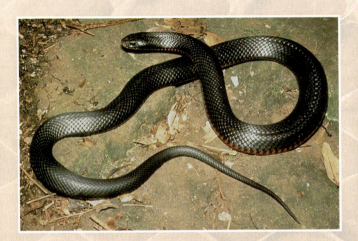

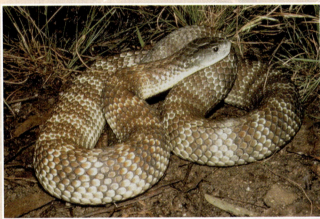

Taipan

Common Death Adder

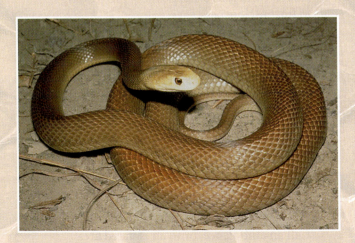

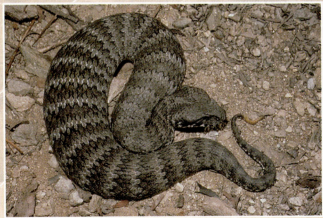

Indicates areas where snakes are found

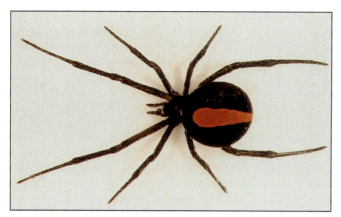

FIGURE 10-6 *The red-back spider.*

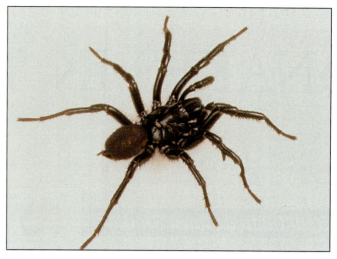

FIGURE 10-7 *The funnel-web spider.*

To give first aid for snake bite follow these guidelines:

1. Use the pressure immobilisation technique for a bite on a limb.

2. Continually monitor the ABC and be prepared to give EAR or CPR if needed.

3. Keep the victim calm, reassured and at total rest.

4. Call an ambulance, or in an isolated area transport the victim to a medical facility immediately. Anti-venom is available for most poisonous snake bites.

5. *Do not* cut the bite to try to drain the venom, *do not* suck or wash the bite, and *do not* apply a tourniquet.

Spider Bites

Red-back spider

The red-back spider has a body length of about 1 cm with a red or orange stripe on the back (Figure 10-6). The venom can be life-threatening for small children or animals.

Symptoms and signs of a red-back spider bite may include:

- pain at the site that spreads to a red, swollen, sweating, hot area

- nausea, vomiting and stomach pain

- heavy sweating

- swollen glands in the armpits or groin area

- pain away from the bite site, for example, on the opposite limb

To give first aid for a red-back spider bite:

1. use an ice pack on the area to lessen the pain

2. continually observe the victim and monitor the ABC

3. call an ambulance immediately, or in an isolated area transport the victim to a medical facility immediately

Do not use the pressure immobilisation technique with this bite because the venom spreads slowly and pressure may increase the pain.

The funnel-web spider

There are many species of funnel-web spider in Australia, but the Sydney funnel-web *(Atrax robustus)* is probably the most dangerous one, being responsible for several deaths. Their webs are rarely seen because they are built underground.

The funnel-web has a large body 3 cm long and, together with its legs, it can cover an adult hand (Figure 10-7). The funnel-web spider is very aggressive and will rise up into a striking position before attacking the prey. Consider a bite from any large, dark-coloured spider to be dangerous regardless of whether it is known to be a funnel-web spider. Give appropriate first aid care immediately.

The symptoms and signs of a funnel-web spider bite include:

- pain, but little other reaction in the bite area

- heavy sweating

- heavy production of saliva; tingling about the mouth

- stomach pain

- altered conscious state, possibly progressing to unconsciousness

- twitching of muscles

- respiratory distress, possibly leading to respiratory arrest

To give first aid for funnel-web spider bites follow these guidelines:

1. Use the pressure immobilisation technique over the bite area if the bite is on a limb.

2. Continually monitor the ABC and be prepared to give EAR or CPR if needed.

3. Keep the victim calm, reassured and at rest.

4. Call an ambulance, or in an isolated area transport the victim to a medical facility immediately.

SPIDERS AND SNAKES

Australian spiders and snakes are among the most lethal in the world. The brown snake genus *(Pseudonaja)* is Australia's most dangerous group of snakes because their venom may cause sudden, unexpected unconsciousness and death.

In years gone by, the treatment for spider and snake bites included cutting through the bite, sucking out the venom and attempting to stop the spread of the venom with a tourniquet. More recently, however, researchers have studied how snake and other venoms spread through the body and have shown that the spread of venom depends on its absorption through the lymphatic system rather than its path directly into the bloodstream.

This research led to the development of the pressure immobilisation technique to slow the spread of venom in the body. Pressure on the bitten area combined with immobilisation of the limb effectively delays the spread of the venom long enough for the victim to reach medical aid and receive **anti-venom.** It is also thought that some venoms become inactive when confined to the area of the bite.

Avoiding the bite or sting by sensible behaviour is still the best approach to poisonous snakes and insects, because death can still occur even with the best medical care. ■

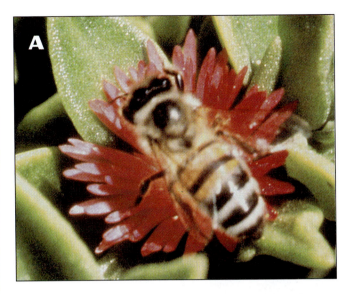

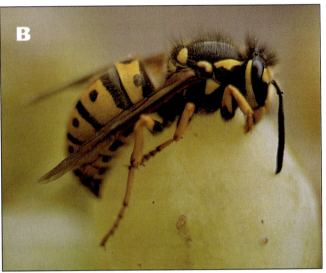

FIGURE 10-8 A *Honey bee.* **B** *European wasp.*

Insect Bites and Stings

Although insect bites and stings are painful, they are rarely fatal. Most insect bites and stings are dangerous only for those who have an allergic reaction, which is more common from bee and European wasp stings. Allergic reactions can occur almost immediately, with a sting in or around the mouth being more serious because the airway may become obstructed by tissue swelling. Australian scorpion stings and ant bites are rarely life-threatening but can cause considerable pain.

Symptoms and signs of insect bites and stings include:

- Pain at the site.
- Swelling and redness around the site.
- Allergic reactions, including itching, rash, swollen eyelids, respiratory distress, altered conscious state.

First aid for an insect bite or sting includes:

1. Use the pressure immobilisation technique immediately if an allergic reaction occurs or the victim is known to be allergic. Call an ambulance or transport the victim to a medical facility without delay.

2. Apply an ice pack or compress to the bite site for pain relief.

3. Monitor the victim's ABC and give EAR or CPR if needed.

Honey bees and European wasps

A sting from a honey bee or European wasp is painful but is life-threatening only in people with a known allergy (see page 172), or in cases where the sting involves the tissues of the mouth or throat.

The honey bee has a single barb to inject venom. This barb separates from the bee's body when it stings. The European wasp is capable of multiple stings and can inject a significant amount of venom (Figure 10-8).

Treatment for both types of stings follows the general principles for any insect sting. In addition, scrape off a bee's stinger sideways with your hand or fingernail, but do not pull or squeeze the venom sac attached to the stinger as this will cause more venom to be injected.

Remember:

For a bee sting, brush or scrape off the barb quickly to stop any more venom being injected

Scorpions, centipedes and bulldog ants

Bulldog ants and scorpions are found in most areas of Australia, while centipedes are less common (Figure 10-9).

Bulldog ants and scorpions inject venom through a sting in the tail and are likely to sting if disturbed or angry. Centipedes inject venom through a bite, but they rarely do so unless they are being handled.

Although the bite or sting from these creatures is painful, it is rarely serious for the victim. First aid treatment consists of applying a cold compress or ice pack over the bite for pain relief. The injured part should also be elevated and supported to assist in the prevention of swelling.

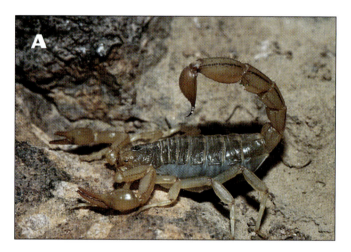

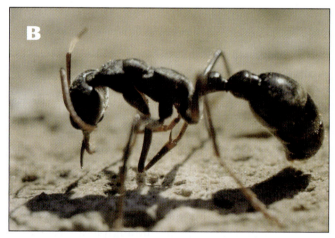

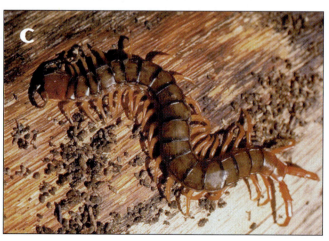

FIGURE 10-9 A *Scorpion.* **B** *Bulldog ant.* **C** *Centipede.*

Tick bites

The Australian paralysis tick, or scrub tick, has poisonous venom which can seriously affect people who are allergic to it. Ticks may attach themselves to the body in any area but typically are found in skin crevices and hairy areas. Ticks can be very small (Figure 10-10).

Symptoms and signs usually develop slowly over several days except in those who develop an allergic reaction. These symptoms and signs include:

- pain or discomfort at the area
- muscle weakness and unsteady walking
- lethargy
- double or blurred vision
- difficulty in swallowing
- difficulty in breathing

An allergic reaction rarely includes swelling around the site, respiratory distress or altered conscious state.

Ticks can also inject infective material as well as toxins. Infections may take some time to develop, for example, Lyme disease and Q fever.

To give first aid for tick bites follow these steps:

1. Remove the tick by levering it out carefully with tweezers. Slide the open blades of sharp tweezers along each side of the tick and lever it outwards. Do not squeeze or pull on the tick as even slight pressure may cause it to inject more venom.

2. Do *not* try to cut out the tick.

3. Check the victim's whole body for additional ticks, including the hair, skin creases and the ears.

4. If allergic reaction occurs or the victim is known to be allergic, use the pressure immobilisation technique immediately and call an ambulance or transport the victim to a medical facility. Anti-venom is available for tick bites.

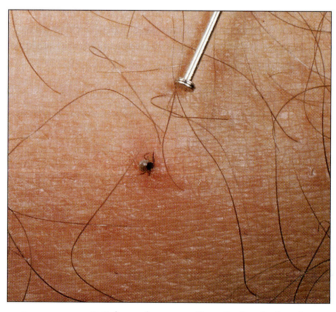

FIGURE 10-10 *A tick can be as small as the head of a pin.*

Jellyfish and Coral Stings

Jellyfish, some corals and other marine life (cnidarians) have stinging capsules, and in some species the venom can be dangerous. In tropical Australian waters these stings can be life-threatening (Figure 10-11).

Cnidarians include a wide variety of marine species. Here they are considered in two groups: cubozoans and bluebottle jellyfish and others. Some hydroids look like plants, and this group of marine life also includes corals and many types of jellyfish. Only someone well experienced with the known species in a given area can be sure whether it is safe to touch any underwater life. Therefore, prevent problems by avoiding contact with all marine life. If contact is made and a sting does occur, only an expert can know for certain the exact species causing the sting. Unless you are certain of the species, treat the sting as a cubozoan sting.

Cubozoans

There are three types of jellyfish in the cubozoan group with potentially life-threatening stings. Although the symptoms and signs of these stings vary, the first aid is the same for all three types.

The box jellyfish (*Chironex fleckeri*) is extremely dangerous to swimmers and is found north of Bundaberg on the east coast, and north of Geraldton on the west coast. The cubozoan jellyfish are square or box-like in shape, whereas other jellyfish are round or dome-shaped (Figure 10-12).

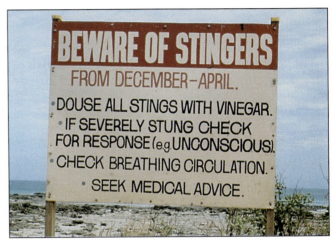

FIGURE 10-11 *A stinger warning sign on a northern beach.*

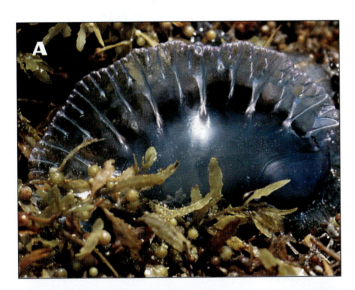

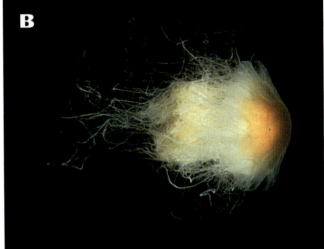

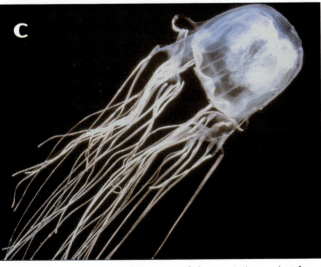

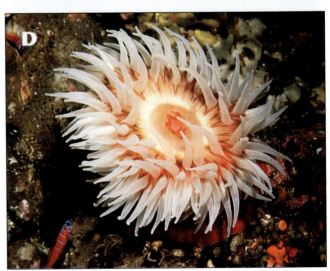

FIGURE 10-12 *The painful stings of these marine animals can cause serious problems.* **A** *Portuguese man-of-war.* **B** *Jellyfish.* **C** *Box jellyfish.* **D** *Sea anemone.*

The symptoms and signs of a **box jellyfish** sting include:

- immediate burning skin pain
- pieces of tentacles clinging to skin
- skin marked in ladder pattern by tentacle stings
- altered behaviour of victim
- respiratory or cardiac arrest in extensive stings involving an area more than 50 per cent of one limb, or its equivalent

The symptoms and signs of the **Irukandji jellyfish** sting occur after a delay of 5 to 40 minutes, and include:

- skin pain
- severe back pain and muscle cramps in chest, abdomen and extremities
- severe headache
- nausea and vomiting
- extensive sweating

The symptoms and signs of the **Jimble** and **Morbakka (Fire Jelly) jellyfish** stings include:

- pain at the sting site which may become severe
- raised red weals on skin and red patches
- rarely, symptoms similar to Irukandji

These stings are serious if the envenomation is extensive from multiple stings. To give first aid for these stings:

1. Prevent the victim from rubbing the stung area.
2. Keep the victim calm, at rest and reassured.
3. Pour vinegar over the stung area (to inactivate the stinging capsules and prevent more envenomation).
4. Use an ice pack or compress on the site to relieve pain. If pain continues after 15 minutes, apply another ice pack.
5. For the stings of Irukandji and box jellyfish, use the pressure immobilisation technique after applying vinegar.
6. Monitor the victim's ABC and call an ambulance. There is an antivenom for box jellyfish stings. Be prepared to give EAR or CPR if needed, and continue until help is available. Sometimes this may be for several hours, although there is still a chance of complete recovery.

Bluebottle jellyfish (Portuguese man-of-war) and other jellyfish, hydroids and corals

Symptoms and signs of a sting by these marine creatures may differ but often include:

- weals on the skin: often white surrounded by a red ring
- pain at the site and in lymph nodes of armpits and groin

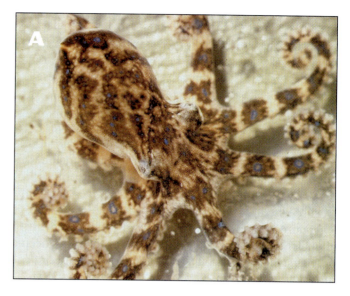

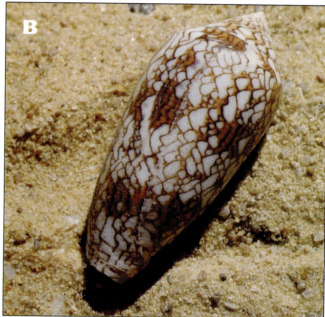

FIGURE 10-13 A *Blue-ringed octopus.* **B** *Cone shell.*

- nausea and vomiting
- headache
- breathing difficulty
- generalised muscle and back pain

These stings are serious, if the envenomation is extensive from multiple stings. To give first aid for stings in this group:

1. Prevent the victim from rubbing the stung area.
2. Keep the victim calm, at rest and reassured.
3. Use an ice pack or compress on the site to relieve pain. If pain continues after 15 minutes, apply another ice pack.
4. Monitor the ABC and call an ambulance if there are any signs of deterioration. Prepare to give EAR or CPR if needed, and continue until help arrives. Sometimes this may be for several hours, although there is still a chance of complete recovery.

Mollusc Bites

Blue-ringed octopus species are found right around the Australian coastline and have a venomous bite which can be life-threatening (Figure 10-13A). Cone shell species in Australia's tropical areas also have poisonous bites when handled or stepped on (Figure 10-13B).

The symptoms and signs of a mollusc bite include:

- relatively painless bite
- numbness of the tongue and lips
- progressive muscle weakness which can lead to respiratory arrest within 30 minutes

To give first aid for a mollusc bite:

1. Keep the victim calm, reassured and at rest.
2. Use the pressure immobilisation technique for the bite area.
3. Call an ambulance, or in isolated area transport the victim to a medical facility immediately.
4. Continually monitor the ABC and be prepared to give EAR if needed. The venom may cause the muscles of respiration to cease functioning, although the heart will continue to beat if EAR is given.

Fish Spine Stings

Stonefish, bullrouts and other fish can inject dangerous venom through their spines when they are handled or stepped on. Stingrays can give a painful sting through the spine on the tail (Figure 10-14).

The symptoms and signs of these stings include:

- severe pain
- swelling, an open wound and discolouration at the site
- panic or irrational behaviour

To give first aid for these stings:

1. If the sting involves a hand or foot, put the stung area in water that is as hot as can be tolerated by the victim. This will help to relieve pain.
2. Call an ambulance, or in an isolated area transport the victim to a medical facility immediately. There is antivenom for stonefish stings.
3. Do not use the pressure immobilisation technique.
4. Do not use ice on a stingray wound as this may prolong the pain.

Platypus Stings

The Australian platypus has poison glands on the back legs (Figure 10-15). When injected, the contents can cause excruciating pain. Although these creatures are shy and are not often seen in the wild, if encountered they should *not* be handled.

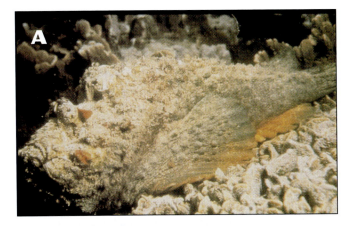

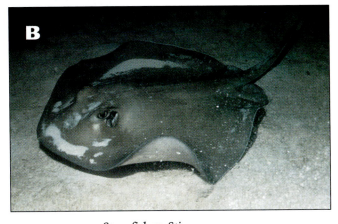

FIGURE 10-14 A *Stonefish.* **B** *Stingray.*

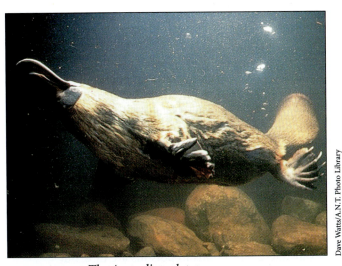

Dave Watts/A.N.T. Photo Library

FIGURE 10-15 *The Australian platypus.*

MARINE STINGER ADVISORY TELEPHONE SERVICE

A medical advisory telephone service is available to assist with information concerning any marine envenomation.

- (08) 222 5116 from within Australia
- (61-8)-224-5116 from outside Australia

Inquiries after hours will be redirected by a taped message. ■

Animal Bites

Animal bites, including the bites of humans, can be dangerous although they are not venomous. Bacteria and viruses live in all animal mouths and can be injected deep into the skin or other tissues with a bite.

The symptoms and signs of an animal bite include:

- puncture wounds or lacerations
- minor or more serious bleeding

If someone is bitten by an animal, try to rescue the victim from the animal without endangering yourself. Do not try to restrain or capture it. The goal of first aid is to prevent infection. Follow these guidelines:

1. *If the wound is minor,* wash it thoroughly with soap and water.
2. Control any bleeding.
3. Watch for later signs of infection.
4. *If the wound is bleeding seriously,* control the bleeding first. Do not try to clean the wound because it will be thoroughly cleaned at a medical facility. Seek immediate medical attention.

If possible, try to remember what the animal looked like and the area in which it was last seen. Call your local council or government emergency number. The operator will contact the appropriate authority, such as animal control or the RSPCA.

Rabies

Rabies is a potentially fatal disease which can be contracted from the bites of infected animals in many countries. Rabies affects both wild and domestic animals. It is not found in Australia, although it could be brought in by a smuggled animal. In such a case, or when bitten in another country, be sure to seek medical attention immediately. Rabies can be confirmed or ruled out by medical examination of the animal, so isolate the biting animal for the authorities if you can do so without danger to yourself.

ANAPHYLAXIS

Severe allergic reactions to poisons are rare, but when one occurs it is truly a life-threatening medical emergency. This reaction is a form of shock called **anaphylaxis.** It occurs as a result of sensitivity of the person to an insect bite or sting or by contact with drugs, medications, foods and chemicals. Anaphylaxis can result from any of the kinds of poisoning described in this chapter.

Symptoms and Signs of Anaphylaxis

Anaphylaxis usually occurs suddenly, within seconds or minutes after contact with the substance. Symptoms and signs can include:

- swelling and redness of skin or other body areas that came in contact with the substance (Figure 10-16)

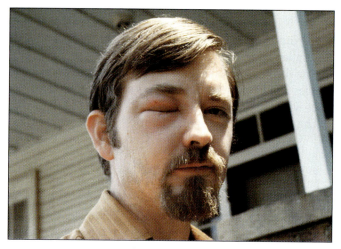

FIGURE 10-16 *In anaphylaxis, the skin usually swells and turns red.*

- hives or rash
- itching
- weakness
- nausea and vomiting
- dizziness
- breathing difficulty, coughing or wheezing— this may progress to an obstructed airway as the tongue and throat swell

Death from anaphylaxis usually occurs only when the victim's breathing is severely impaired.

Care for Anaphylaxis

If an unusual inflammation or rash is noticeable immediately after contact with a possible source, it could be an allergic reaction. Follow these guidelines for first aid:

1. Observe the person carefully because any allergic reaction can develop into anaphylaxis.
2. If the poisonous substance is on the skin, wash it off with water; if the substance has been inhaled, remove the victim from the area if it is safe to do so.
3. Assess the person's airway and breathing. If the person has any breathing difficulty or complains that their throat feels as if it is closing, call an ambulance immediately. Help the victim into the most comfortable position for breathing.
4. Monitor the ABC and offer reassurance.

People who know they are extremely allergic to certain substances usually try to avoid them, although this is sometimes impossible. These people may carry prescribed medication in the form of a tablet, puffer or injection, in case they have a severe allergic reaction.

If you think you are allergic to a substance, your doctor can arrange tests to establish your level of sensitivity. Desensitisation may be available for those proven to be allergic.

A BEE STING

Paul had been stung by a bee on two occasions while at school. The first sting was red and painful for a while but quickly subsided. The second sting two years later was more severe, with an itchy rash on his trunk, an asthma-like wheeze, a rising pulse rate and a gradually increasing swelling of his face, mouth and throat. He was at school at the time. His high school teacher recognised that he was showing signs of an allergic reaction to bee venom, so she immediately drove him to the nearest doctor for treatment. After a couple of injections he improved rapidly and was allowed to go home to recover from his ordeal.

The doctor sent Paul for an allergy blood test, and the result showed a high level of antibodies in his system, which meant that another bee sting could be fatal. He was advised to have a course of desensitisation injections over the next few months to build up his protection against bee venom. Although unhappy about the treatment, Paul agreed and started the course.

When the course finished some months later, a further blood test showed that the antibody level had returned to normal. However, Paul's doctor gave him some small tablets to carry at all times and told him to put one under his tongue if he was ever stung by a bee. Although not expecting any problems, Paul carried a couple of the tablets in a special airtight container and kept them in his car once he started work as a tree lopper.

One day Paul was cutting down a diseased gum tree from a cherry picker 30 metres above the ground. Resting between cutting branches, Paul stood with his hand on the side of the cherry picker box and suddenly felt a sharp, burning pain on the back of his hand. When he realised that it was a bee which had just stung him, he shouted down to his mates to lower the cherry picker and get his emergency medication from his car. He quickly put the tablet under his tongue and was driven at speed to a nearby clinic for emergency treatment. The tablet worked, and Paul made a rapid recovery after minor medical treatment.

He does not want to change his occupation because he loves the outdoor life. However, he now carries his medication in the form of an adrenaline puffer which he keeps with him at all times. He knows that he can take 1 to 2 puffs almost immediately if he is ever stung again, and he now feels much safer when he sees bees around a tree on which he is working. ■

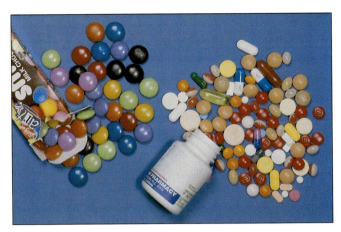

FIGURE 10-17 *To a child, poisonous medications can look like lollies.*

POISONING PREVENTION

The best approach to poisoning emergencies is to prevent them from occurring in the first place. This is a simple principle, but often people do not take enough precautions. Of all the child poisoning cases reported, the vast majority occurred when the child was under the direct supervision of a parent or guardian.

Many substances commonly found in or around the house are poisonous. Children are especially vulnerable to these because of their tendency to put everything in their mouths.

When giving medication to a child, do so carefully. Medicines are not lollies and should never be called lollies to entice a child to take them. Cough syrup looks like a soft drink to children, and many coated medicine tablets look and taste like lollies (Figure 10-17). Some children's medicine has a pleasant sweet flavour so that children will take it more easily. When giving any of these substances, make it clear to the child that this is medicine. Take care also to keep the medication out of reach and in the original container. In addition, never take medicine in front of children as they may copy your actions.

By following these general guidelines, you will be able to prevent many poisoning emergencies:

- Keep all medications and household products well out of the reach of children. Special devices are available to keep children from opening cupboards. Use these or other methods to keep children from reaching any substances which can poison them. Consider all household or pharmacy products to be potentially harmful. Specific information about safety devices can be obtained from the Child Accident Prevention Foundation of Australia office, or Children's Hospital in your capital city. The box on the next page lists some poisonous substances commonly found in or around the home.

- Use childproof safety caps on containers of medication and other potentially dangerous products.

- Keep products in their original containers with the labels in place.

SOME POISONOUS SUBSTANCES

Household products and medications

- Acids
- Ammonia
- Aspirin
- Bleach
- Cosmetics
- Dishwasher detergent
- Drain cleaner
- Heating fuel
- Iodine
- Kerosene
- Lighter fluid
- Mineral turpentine
- Paint
- Petrol
- Rat poison
- Rust remover
- Strong detergents
- Toilet bowl cleaners
- Weed killers

Plants

- Arum lily
- Castor oil plant
- Deadly nightshade *(when unripe)*
- Dieffenbachia
- Elderberry *(if not cooked)*
- Foxglove
- Holly berries
- Laburnum
- Lantana
- Lily of the valley
- Mistletoe berries *(European variety)*
- Mushrooms and toadstools
- Oleander
- Poinsettia
- Potato vines
- Rhododendron
- Rhubarb leaves
- Rhus tree

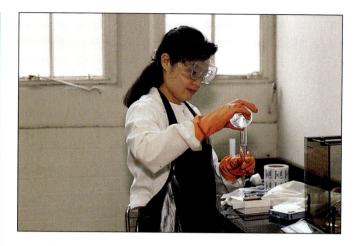

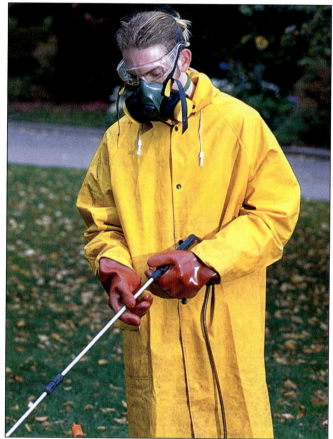

FIGURE 10-18 *Wear proper clothing for any activity which may put you into contact with a poisonous substance.*

- Use poison symbols to identify dangerous substances and teach children what the symbols mean.

- Dispose of outdated products by returning unused portions to the local supplier. Do not tip them down the sink or toilet.

- Use potentially dangerous chemicals only in well-ventilated areas, or substitute less dangerous ones whenever possible.

- If spraying chemicals such as pesticides or weedicides, use the least toxic substance available for the job. Choose a day when there is little or no wind, and keep children out of the area.

- Wear gloves, face mask and protective eyewear, and be sure to follow the manufacturer's directions (Figure 10-18).

Preventing bites and stings from insects, spiders, ticks or snakes is the best protection against the transmission of injected poisons. When in bushy or grassy areas, follow these general guidelines to prevent bites and stings:

- Wear long-sleeved shirts and long pants.

- Tuck your pant legs into your socks or boots; tuck your shirt into your pants.

- Wear light-coloured clothing to make it easier to see tiny insects or ticks.

- Use a rubber band or tape the area where pants and socks meet so that nothing can get under the clothing.

- When hiking in the bush, stay in the middle of the track. Avoid undergrowth and tall grass.

- Wear sturdy hiking boots.

- If you come across a snake, do not disturb it, and be careful because there may be others nearby.

- If in a tick-infested area:

  —Inspect yourself carefully for insects or ticks after being outdoors, or have someone else do it. If you are outdoors for a long period of time, check yourself several times during the day.

Check especially in hairy areas of the body (back of the neck and the scalp).

—If you have pets that go outdoors, spray them with repellent made for your type of pet. Apply the repellent according to the label, and regularly check your pet for ticks.

If you plan to be in a grassy or wooded area for a length of time, or if you know the area is highly infested with insects or ticks, you may want to use a repellent. Diethyltolusmide (DEET) is an active ingredient in many skin-applied repellents which are effective against ticks and other insects. Repellents containing DEET can be applied on exposed areas of skin and clothing. However, public health authorities advise consumers to choose a repellent with the lowest possible concentration of DEET, especially to use on children, who have a higher risk of a toxic reaction. Insecticides containing permethrin (another common insecticide) should be used only on clothing.

If you use repellents, including those for flies, mosquitos and other insects, follow these general rules:

- Keep all repellents out of the reach of children.
- To apply repellent to the face, first spray it on your hands and then apply it from your hands to your face. Avoid sensitive areas such as the lips and the eyes.
- Never spray insecticides not intended for human use on your skin.
- Never use repellents on a wound or irritated skin.
- Never put repellents on children's hands because they may put them in their eyes or mouth. Apply repellents to a child's clothing rather than directly onto the skin, to reduce the risk of toxic reaction.
- Use repellents sparingly. One application will last four to eight hours. Heavier or more frequent applications will not increase effectiveness.
- Wash treated skin with soap and water and remove treated clothing after you come indoors.
- If you suspect you are having a reaction to a repellent, wash the treated skin immediately and call your doctor.

Summary

- Poisonings can occur in one of four ways: ingestion, inhalation, absorption and injection.
- For suspected poisonings, call your Poisons Information Centre (PIC) and/or your local emergency number for advice.
- The general care of poisoning includes:
  —surveying the scene for safety and clues about the poisoning
  —removing the victim from the source of the poison
  —carrying out a primary survey and care for unconsciousness following the Basic Life Support flow chart (see page 35)
  —with a conscious victim, conducting a secondary survey for more information
  —calling the PIC or emergency number and following their directions
  —not giving the victim anything to eat or drink unless advised to do so by the medical authority
- Other first aid is specific for the type of poisoning and the toxin or venom. When in doubt, call the PIC.
- The best way to avoid poisoning is to take steps to prevent it.

Answers to Application Questions

1. Identification of a suspected poison is often difficult, and treatment for poisoning can vary substantially depending on what the poisonous substance is, how much has been taken and the condition of the victim. The Poisons Information Centre in each state and territory has access to current information on most poisonous substances, drugs, medications, etc. and can assist you in identifying the poison. The professional officer you speak to will be able to advise the best first aid care to give, based on the type of poison and the size, age and weight of the victim.

2. The pressure immobilisation technique works by limiting the spread of venoms through the body.

The pressure reduces the flow of lymph, which carries the poison from the site. However, this technique only slows the spread of the poison until the victim reaches medical attention: it does not stop the poisoning. With some slow-moving venoms, such as that of the red-back spider, there is ample time for the victim to reach medical aid before serious symptoms and signs occur. For a red-back spider bite, the pressure immobilisation technique unnecessarily increases the pain the victim feels as the area swells, when the venom is generally not life-threatening. Swelling in these instances can often be severe.

Study Questions

1. *Match each term with the correct definition.*

   a. Absorbed poison.
   b. Anaphylaxis.
   c. Ingested poison.
   d. Inhaled poison.
   e. Injected poison.
   f. Antivenom.
   g. Poisons Information Centre (PIC).
   h. Pressure immobilisation technique.

   _____ A treatment using antibodies against specific poisons in venom.
   _____ A poison introduced into the body through bites, stings or a hypodermic needle.
   _____ A life-threatening allergic reaction.
   _____ A centre staffed by professionals who can tell you how to provide care in a poisoning emergency.
   _____ A poison that is swallowed.
   _____ A poison that enters the body through contact with the skin.
   _____ A bandage on the site of a bite or sting to slow the spread of the venom.
   _____ A poison that enters the body through breathing.

2. **List at least six common symptoms and signs of poisoning.**

3. **List at least four factors that determine the severity of a poisoning.**

4. **List the steps of the pressure immobilisation technique.**

5. **Describe at least four ways to prevent bites and stings.**

6. **List at least four rules for using any repellent.**

7. *Describe how to care for a person who has spilled a poisonous substance on the skin.*

8. *You suspect a man has swallowed poison. You should first:*
   a. give him something to drink
   b. induce vomiting
   c. call your local Poisons Information Centre
   d. assist him to lie down.

9. *In caring for the victim of an inhaled poison, you should:*
   a. be sure the area is safe for you to enter
   b. remove the victim from the source of the poison if it is safe to do so
   c. monitor the ABC
   d. call the Poisons Information Centre or an ambulance.
   e. All of the above.

10. *In caring for a bee sting, you should:*
   a. remove the remaining stinger barb by scraping it from the skin
   b. remove a remaining stinger barb using tweezers
   c. wash the sting site, then cover it.
   d. a and c.

11. *When spending time outdoors in scrubland or tall grass, to prevent bites and stings you should:*
   a. stay on established tracks and trails
   b. wear sturdy walking shoes
   c. tuck pant legs into boots or socks.
   d. All of the above.

12. *You and a friend are bushwalking and your companion is stung by a European wasp. You provide first aid. Your friend appears to be fine. When you ask how she feels, she responds, "Fine, but I'm just a little worried. My father is allergic to wasp stings and I don't know if I am or not." List at least four symptoms or signs that would tell you if your friend needs further care.*

Answers are in Appendix A (page 362).

Applying a Pressure Immobilisation Bandage

The victim has been bitten by a snake on the lower leg. She is not sure but thinks it was the venomous tiger snake. An ambulance has been called but may not arrive for 30 minutes. You have the victim lying calmly on the ground.

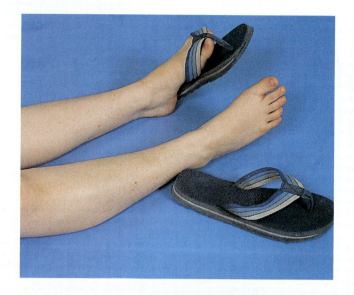

Apply a pressure bandage over the bite area

- Use a crepe roller bandage over the bite area to apply firm pressure.
- Tie or tape bandage in place.

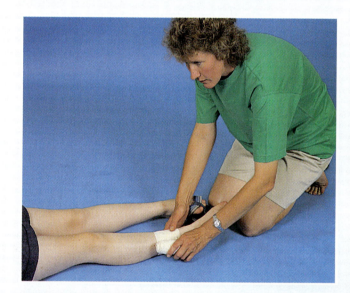

Apply a second bandage upward on the extremity

- Bandage the leg upward from the toes to above the knee.
- Bandage the leg as high as you can.
- Secure the end of the bandage.

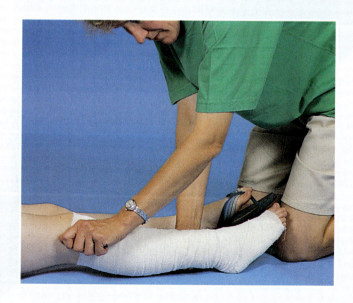

PRACTICE GUIDE

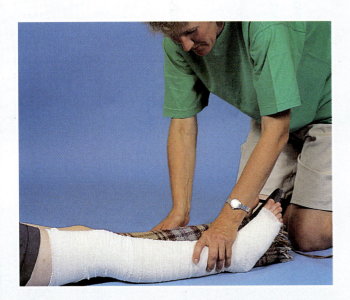

Apply a padded splint to immobilise the leg

- Apply an improvised splint which extends well above the bandaged area.
- Secure the splint in place with 2 or more ties over padding where there are joints.

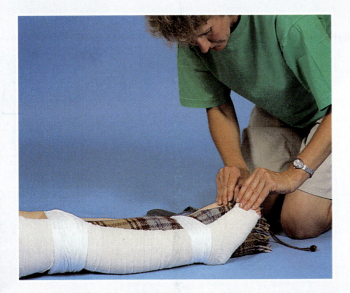

Check the victim's toes to ensure circulation has not been cut off

- Look for discolouration of the skin on the foot and toes.
- Ask the victim if the foot feels cold or numb.

If the circulation is not restricted ...

- Keep the victim at rest and wait for the ambulance.

If the victim's circulation is restricted ...

- Loosen the bandage slightly, but maintain pressure over the bite site.

Monitor the victim until the ambulance arrives

- Monitor the conscious state and check the ABC.
- Be prepared to give EAR or CPR if needed.

PRACTICE GUIDE

Exposure to Heat and Cold

IN ORDER TO FUNCTION properly, body temperature must be maintained within a narrow range of approximately 36 to 39 °C. Exposure to heat and cold may cause a wide range of serious injuries and illnesses, some of which can be life-threatening. Extreme heat can cause burns, and even normal environmental heat can cause heat illnesses or an emergency such as heat stroke. Cold extremes can cause frostbite, cold burns and the life-threatening emergency of hypothermia.

This chapter outlines how to recognise the symptoms and signs of heat and cold injuries and illnesses, and what care to provide.

For Review

A basic understanding of the functions of the circulatory system, skin, the inter-relationship of the body systems (Chapter 2) and a knowledge of how to care for shock (Chapter 6) will help your understanding of the chapter.

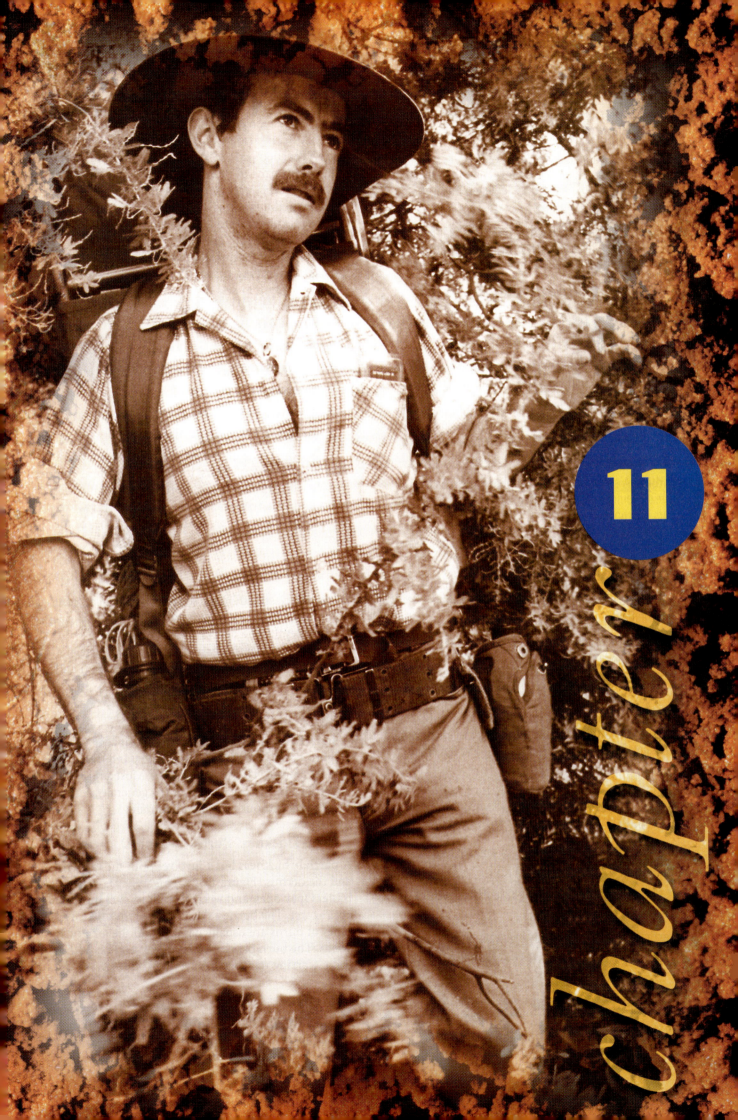

chapter

11

Key Terms

Burn: An injury to the skin or other body tissues caused by heat, chemicals, electricity or radiation.

Critical burn: Any burn that is potentially life-threatening, disabling or disfiguring; a burn requiring medical attention.

Cryogenic *(cry-o-jen-ic)* **burn:** A cold burn that results from contact with a substance such as liquid oxygen, liquid nitrogen or snow and ice; similar to frostbite.

Dehydration: Excessive loss of water from the body's tissues which leads to a disturbance in the balance of essential electrolytes; may follow any condition in which there is rapid depletion of body fluids.

Dressing: A pad placed directly over a wound to absorb blood and other body fluids and to prevent infection.

Electrolytes *(e-lec-tro-lites)*: Elements or compounds found in blood and tissue fluids, e.g. potassium, sodium and chloride. Proper quantities and a balance among them are essential for normal metabolism and function.

Frostbite: A serious condition in which body tissues freeze, commonly at the extremities, in the fingers, toes, ears and nose.

Full-thickness burn: A burn injury involving both layers of skin and underlying tissues; skin may be charred.

Heat exhaustion: A form of shock, due to depletion of body fluids resulting from overexposure to a hot environment.

Heat stroke: A life-threatening condition that develops when the body's temperature regulating and cooling mechanisms are overwhelmed and body systems begin to fail.

Hypothermia *(hy-po-ther-mee-a)* A life-threatening condition in which the body's warming mechanisms fail to maintain normal body temperature and the entire body cools to 35°C or lower.

Partial-thickness burn: A burn injury involving both layers of skin; characterised by red, wet skin and blisters.

Scald: A burn caused by exposure of the skin to a hot liquid or vapour.

Soft tissue: Body structures that include the layers of skin, fat and muscles.

Superficial burn: A burn injury involving only the top layer of skin; characterised by red, dry skin.

BURNS

Burns are a type of **soft tissue** injury caused primarily by heat. Burns also can occur when the body is exposed to certain chemicals, electricity, extreme cold or solar and other forms of radiation.

When a burn occurs, the heat first destroys the epidermis, the top layer of skin. If the burn progresses, the dermis, the second layer, is injured or destroyed. Burns break the skin and thus can cause infection, fluid loss and loss of temperature control. Deep burns can damage underlying tissues. Burns also can damage the respiratory system and the eyes.

The severity of a burn depends on:

- the temperature of the object or gas causing the burn
- the length of exposure to the source
- the location of the burn
- the extent of the burn
- the victim's age and medical condition

The people most at risk of severe burns are those over 60 and under 5 years, because their skin is thinner. People with chronic medical problems, malnutrition, heart and kidney problems are also more at risk, especially if they are exposed to the burn source for a longer period.

Types of Burns

Burns are classified by the source, such as heat, cold, chemicals, electricity or radiation. They are also classified by depth. The deeper the burn, the more severe it is. The three depth classifications are superficial (first degree), partial-thickness (second degree) and full-thickness (third degree).

Superficial Burns (First Degree)

A **superficial burn** involves only the top layer of skin (Figure 11-1). The skin is red and dry, and the burn is usually painful. The area may swell. Most sunburns are superficial burns. Superficial burns generally heal in 5 to 6 days without permanent scarring.

Partial-Thickness Burns (Second Degree)

A **partial-thickness burn** involves both the epidermis and the dermis (Figure 11-2). This injury is red and blisters may open and weep clear fluid, making the skin appear wet. The burned skin may look mottled. These types of burns are usually painful, and the area often swells. The burn usually heals in 3 or 4 weeks, although some scarring may occur.

Full-thickness Burns (Third Degree)

A **full-thickness burn** destroys both layers of skin, as well as any or all of the underlying structures—fat, muscles, bones, blood vessels and nerves (Figure 11-3).

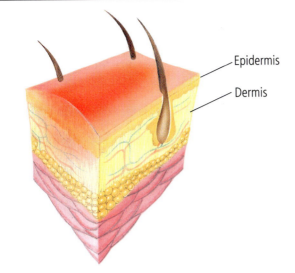

Epidermis

Dermis

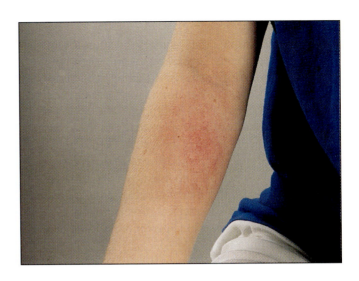

FIGURE 11-1 *A superficial (first degree) burn.*

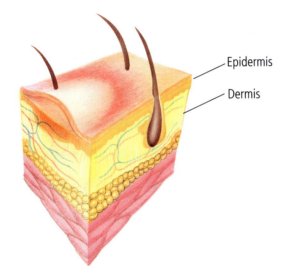

Epidermis

Dermis

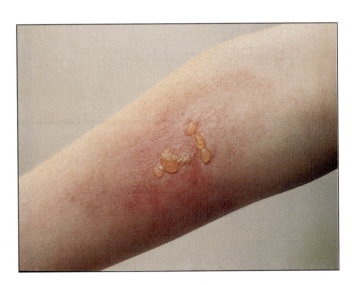

FIGURE 11-2 *A partial (second degree) burn.*

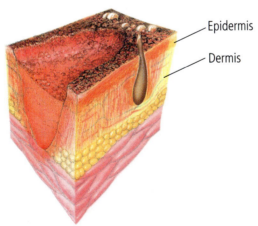

Epidermis

Dermis

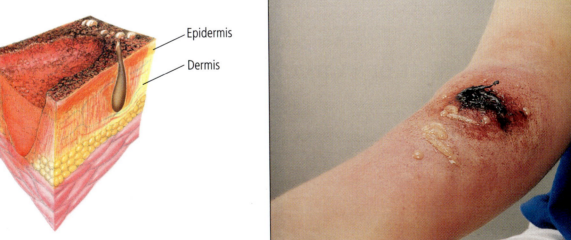

FIGURE 11-3 *A full-thickness (third degree) burn.*

These burns may look brown or charred (black), with the tissues underneath sometimes appearing white. They can be either extremely painful or relatively painless if the burn has destroyed nerve endings in the skin. Full-thickness burns are life-threatening. When burns are open the body loses fluid, and the victim is likely to go into shock. These burns are also highly prone to infection. Scarring occurs and may be severe. Many full-thickness burn sites eventually require skin grafts.

Identifying Critical Burns

A **critical burn** is one that requires the attention of medical professionals. Critical burns are potentially life-threatening, disfiguring or disabling. Knowing whether you should call an ambulance or seek medical aid for a burn injury is often difficult.

It is not always easy or possible to assess the severity of a burn immediately after the injury. Even superficial burns to large areas of the body or to certain body parts can be critical. A person with burns to a large area of the body is more likely to suffer shock due to the increased fluid loss. Hospitals and medical professionals use various methods to assess the percentage of body area affected by a burn (Figure 11-4).

You cannot judge severity by the pain the victim feels because nerve endings may be destroyed. Call an ambulance immediately for assistance for burns which:

- have caused the victim to have difficulty in breathing
- affected more than one body part
- are to the head, neck, hands, feet or genital area
- are either partial-thickness or full-thickness burns involving a child or an elderly person
- are the result of chemicals, explosions or electricity

Most burns caused by flames or hot oil require medical attention, especially if the victim is under

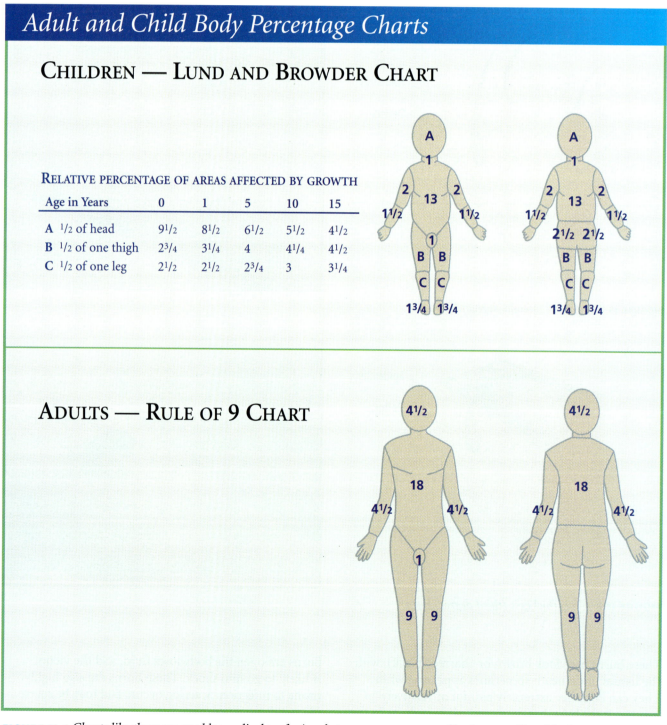

Adult and Child Body Percentage Charts

CHILDREN — LUND AND BROWDER CHART

RELATIVE PERCENTAGE OF AREAS AFFECTED BY GROWTH

Age in Years	0	1	5	10	15
A 1/2 of head	9 1/2	8 1/2	6 1/2	5 1/2	4 1/2
B 1/2 of one thigh	2 3/4	3 1/4	4	4 1/4	4 1/2
C 1/2 of one leg	2 1/2	2 1/2	2 3/4	3	3 1/4

ADULTS — RULE OF 9 CHART

FIGURE 11-4 *Charts like these are used by medical professionals to assess percentage of body area affected by burns.*

or over 60 years of age. Hot oil is slow to cool and difficult to remove from the skin. Burns which involve hot liquid or flames contacting clothing also will be serious, because clothing prolongs the heat contact with the skin. Some synthetic fabrics melt and stick to the body. They may take longer to cool than the soft tissues. Although these burns may appear minor at first, they can continue to deteriorate over a period of time.

Care for Burns

As you approach the victim, decide if the scene is safe. Look for fire, smoke, fallen electrical wires and warning signs for chemicals or radiation. If the scene is unsafe, call the emergency services number and wait for fire or ambulance personnel to arrive.

If the scene is safe, approach cautiously. Carry out a primary survey and call for an ambulance if necessary. Pay close attention to the victim's airway. Note burns around the mouth or nose or the rest of the face which may indicate that air passages or lungs have been burned (Figure 11-5). If you suspect a burned airway or burned lungs, continually monitor breathing. Air passages may swell, impairing or stopping breathing.

As you conduct a secondary survey, look for additional signs of burn injuries. Look also for other injuries, especially if there was an explosion or electric shock. Remember, *burns do not bleed*—any bleeding indicates the presence of another injury.

If burns are evident, follow these four basic care steps:

1. Cool the burned area.
2. Cover the burned area.
3. Prevent infection.
4. Minimise shock.

Even after the source of heat has been removed, soft tissue will continue to burn for minutes afterwards, causing more damage. Therefore, it is essential to cool any burned areas immediately with large amounts of cool water for up to 20 minutes (Figure 11-6A). Use whatever resources are available—a bucket, shower or garden hose. Remove any loose clothing from the area (Figure 11-6B). Do not try to remove any clothing that is sticking to skin. Remove any rings, watches or other jewellery as quickly as possible before swelling occurs.

You can apply soaked towels, sheets or other wet cloths to a burned face or other area which cannot be immersed. Be sure to keep these compresses cool by adding more water, otherwise, they will quickly absorb the heat from the skin's surface.

Allow plenty of time for the burned area to cool. If pain continues or if the edges of the burned area are still warm to the touch when the area is removed from the water, continue cooling.

Burns often expose sensitive nerve endings. Cover the burned area to keep out air and help reduce pain (Figure 11-6C). Use dry, sterile dressings if possible, and loosely bandage them in place. The bandage should

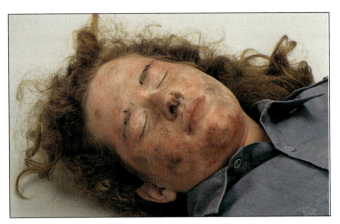

FIGURE 11-5 *Facial burns may indicate that air passages or lungs have been burned.*

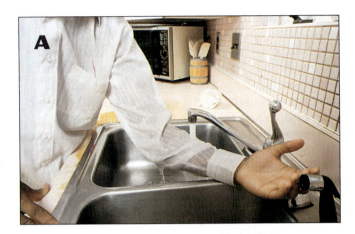

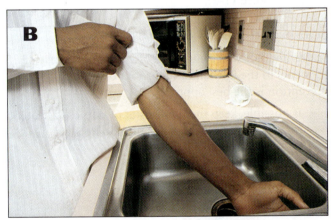

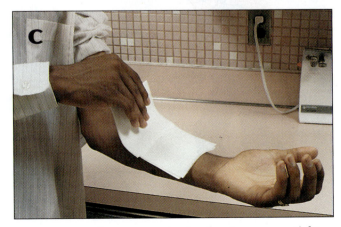

FIGURE 11-6 A *Large amounts of cool water are essential to cool burned areas.* **B** *Remove any loose clothing covering the burned area.* **C** *Cover the burned area.*

not put pressure on the burn surface. If the burn covers a large area of the body, cover it with clean, dry sheets or other non-fluffy cloth.

Covering the burn also helps to prevent infection. Do not put ointments, butter, oil or other commercial or home remedies on blisters or full-thickness burns or on any burn that will receive medical attention. Oils and ointments seal in heat and do not help in the relief of pain. Other home remedies can contaminate open skin areas, causing infection. Do not break blisters. Intact skin helps prevent infection.

For small superficial burns and burns with open blisters which are not sufficiently severe or extensive to require medical attention (e.g. smaller than a 20c piece), care for the burned area as for an open wound. Keep the area clean and dry, and watch for signs of infection. For children, any burns larger than the size of the child's own palm should be seen by a doctor.

Full-thickness burns can cause shock as a result of pain and loss of body fluids. Lie the victim down unless there are signs of breathing difficulty. Raise the burned area above the level of the heart if possible. Burn victims tend to get cold, so help the victim to maintain body temperature by covering with a sheet or light blanket.

If you are alone and your clothing catches on fire, follow the simple guide of "Stop, drop and roll". Stop whatever you are doing, drop to the ground, and roll until the flame is out. Children should be taught this procedure as soon as they are old enough to understand it (Figure 11-7).

Scalds and Hot Water Burns

Scalds and hot water burns are often the result of accidents in the kitchen or bathroom of a home. Prevention is the best approach:

- If possible, keep the thermostat of domestic heaters turned down and the water not too hot.

> ### DOS AND DONT'S OF BURN CARE
>
> **Dos**
> - Cool burns by flushing with cool water.
> - Remove rings and jewellery.
> - Cover the burn with a dry, sterile dressing.
> - Take steps to minimise shock.
>
> **Dont's**
> - Apply ice directly to burns.
> - Touch burns with anything except sterile or clean dressings; do not pull clothes over any burned area.
> - Remove pieces of cloth that stick to a burned area.
> - Try to clean a full-thickness burn.
> - Break blisters.
> - Use any kind of oil or ointment on severe burns.
> - Use cotton wool or other fluffy material on burns. ▪

- Don't leave young children alone in the bathroom or kitchen.
- Turn the handles of saucepans on the stove so that a child cannot reach them, and keep appliance cords tucked away.

Treat scalds by removing any clothing as quickly as possible because it traps the heat. Cool the area with water and treat as for any other burn.

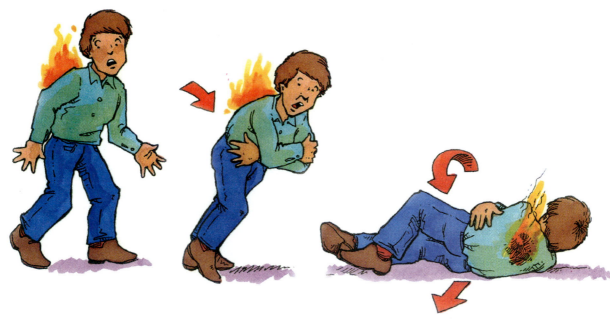

FIGURE 11-7 *If you are alone and your clothing catches on fire, stop, drop and roll.*

Special Situations

Chemical burns

Chemical burns are common in industrial settings but also occur in the home. Cleaning solutions, such as household bleach, drain cleaners, toilet bowl cleaners, paint strippers and lawn or garden chemicals often contain caustic chemicals, which destroy tissues. Typically, burn injuries result from chemicals which are strongly acid or alkaline. These substances can quickly injure the skin. As with heat burns, the stronger the chemical and the longer the contact, the more severe the burn. The chemical will continue to burn as long as it is on the skin. You must remove the chemical from the body as quickly as possible and call an ambulance. Some chemicals such as dishwasher crystals are activated by water, so brush off as much of the chemical as possible before flushing with water.

Flush the burn with large amounts of cool, running water (Figure 11-8). Continue flushing for 20 to 30 minutes. Do not use too much water pressure from a hose; the force may further damage burned skin. Help the victim remove contaminated clothes, and take steps to minimise shock. If an eye is burned by a chemical, keep flushing the affected eye until ambulance personnel arrive (Figure 11-9). Ensure that water flushes underneath the eye lids.

Electrical burns

The human body is a good conductor of electricity. When someone comes into contact with electricity from a power line, a malfunctioning household appliance, lightning or some other source, the electricity is conducted through the body. Some body parts, such as the skin, resist the electrical current. Resistance produces heat, which can cause burn injuries (Figure 11-10). The severity of an electrical burn depends on the type and amount of contact, the current's path through the body, and how long the contact lasted. Electrical burns are often deep, and the victim will have both an entrance and an exit wound. Although these wounds may look superficial, the tissues below may be severely damaged.

Electrical injuries cause other problems in addition to burns. Electricity can make the heart beat erratically or even stop. Respiratory arrest may occur. Suspect a possible electrical injury if you hear a sudden loud pop or bang and/or see an unexpected flash.

The symptoms and signs of electrical injury include:

- unconsciousness
- dazed, confused behaviour
- obvious burns on the skin surface
- breathing difficulty
- weak, irregular or absent pulse
- burns both where the current entered and where it left the body, often on the hand or foot

Never approach a victim of an electrical injury until you are sure the power is turned off. If there is a fallen

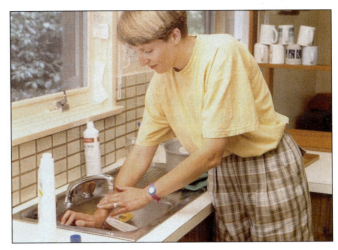

FIGURE 11-8 *Flush a chemical burn with cool, running water.*

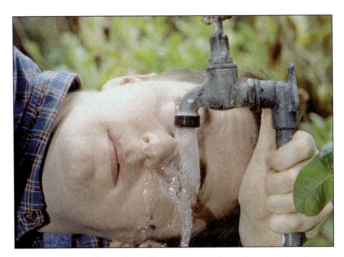

FIGURE 11-9 *Flush the affected eye with cool water in the case of a chemical burn to the eye. Keep the affected eye lower to prevent contamination of the unaffected eye. Some facilities may have special eyewash stations.*

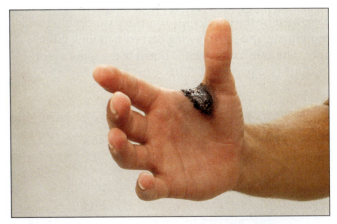

FIGURE 11-10 *An electrical burn may severely damage underlying tissues.*

power line, *wait for the emergency services to turn off the power* and stay at least 6 metres away. Electricity can travel through water easily, and even a heavy dew can assist its passage for several metres. If people are in a car with a fallen wire across it, shout to tell them to stay in the vehicle, because they are safely insulated inside the car.

To care for a victim of an electrical injury, make sure the scene is safe. Call emergency services and ambulance personnel immediately. Carry out a primary survey. The victim may have breathing difficulties or be in cardiac arrest. Give care for any life-threatening conditions.

In the secondary survey, look for two burn sites, and cool them by flushing with water. Cover any burn injuries with a dry, sterile dressing and give care for shock.

With a victim of a lightning strike, look for life-threatening conditions such as respiratory or cardiac arrest. If unconscious, turn the victim onto the side and follow the Basic Life Support flow chart (see page 35). Any burns are a lesser problem. The victim may also have fractures.

Radiation burns

Both the solar radiation of the sun and other types of radiation can cause burns. Solar burns are similar to heat burns; usually they are mild but can be painful (Figure 11-11). They may blister, involving more than one layer of skin. Care for sunburn as you would any other burn. Cool the burn and protect the burned area from further damage by staying out of the sun.

People are rarely exposed to other types of radiation unless working in special settings such as certain medical, industrial or research settings. If you work in such a setting, you will be informed of the precautions you should take to prevent overexposure. Training is also provided to teach you how to prevent and respond to such emergencies.

Cryogenic Burns

Cryogenic burns, or cold burns, can result from contact with extremely cold substances such as ice, liquid oxygen and liquid nitrogen. These injuries most commonly occur in occupational settings and can be prevented by the correct use of protective clothing and equipment, and by following correct handling guidelines. The care for cryogenic burns is the same as for frostbite (see pages 192–93).

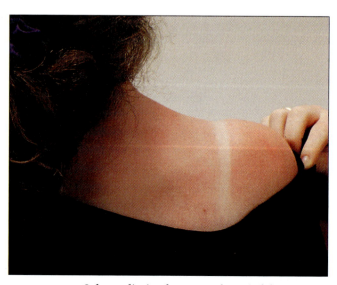

FIGURE 11-11 *Solar radiation burns can be painful.*

EXTREMES OF TEMPERATURE

The human body is equipped to withstand extremes of temperature. Usually, its mechanisms for regulating body temperature work very well. However, when the body is overwhelmed by extremes of heat and cold, illness occurs.

Extreme temperatures can occur anywhere, both indoors and outdoors, but a person can develop a heat- or cold-related illness even if temperatures are not extreme. The effects of humidity, wind, clothing, living and working environment, physical activity, age and an individual's health are all factors in heat- and cold-related illnesses.

Illnesses caused by exposure to temperature extremes are progressive and can become life-threatening. Once the signs of a heat- or cold-related illness begin to appear, a victim's condition can rapidly deteriorate and lead to death. If the victim shows any of the signs of sudden illness, the environmental conditions should alert you to look for the presence of a heat- or cold-related illness and the need to give the appropriate care. Immediate care can prevent the illness from becoming life-threatening.

In this section you will learn how extremes of heat and cold affect the body, how to recognise temperature-related emergencies and how to provide care.

How Body Temperature Is Controlled

Body temperature must remain constant for the body to work efficiently. Normal body temperature is 37°C. Body heat is generated primarily through the conversion of food to energy. Heat is also produced by muscle contractions, as in exercise or shivering.

Heat always moves from warm areas to cooler ones. Because the body is usually warmer than the surrounding air, it tends to lose heat to the air. The body maintains its temperature by constantly balancing heat loss with heat production (Figure 11-12). The heat produced in routine activities is usually enough to balance normal heat loss.

When body heat increases, the body loses heat through the skin. Blood vessels near the skin dilate, or widen, to bring more warm blood to the surface. Heat then escapes and the body cools (Figure 11-13A).

The body is also cooled by the evaporation of sweat. When the air temperature is very warm, dilation of blood vessels is a less effective means of removing heat. Therefore, sweating increases. When the humidity is

BEFORE THE DOWN JACKET

The goose bump had a prehistoric purpose. In early humans, the goose bump caused body hair to rise and trap a protective layer of warm air around the body. ∎

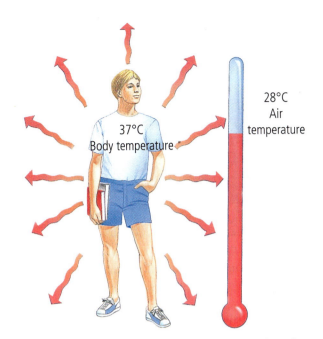

FIGURE 11-12 *Because the body is usually warmer than the surrounding air, it tends to lose heat to the air.*

high, sweat does not evaporate as quickly; it stays longer on the skin and has little or no cooling effect.

When the body reacts to cold, blood vessels near the skin constrict and move warm blood to the centre of the body. This maintains the "core" temperature around the vital organs at a constant 37°C. Less heat escapes through the skin, and the body stays warm (Figure 11-13B). When constriction of blood vessels fails to keep the body warm, shivering results. Shivering produces heat through muscle action.

Three main factors can affect how well the body maintains its temperature: air temperature, humidity and wind. Humidity and wind multiply the effects of heat or cold. Extreme heat or cold accompanied by high humidity hampers the body's ability to effectively maintain temperature. A cold temperature combined with a strong wind rapidly cools exposed body parts. The combination of temperature and wind speed form what is called the "wind chill factor".

Other factors, such as the clothing you wear, how often you take breaks from exposure to extreme temperature, how much and how often you drink water, your food intake and how intense your activity is, also affect how well your body manages extremes of temperature. These are all factors you can control to prevent illnesses related to heat or cold.

People at Risk of Heat- or Cold-related Illnesses

People most at risk of heat or cold illnesses include:

- those under the influence of alcohol
- those seriously injured, such as with burns
- those who work or exercise strenuously outdoors
- elderly people
- young children
- those with health problems, especially vomiting and diarrhoea
- those who have had a heat- or cold-related illness in the past
- those who have cardiovascular disease or other conditions that cause poor circulation
- those who take medication to eliminate water from the body (diuretics)
- those suffering from malnutrition
- an immobilised or trapped person

Usually people seek relief from an extreme temperature before they begin to feel ill. However, some

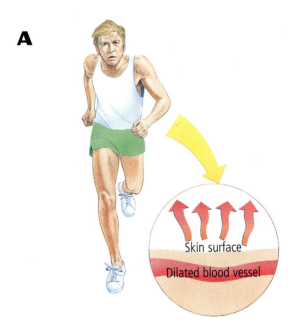

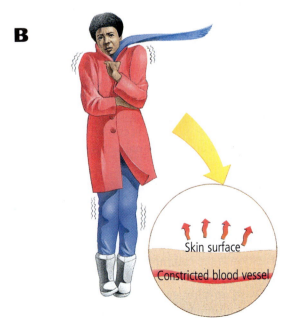

FIGURE 11-13 A *Your body loses heat by dilating the blood vessels near the skin's surface.* B *The body conserves heat by constricting the blood vessels near the skin.*

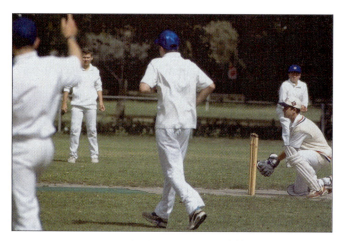

FIGURE 11-14 *In certain situations, it is difficult to escape temperature extremes.*

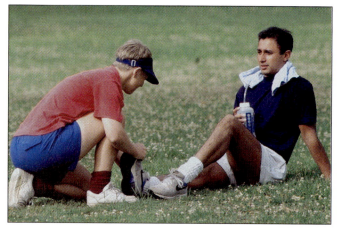

FIGURE 11-15 *Resting, lightly stretching the affected muscle and replenishing fluids is usually enough for the body to recover from muscular cramps.*

people do not or cannot easily escape these extremes (Figure 11-14). Athletes and those who work outdoors often keep working even after they develop the first symptoms and signs of illness, which they may not even recognise.

HEAT-RELATED CONDITIONS

Heat exhaustion and **heat stroke** are conditions caused by over-exposure to heat. Muscular cramps can be related to activity in hot conditions but are quite separate.

Muscular Cramps

Muscular cramps are painful spasms of skeletal muscles. The exact cause is not known, although the cramps develop fairly rapidly and usually occur after heavy exercise or work outdoors in warm or even moderate temperatures.

Follow these guidelines to care for muscular cramps:

1. Help the victim to rest comfortably in a cool place.

2. Provide cool water, because rest and clear fluids are usually all the body needs to recover.

3. Lightly stretch the muscle and gently massage the area (Figure 11-15).

4. Do not give the victim salt tablets or salt water. Ingesting high concentrations of salt, whether in tablet or liquid form, can hasten the onset of heat-related illness. There is enough salt in the daily diet, and any additional salt increases tissue **dehydration.**

It is essential to drink plenty of fluids during and after physical activity.

Heat Exhaustion

Heat exhaustion is the common form of heat-related illness. It typically occurs after long periods of strenuous exercise or work in a hot environment. Although heat exhaustion is commonly associated with athletes, it also affects firefighters, construction workers, factory workers and others who wear heavy clothing in a hot, humid environment.

Heat exhaustion is an early indication that the body's temperature-regulating mechanism is becoming over-whelmed. The victim loses fluid through sweating, which decreases the blood volume. Blood flow to the skin increases, reducing blood flow to the vital organs. Because the circulatory system is affected, the person develops mild shock.

The symptoms and signs of heat exhaustion include:

- normal or below normal skin temperature
- cool, moist, pale skin progressing to red skin
- headache
- nausea
- dizziness and weakness
- exhaustion
- sweating
- rapid, weak pulse

Heat exhaustion in its early stage can usually be reversed with prompt care. Often the victim feels better after resting in a cool place and drinking cool water. If heat exhaustion progresses, however, the victim's condition worsens. The body temperature continues to climb and the victim may vomit and begin to show changes in the level of consciousness.

Care for Heat Exhaustion

1. Encourage the victim to rest lying down with the legs slightly raised. Loosen any tight clothing.

2. If fully conscious, give small drinks of cold water to drink. If the victim is vomiting and unable to take any fluids, arrange for urgent medical treatment.

3. If unconscious, position the victim on the side and care for the airway, breathing and circulation following the Basic Life Support flow chart (page 35).

1 *Explain why some people feel "faint" in hot weather.*

Heat Stroke

Heat stroke is the least common and most severe heat emergency. Heat stroke develops when the body systems are overwhelmed by heat and begin to stop functioning. Sweating stops because body fluid levels are low. When sweating stops, the body cannot cool itself effectively, and body temperature rapidly rises. It soon reaches a level at which the brain and other vital organs, such as the heart and kidneys, begin to fail. If the body is not cooled, convulsions, unconsciousness and death will result.

Heat stroke is a serious medical emergency. You must recognise the signs of this heat-related illness and provide care immediately.

The signs of heat stroke include:

- high body temperature (often as high as 40°C)
- red, hot, dry skin
- progressive deterioration in the conscious state
- full, bounding pulse
- rapid, shallow, noisy breathing

Someone with heat stroke may at first have a strong, rapid pulse, as the heart works hard to rid the body of heat by dilating blood vessels and sending more blood to the skin. As consciousness deteriorates, the circulatory system begins to fail and the pulse becomes weak and irregular. Without prompt care, the heat stroke victim will die.

Caring for Heat-Stroke

When any symptoms and signs of sudden illness develop and you suspect the illness is caused by overexposure to heat, follow these general care steps immediately:

1. Stop the person from continuing any activity.
2. Cool the body.
3. Give cool, clear fluids if the victim is fully conscious.
4. Minimise shock.
5. Seek urgent medical care.

When you recognise heat-related illness in its early stages, you can usually reverse it. Remove the victim from the hot environment and give the victim frequent drinks of cool water. Moving the victim out of the sun or away from the heat allows the body's own temperature-regulating mechanism to recover, cooling the body more quickly. Remember, it is important that the victim be

THE DANGER OF HEAT

Who would have thought that going for a run on a hot day could severely disable and almost kill a fit athlete? John Jacobsen, like most young men, would never have anticipated what happened to him that summer afternoon.

An 8-kilometre fun run was scheduled outside a small town in New South Wales. John and two friends who had raced together in the past registered for the run. The day became much hotter than expected, and when the temperature rose to 42°C, the run was cancelled. John and his friends decided to run the course anyway. They drank water before they started but did not bother to take water with them or arrange for it along the way, a nearly fatal mistake.

John was running hard and was well out in front. He ignored the symptoms of heat exhaustion and then heat stroke. He did not stop for water or to cool off, and kept running when he became delirious and incapable of rational thought, unaware of the horrifying things happening in his body. He collapsed less than an hour from the start.

John's body had become severely overheated and extremely dehydrated, resulting in muscle tissue in his legs dying and liquefying. The dying muscles released toxins that thickened his blood, causing additional injury throughout his body, including brain and lung damage and kidney failure. Unconscious, he was packed in cold, wet towels while being driven by ambulance to the closest hospital.

At one point John's heart stopped—he was fortunate it was restarted. Later, one leg had to be amputated at the buttock because of gangrene. For eight weeks he was on dialysis because of kidney failure. The extent of the brain damage is not yet known. After six months of constant medical care, he still cannot get out of bed by himself. Many months of rehabilitation lie ahead. Yet he knows he is lucky to be alive.

Sports physicians say John's case is rare, but less extreme cases of injury caused by heat are more common. The key is prevention. Prepare ahead of time for any necessary activity in the heat, by, among other things, ensuring adequate hydration by drinking lots of water the day before the activity as well as during it. Never ignore the body's warning signs to stop and cool off. ■

persuaded to stop all activity, as the person may be beyond the point of making a rational decision.

Loosen any tight clothing and remove clothing soaked with perspiration. Apply cool, wet cloths, such as towels or sheets, to the skin and fan the victim to increase evaporation. Continue cooling the victim until the body temperature falls to 38°C.

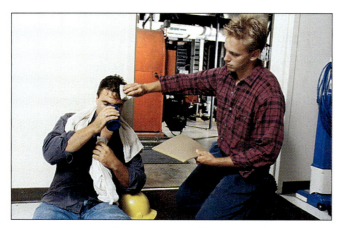

FIGURE 11-16 *For the early stages of heat-related illness, apply cool, wet cloths and fan the victim to increase evaporation. Give the victim cool water to drink.*

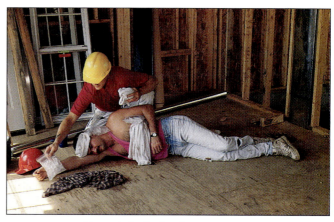

FIGURE 11-17 *To cool the body of a victim of heat-related illness, cover with cool, wet towels and apply ice packs to groins and armpits.*

If the victim is conscious, drinking cool water slowly will help replenish the vital fluids lost through sweating (Figure 11-16). The victim is likely to be nauseated, and water is less likely than other fluids to cause vomiting and is more quickly absorbed into the body from the stomach. Do not let the victim drink too quickly. Give half a glass (100ml) about every 15 minutes. Let the victim rest in a comfortable position, and watch carefully for changes in the victim's condition. A victim of heat-related illness should not resume normal activities the same day.

When to Call an Ambulance

Refusing water, vomiting and changes in the victim's conscious state are signs that the victim's condition is worsening. Call an ambulance immediately if you have not already done so. If the person vomits, stop giving fluids and position the victim on the side. Make sure the airway is clear. Monitor the ABC and check vital signs. Keep the victim lying down and continue to cool the body.

A change in the conscious state is the first reliable sign that a victim's condition is deteriorating. If you observe changes in the conscious state, cool the body by any means available. Soak towels or sheets and apply them to the victim's body. If you have ice packs or cold packs, place them on each of the victim's wrists and ankles, on the groin, in each armpit and on the neck to cool the large blood vessels (Figure 11-17). Do not apply rubbing alcohol, which closes the skin's pores and prevents heat loss. Maintain an open airway and monitor the ABC. Immersing the victim in a bath of cool water is not a good idea because doing so may cause additional problems, including abnormal heart rhythms. A person with heat stroke may experience respiratory or cardiac arrest. Be prepared to give EAR or CPR.

COLD EMERGENCIES

Frostbite and **hypothermia** are two types of cold emergencies. Frostbite occurs in body parts exposed to the cold. Hypothermia is a general body cooling which develops when the body can no longer generate sufficient heat to maintain normal body temperature.

Frostbite

Frostbite is the freezing of body tissues. It usually occurs in exposed areas of the body, depending on the air temperature, length of exposure and the wind. Frostbite can affect superficial or deep tissues. In superficial frostbite, the skin is frozen but the tissues below are not. In deep frostbite, also called freezing, both the skin and underlying tissues are frozen. Both types of frostbite are serious. The water in and between the body's cells freezes and swells. The ice crystals and swelling may damage or destroy the cells. Frostbite can cause the loss of fingers, hands, arms, toes, feet and legs.

The symptoms and signs of frostbite include:

- lack of feeling in the affected area
- skin that appears waxy
- skin that is cold to the touch
- skin that is discoloured (flushed, white, yellow, blue)

Care for Frostbite

When caring for frostbite, handle the area gently. Never rub an affected area as this will cause further damage because of the sharp ice crystals in the skin. Follow these steps:

1. Take the victim to shelter before gently removing any clothing or covering from the affected area.

2. Immediately rewarm the affected parts by skin-to-skin heat transfer from a warm part of yourself or the person; for example, place frostbitten hands in the victim's own armpits, or frostbitten feet into your armpits. Cover frostbitten ears, nose or face with warm hands until colour and sensation return.

3. As an alternative, rewarm the area gently by soaking the affected part in warm water if possible (Figure 11-18A). Test the water temperature yourself, because if the temperature is uncomfortable to your touch the water is too warm.

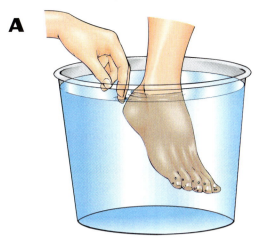

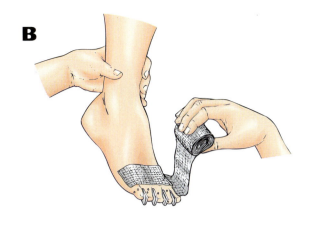

FIGURE 11-18 A *Warm the frostbitten area gently by soaking it in water. Do not allow the frostbitten area to touch the container.* **B** *After rewarming, wrap the area with a dry, sterile dressing. If fingers or toes are frostbitten, place dry material between them.*

4. Lightly cover the area with soft dressings. If fingers or toes are frostbitten, place soft material such as cotton or tissues between them (Figure 11-18B). Avoid breaking any blisters.

5. Raise the affected parts to help reduce pain and swelling.

6. Seek medical attention as soon as possible.

Hypothermia

In hypothermia, the entire body cools when its warming mechanisms fail. The victim will die if not given adequate care. In hypothermia, body temperature drops below 35°C, which will not register on a normal thermometer. As the body temperature cools to below 28°C, the heart begins to beat erratically and eventually stops. Death then occurs.

The symptoms and signs of hypothermia include:

- Shivering (which may be absent in later stages).
- Slow, irregular pulse.
- Numbness.
- Glassy stare.
- Apathy and decreasing levels of consciousness.
- Abnormal co-ordination, trouble walking.

The air temperature does not have to be below freezing for people to develop hypothermia. Elderly people in poorly heated homes, particularly people with poor nutrition and who get little exercise, can develop hypothermia at higher temperatures. The homeless and the ill are also at risk. Certain substances, such as alcohol and barbiturates, can also interfere with the body's normal response to cold, causing hypothermia to occur more easily. Medical conditions such as infection, insulin reaction, stroke and brain tumour also make a person more susceptible. Anyone remaining in cold water or wet clothing for a prolonged time may also easily develop hypothermia.

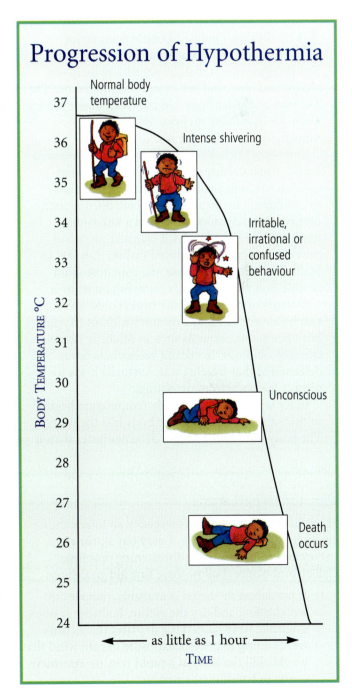

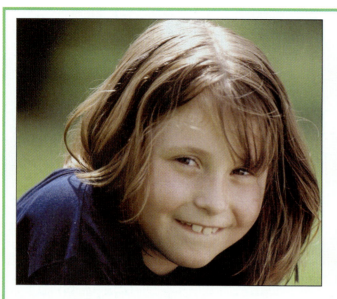

AN ICY RESCUE

Rescuers who pulled Michelle from an icy creek near her home thought she was dead. The child's eyes stared dully ahead, her body was chilled and blue, and her heart had stopped beating. The two-and-a-half year old had been under the icy water for more than an hour. By all basic measurements of life, she was dead.

Years ago, Michelle's family would have prepared for her funeral. Instead, paramedics performed CPR on Michelle's still body as they rushed her to a children's medical centre, where doctors took over her care. Doctors there used a heart-lung machine for Michelle, which warmed the blood, provided oxygen and removed carbon dioxide. As Michelle's temperature rose, the comatose child gasped. Soon her heart was pumping on its own.

Doctors once believed the brain could not survive more than 5 to 7 minutes without oxygen, but miraculous survivals such as Michelle's have changed opinions. Ironically, researchers have determined that freezing water actually helps to protect the body from drowning.

In icy water, a person's body temperature begins to drop almost as soon as the body hits the water. The body loses heat in water 32 times faster than it does in the air. Swallowing water accelerates this cooling. As the body's core temperature drops, so does the metabolic rate drop. Activity in the cells almost comes to a standstill, and they require very little oxygen. Any oxygen left in the blood is diverted from other parts of the body to the brain and heart.

This state of suspended animation allows humans to survive underwater four to five times longer than doctors once believed was possible. Nearly 20 cases of miraculous survivals have been documented in medical journals, although unsuccessful cases are rarely described. Most cases involve children who were 15 minutes or longer in water temperatures of 5°C or less. Children survive better because their bodies cool faster than adult bodies.

Researchers once theorised that the physiological responses were caused by a "mammalian dive reflex" similar to a response found in whales and seals. They believed the same dive mechanism which allowed whales and seals to stay underwater for long periods of time was triggered in drowning humans. However, experiments have failed to support the idea, and many researchers now say that the best explanation for the slowdown is simply the body's response to extreme cold.

After being attached to the heart-lung machine for nearly an hour, Michelle was moved into an intensive care unit. She stayed in a coma for more than a week. She was blind for a short period, and doctors weren't sure she would recover. But slowly she began to respond. First she smiled when her parents came into the room, and soon she was talking like a two-and-a-half year old again. After Michelle left the hospital, she suffered a tremor from nerve damage, but she was one of the lucky ones—eventually she regained her sight, full balance and co-ordination.

Although breakthroughs have saved many lives, parents still must be vigilant around their children and others near water. Most near-drowning victims are not as lucky as Michelle. One out of every three survivors suffer neurological damage. There is no substitute for close supervision.

Care for Hypothermia

Hypothermia is a medical emergency, so follow the emergency action principles. Carry out a primary survey and care for any life-threatening problems. Call an ambulance. Follow these first aid guidelines:

1. If insulation or shelter is available, remove any wet clothing and dry the victim. If shelter is not available, wrap something dry over the victim's wet clothing to prevent exposure to cold wind that would chill the body at a rapid rate. Be extremely gentle in handling the person.

2. Warm the body gradually by wrapping the victim in blankets or putting on dry clothing and removing them to a warm environment. If available, apply hot water bottles, heating pads (if the victim is dry) or other heat sources to the armpits and groins. Keep a barrier, such as a blanket, towel or clothing, between the heat source and the victim to avoid burning the skin. If no other heat source is available, the rescuer's own body heat may be used.

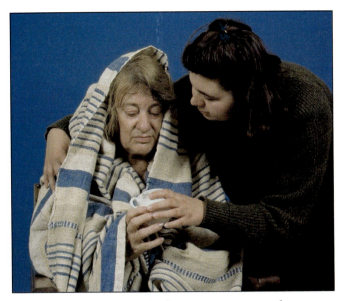

FIGURE 11-19 *For a hypothermia victim, rewarm the body gradually.*

3. If the victim is alert, give the victim warm liquids to drink (Figure 11-19).

4. Do not warm the victim too quickly, for example, by immersing the victim in warm water. Rapid rewarming of the whole body can cause the onset of dangerous heart rhythms.

In cases of severe hypothermia, the victim may be unconscious, breathing may have slowed or stopped and the pulse may be slow and irregular. The body may feel stiff as the muscles become rigid. Monitor the ABC, give EAR if necessary, and continue to warm the victim until ambulance personnel arrive. Be prepared to start CPR and continue until help arrives.

Hypothermia in Infants

Infants more commonly suffer from hypothermia because their body temperature regulating systems are not well developed. You cannot judge whether the infant has hypothermia from appearance alone, because the infant may look very healthy, with pink hands, feet and face. The following changes in behaviour are the signs of hypothermia:

- when the infant is unusually quiet
- when the infant seems limp and drowsy
- when the infant refuses food.

The first aid for infants with hypothermia is the same as for adults.

Consuming alcohol usually makes a person feel warmer. Would you recommend that people drink alcohol in moderation on a cold day to keep warm? Why or why not?

SUMMARY OF FIRST AID FOR HEAT AND COLD EMERGENCIES

COLD EMERGENCIES

Frostbite

- Cover affected area.
- Handle gently; never rub.
- Soak affected part in warm water.
- Do not let affected part touch the bottom or sides of the container.
- Keep the affected part in water until it is pink and warm.
- Cover with dry, soft, clean dressing.

Hypothermia

- Call an ambulance.
- Try to find shelter; protect the victim from wind chill.
- Warm the body gradually by wrapping it in blankets or putting on dry clothing, or by using body heat.
- Apply available heat sources (covered hot water bottle or heating pad) to armpits or groin area if the victim is dry, but not to extremities; use rescuer's body heat if necessary.
- Give warm liquids to an alert victim.
- Do not rewarm the victim too quickly.
- Handle gently.

HEAT EMERGENCIES

Muscular Cramps

- Help the victim to rest in a cool place.
- Give the victim cool water.
- Stretch the muscle and massage the area.

Heat-Related Illness

- Help the victim to rest in a cool place.
- Give the victim cool water.
- Monitor the victim's condition for signs of deterioration.
- Loosen tight clothing.
- Remove perspiration-soaked clothing.
- Apply cool, wet cloths to skin, and fan the victim.
- Monitor the condition carefully.
- Call an ambulance immediately.
- Cool the body by any means available:
  —wet towels or sheets
  —ice packs to armpits and/or groins.
- Monitor the ABC.
- Be prepared to perform EAR or CPR.

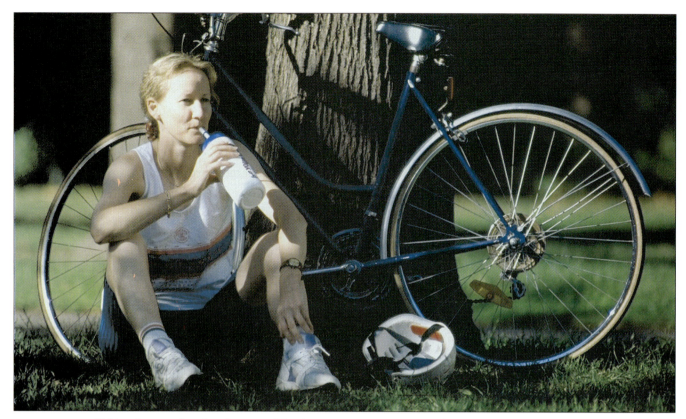

FIGURE 11-20 *Taking frequent breaks when exercising in extreme temperatures allows your body to readjust to normal body temperature.*

PREVENTING HEAT AND COLD EMERGENCIES

Generally, illnesses caused by overexposure to extreme temperatures are preventable. To prevent heat or cold emergencies from happening to you or anyone you know, follow these guidelines:

- Avoid being outdoors in the hottest or coldest part of the day.
- Change your activity level according to the temperature.
- Take frequent breaks.
- Dress appropriately for the environment.
- Drink large amounts of fluids.
- Consume regular, nutritious meals.

The easiest way to prevent illness caused by temperature extremes is to avoid being outside during the part of the day when temperatures are most intense. For instance, if you plan to work out-of-doors in hot weather, plan your activity for the early morning and evening hours when the sun is not as strong. Likewise, if you must be out-of-doors on cold days, plan your activities for the warmest part of the day.

Not everyone can avoid extremes of temperature however. Often work or other situations require exposure to extreme conditions. But you can take additional precautions such as changing your activity level and taking frequent breaks. For instance, in very hot conditions, exercise only for brief periods then rest in a cool, shaded area. Frequent breaks allow your body to readjust to normal body temperature, enabling it to better withstand brief periods of exposure to extremes of temperature (Figure 11-20). Avoid heavy exercise during the hottest or coldest part of the day. Extremes of temperature promote fatigue, which hampers the body's ability to adjust.

Always wear clothing appropriate to the environmental conditions and your activity level. When possible, wear light coloured cotton clothing in the heat. Cotton absorbs perspiration and lets air circulate through the material. This lets heat escape and perspiration evaporate, cooling the body. Light coloured clothing reflects the sun's rays.

When you are in the cold, wear layers of clothing made of tightly woven fibres, such as wool, that trap warm air against your body. Wear a head covering in both heat and cold. A hat protects the head from the sun's rays in the summer and prevents heat from escaping in the winter. Also protect other areas of the body, such as the fingers, toes, ears and nose from cold exposure by wearing protective coverings.

Whether in heat or cold, always drink enough fluids and eat regularly. Drinking plenty of fluids is the most important thing you can do to prevent heat- or cold-related illnesses. Just as you would drink cool fluids in the summer, drink warm fluids in the winter. Cool and warm fluids help the body maintain a normal temperature. If cold or hot drinks are not available, drink plenty of plain water. Do not drink beverages containing caffeine or alcohol, which hinder the body's temperature-regulating mechanism. In a cold environment, eating regular meals supplies your body with enough fuel for your activity.

Summary

Burns

- Burn injuries damage the layers of the skin and sometimes internal structures as well.

- When caring for a burn victim, first ensure your own safety by making sure the scene is safe, and follow the emergency action principles.

- Follow the basic steps of burn care:

  —Call an ambulance for serious burns.

  —Cool the burned area with water to minimise additional tissue destruction.

  —Keep air away from the burned area by covering it with dry, sterile dressings or dry, clean sheets or other cloth.

  —Take steps to prevent infection.

  —Maintain the victim's body temperature to minimise shock.

  —Check for inhalation injury if the person has a heat or chemical burn. With electrical burns, check carefully for additional problems such as breathing difficulty, cardiac problems and fractures.

Exposure to heat and cold

Overexposure to extreme heat and cold may cause a person to become ill. The severity of illness depends on factors such as physical activity, clothing, wind, humidity, working and living conditions and the person's age and physical condition.

- Heat cramps may indicate a person is in the early stage of a heat-related illness.

- For heat exhaustion and heat stroke, urge the victim to stop physical activity, cool the victim appropriately and call an ambulance.

- Frostbite and hypothermia are both serious cold-related conditions, and the victim of either needs medical care.

- For both hypothermia and frostbite, rewarm the victim appropriately.

Answers to Application Questions

1. In an effort to cool the body, blood flow to the skin is increased, bringing warm blood to the surface and allowing heat to escape. As more blood flows to the skin, blood flow to vital organs, such as the brain, is reduced. This reduction of blood flow causes a lack of oxygen-rich blood in the brain, creating a temporary decline in the level of consciousness and making the person feel weak and dizzy, or faint. A person who feels faint should lie down and rest in a cool place and sip cool water.

2. Although consuming alcohol makes you feel warm, it actually decreases body temperature. When you drink alcohol, blood vessels dilate and blood flow to the skin increases, causing the loss of body heat through the skin. Therefore, alcohol should not be consumed on a cold day in an attempt to keep warm.

Study Questions

1. *Match each term with the correct definition.*

    a Cryogenic burn.

    b Critical burn.

    c Radiation burn.

    d Superficial burn.

    e Partial-thickness burn.

    f Full-thickness burn.

    _____ Any burn that is potentially life-threatening, disabling or disfiguring.

    _____ A burn that destroys skin and underlying tissues.

    _____ A burn caused by contact with an extremely cold substance.

    _____ A burn caused by the sun or other sources.

    _____ A burn which damages only the top layer of skin.

    _____ A burn that destroys the skin but not the tissues underneath.

2. *List four causes of burn injury.*

3. *List three types of burn injury.*

4. *In caring for an electrical burn injury, you must first:*

    a. remove the victim from the power source

    b. do a primary survey

    c. make sure the power source is turned off

    d. look for two burn sites

5. *Burns that require professional medical attention:*

    a. cover more than one body part

    b. are those resulting from electricity, explosions or chemicals

    c. are burns whose victims are having difficulty breathing.

    d. a and c.

    e. a, b and c.

6. *The laboratory technician at the lab bench near you has spilt a corrosive chemical and you can see reddening of the lower arm and hand. You should first:*

    a. remove the chemical with a clean cloth

    b. put a sterile dressing over the burn site

    c. flush the burn with water

    d. have the victim remove contaminated clothes

7. *Match each term with the correct definition.*

a. Frostbite.

b. Muscular cramps.

c. Heat exhaustion.

d. Heat stroke.

e. Hypothermia.

_____ A shock caused by strenuous work or exercise in a hot environment. Symptoms and signs include cool, moist, pale or red skin; headache; nausea; and dizziness.

_____ A life-threatening body cooling that develops when the body's warming mechanisms fail to maintain normal body temperature.

_____ A life-threatening condition that develops when the body's cooling mechanism fails.

_____ The freezing of body tissues caused by overexposure to cold.

_____ Painful spasms of skeletal muscles that develop following heavy exercise or work outdoors in warm or moderate temperatures.

Use the following scenario to answer questions 8 to 10.

You and your mother are working in the yard. It is a sunny, humid day. Your mother is wearing her usual gardening outfit, which includes a floppy hat and a white cotton shirt. You are wearing a navy blue tank top and a pair of jeans.

You have been working for nearly 2 hours when you feel a sudden chill. You shake it off and continue working. While your mother has gone inside, you take a drink of her water. Although she has had several glasses, you have not really felt thirsty and have not had anything to drink.

When your mother returns, she notices you look pale and are sweating heavily. She asks how you feel. You reply that you feel weak. In fact, you also feel a little nauseated and dizzy.

Your mother insists that you stop working and go inside or at least sit in the shade for a while. As you stand up to move to the shade, you feel dizzy and weak.

8. *List the symptoms and signs of heat exhaustion you find in the scenario.*

9. *List the actions you could have taken to prevent heat exhaustion.*

10. *Now that you are out of the sun, what care should your mother give?*

Use the following scenario to answer questions 11 and 12.

You and a friend have been skiing all morning. The snow is great, but it is really cold. Your friend has complained of freezing hands and feet for the last half hour or so and has now lost all sensation in the fingers and toes. You decide to return to the ski lodge. Once inside, you help your friend to remove mittens and ski boots, and notice waxy and white fingers which feel very cold to touch.

11. *List the symptoms and signs of frostbite you find in the scenario.*

12. *How would you care for your friend's hands and feet?*

Answers are in Appendix A (page 362).

Wounds

A **WOUND** is an injury to the skin, sometimes also injuring underlying muscle and other organs. Wounds may bleed profusely or little, and may involve extensive or minor damage to the skin and other tissues. Wounds in different body areas require different attention. All wounds that include a break in the skin put the body at risk of infection; thus, all wounds require first aid.

This chapter outlines how to care for a major wound which requires medical treatment and a minor wound which you may treat yourself.

For Review

A basic understanding of the structure of the skin and the circulatory system, the inter-relationship of the body systems (Chapter 2), how to control bleeding (Chapter 5) and how to care for shock (Chapter 6) will help your understanding of the chapter.

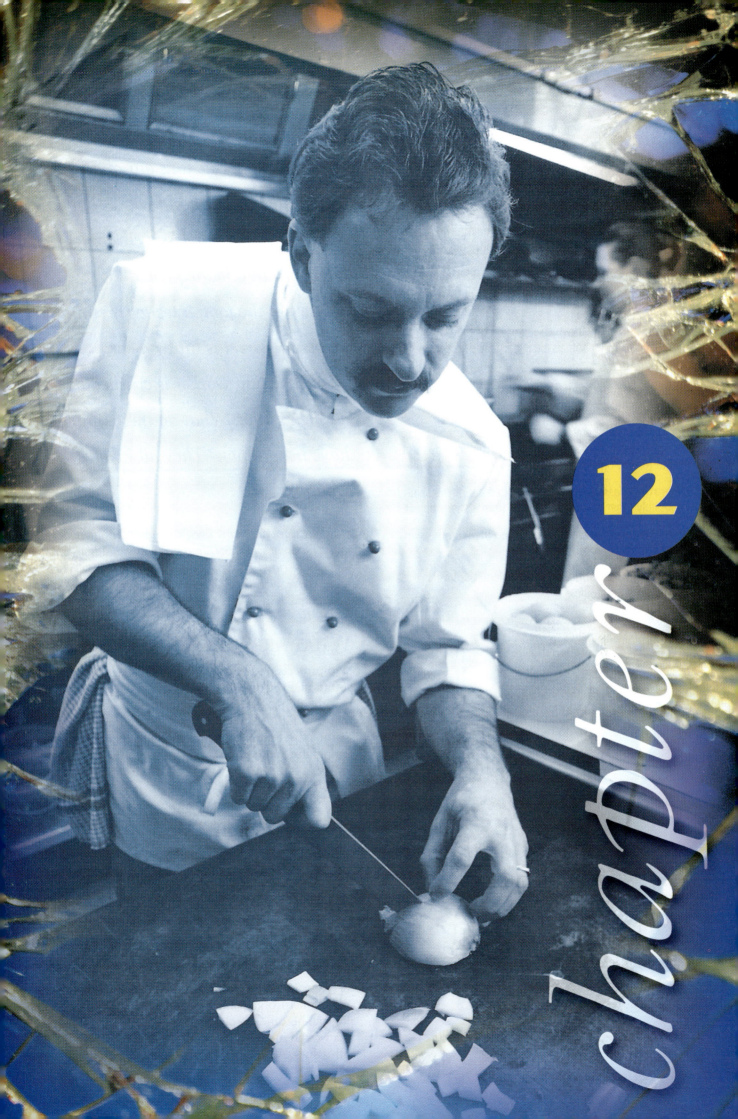

12

chapter

Key Terms

Abrasion: An open wound in which the skin has been rubbed or scraped away; often called a graze.

Amputation: An injury in which an appendage, such as a finger or toe, arm or leg, has been completely severed from the body.

Antiseptic: A substance which helps to limit the growth and spread of micro-organisms in and around a wound.

Asepsis *(ay-sep-sis):* Protection against infection by using sterile techniques in wound cleaning and other procedures.

Avulsion: An injury in which a portion of the skin and sometimes other soft tissue is partially or completely torn away.

Closed wound: A wound in which soft tissue damage occurs beneath unbroken skin.

Disinfectant: A chemical used to destroy harmful micro-organisms; it is stronger than an antiseptic and is not safe for use on human skin.

Laceration *(lass-e-ray-shon):* A jagged cut of the skin and possibly other soft tissue, usually from a sharp object.

Open wound: A wound resulting in a break in the skin surface.

Soft tissue: Body structures that include the layers of skin, fat and muscles.

Wound: An injury to the skin which sometimes involves underlying soft tissues.

A toddler scrapes her knee while learning to run; a child needs stitches in his chin after he falls out of a tree; a woman cuts her hand while chopping wood; a farmer carelessly climbing over a fence with a loaded rifle shoots himself in the foot; a teenager running across the street is hit by a car; a construction worker is crushed by a fallen girder. What do these injuries have in common? They all involve wounds.

In our work and daily lives, wounds occur often and in many different ways. Fortunately, most wounds are minor and can be cared for easily. Some wounds, however, are more severe, bleed heavily and require immediate medical attention.

WHAT ARE WOUNDS?

Skin protects underlying body structures, including **soft tissues** (Figure 12-1). In Chapter 2, you learned that the skin is the largest single organ of the body and that without it the body could not function. It provides a protective barrier for the body, helps regulate body temperature and, through the nerves in the skin, sends important information about the environment to the brain.

The skin has two layers. The outer layer of skin, the epidermis, provides a barrier to bacteria and other organisms which can cause infection. The deeper layer, called the dermis, contains the important structures of the nerves, the sweat and oil glands and the blood vessels. The skin is well supplied with blood vessels and nerves; therefore, most superficial injuries are likely to bleed and be painful. Beneath the skin lies a layer of fat, and beneath the fat layer lie the muscles.

Any injury to the skin or soft tissues beneath threatens the body. Injuries causing breaks in the skin carry great risk of infection. Because the skin tends to collect micro-organisms, injuries involving breaks in the skin can become infected unless properly cared for.

A wound includes injury to the skin or underlying soft tissues. Wounds can be either closed or open.

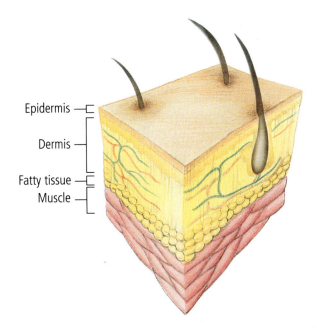

FIGURE 12-1 *Layers of skin, fat and muscle form a protective soft tissue layer for the body.*

Closed Wounds

A wound is called a **closed wound** when the damage occurs beneath the surface of the skin, leaving the outer layer intact. The simplest closed wound is a bruise, also called a contusion. Bruises result when the body is subjected to a force, such as when you bump your leg on a table or chair, which results in damage to soft tissue layers and vessels beneath the skin, causing internal bleeding.

Open Wounds

A wound is called an **open wound** if there is a break in the skin's outer layer. Open wounds usually result in external bleeding. The break can be as minor as a scrape of the surface layer of skin or as severe as a deep penetration into or through the body. The amount of bleeding depends on the severity of the injury. However, any break in the skin provides an entry point for disease-producing micro-organisms.

Types of Wounds

Wounds are classified according to the type of damage done to the skin and tissues below, which depends on the forces or objects that caused the injury. The chart on pages 204 to 207 illustrates and describes the main types of wounds.

1 *Why is an open wound often more serious than a closed wound?*

CARE OF MAJOR WOUNDS

When caring for any open wound, you need to first decide whether the wound is major or minor. Consider a wound to be minor only if damage to the skin is superficial, bleeding is minimal and stops quickly, and the wound is smaller than 2.5 centimetres. Consider all other wounds to be major wounds requiring immediate medical attention.

Although the general principles of care are the same for all major wounds, the specific first aid depends on the type of wound and, in some cases, its location on the body.

Follow these principles of care for all major wounds:

1. Put a dressing on the wound and control the bleeding (Figure 12-2). Chapter 5 describes how to use pressure dressings and other techniques to control bleeding.

2. Call an ambulance or otherwise get the victim to medical attention immediately.

3. Once bleeding has been controlled, do not remove the dressing, because bleeding can easily start again.

4. Do not try to clean the wound. Hospital or medical personnel will clean the wound and take other necessary measures to prevent infection.

5. If the bleeding is severe, be prepared also to treat the victim for shock.

In addition to this general care, different types of wounds require specific care as described in the following sections.

Remember:
Never apply pressure over a fracture.

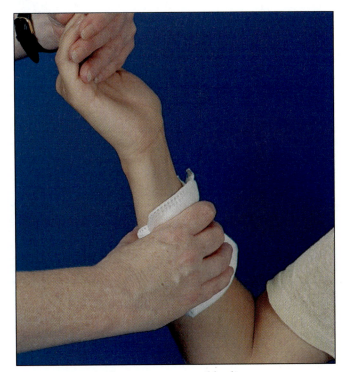

FIGURE 12-2 *Apply pressure to stop bleeding.*

TYPES OF WOUNDS

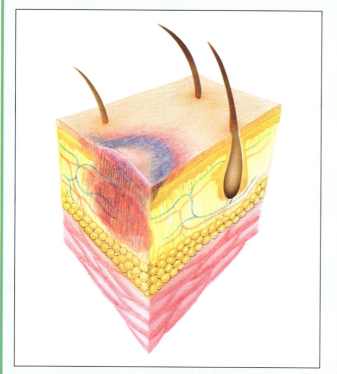

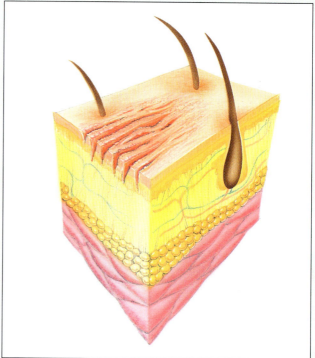

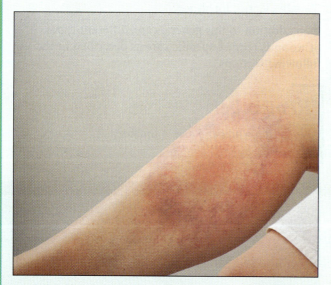

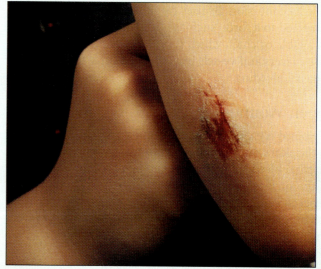

Bruise (Contusion)

A bruise, or contusion, is an injury to soft tissue layers and vessels beneath the skin, causing internal bleeding. When blood and other fluids seep into the surrounding tissues, the area discolours and swells. The amount of discolouration and swelling varies depending on the severity of the injury. At first, the area may only appear red. Over time more fluid leaks into the area, which turns dark red or purple. Violent forces can cause more severe soft tissue injuries involving larger blood vessels and the deeper layers of muscle tissue. These injuries can result in profuse bleeding beneath the skin.

Abrasion

An abrasion is the most common type of open wound. It is characterised by skin which has been rubbed or scraped away. This often occurs when a child falls and scrapes a hand or knee. An abrasion is sometimes called a carpet burn, gravel rash or strawberry. The scraping away of the outer skin layers exposes sensitive nerve endings, so an abrasion is usually painful. Bleeding is usually not severe, because only the small capillaries are affected. Because of the way the injury occurs, dirt and other matter can become embedded in the skin, making it especially important to clean the wound thoroughly.

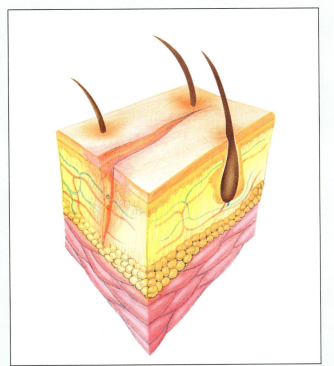

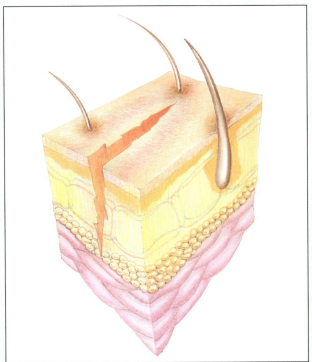

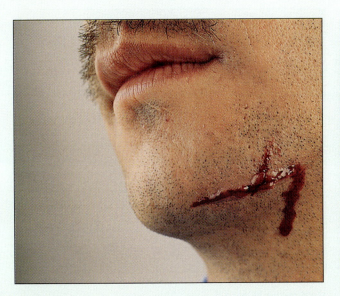

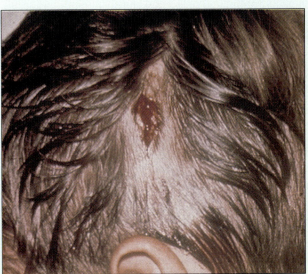

Incision

An incision is a cut, usually from a sharp object, with smooth edges. Incisions are commonly caused by sharp-edged objects such as knives, scissors or broken glass. Deep incisions can affect the layers of fat and muscle, damaging both nerves and blood vessels. Incisions usually bleed profusely, depending on the structures involved. Nerves may also be injured.

Laceration

A laceration is like an incision but has jagged edges. Lacerations are commonly caused by sharp-edged objects but can also result when a blunt force splits the skin. This often occurs in areas where bone lies directly under the skin's surface, such as the chin. Like incisions, deep lacerations can affect the layers of fat and muscle. Both nerves and blood vessels may be damaged and severe bleeding may occur.

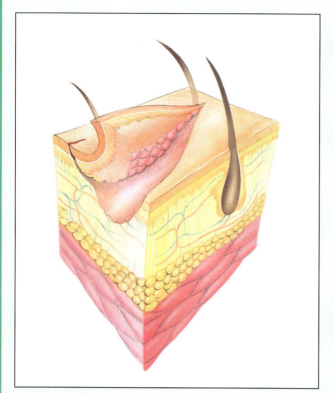

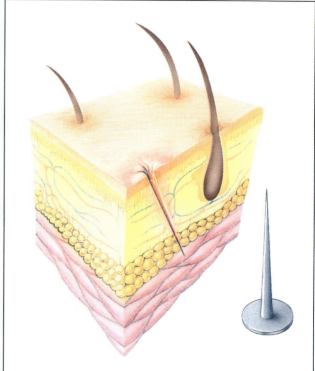

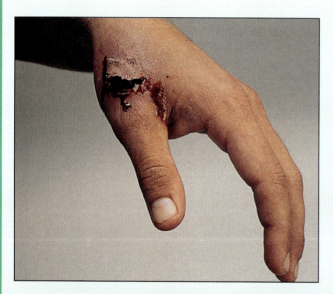

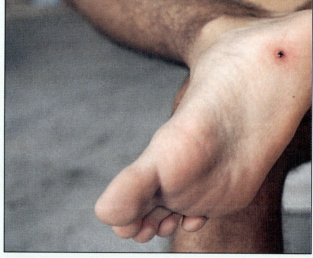

Avulsion

An avulsion is an injury in which a portion of the skin and sometimes other soft tissues are partially or completely torn away. A partially avulsed piece of skin may remain attached but hang like a flap. Bleeding is usually significant because avulsions often involve deeper soft tissue layers. Sometimes a force is so violent that a body part, such as a finger, may be severed. An appendage that is severed is called an amputation. Although damage to the tissue is severe, bleeding is usually not as bad as you might expect. The blood vessels usually constrict and pull in at the point of injury, slowing bleeding and making it relatively easy to control with direct pressure. Often a completely severed body part can be successfully reattached with surgery.

Puncture Wound

A puncture wound results when the skin is pierced with a pointed object such as a nail, a piece of glass, a splinter, a knife, a bullet or an animal bite. The skin usually closes around the penetrating object, therefore external bleeding is generally not severe. However, internal bleeding can be severe if the penetrating object damages major blood vessels or internal organs. Puncture wounds are also potentially dangerous because they readily become infected. Objects penetrating the soft tissues carry micro-organisms that cause infections.

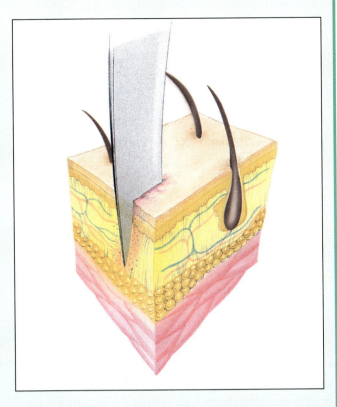

TETANUS

Of particular danger is the possibility of infection with tetanus, a micro-organism which is commonly found in soil, particularly where fertilisers or animal excrement is present. Tetanus produces a powerful poison which enters the nervous system and affects specific muscles; for example, jaw muscles contract causing "lockjaw." Once tetanus reaches the nervous system its effects are serious and may be life threatening. Therefore, people working outdoors or in areas where the tetanus bacillus is prevalent should keep their tetanus immunisations up to date. ■

2 *Why is tetanus immunisation important?*

Abrasions

Abrasions are usually minor wounds with slight bleeding that soon stops on its own. Cleaning and covering the wound with a non-adherent dressing may be the only care needed (see the later section on minor wounds).

However, the risk of infection with a larger abrasion necessitates medical attention. In this case, apply a sterile non-adherent dressing or pad after cleaning the wound, and bandage it in place. The victim should seek prompt medical advice.

Blast Wounds

Blast wounds result from an explosion such as may occur with the ignition of fumes accumulating in an industrial setting or home. Blasts create a high pressure wave which impacts on the body and may injure the lungs and other organs. The blast also may result in flames or flying debris, which can cause additional injury such as fractures and burns.

The symptoms and signs of a blast injury may include coughing up frothy blood-tinged fluid, possible bleeding from the ears, multiple soft tissue injuries, possible fractures and the symptoms and signs of shock.

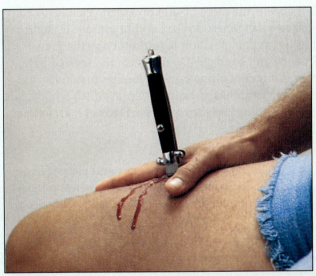

Embedded Object

An object that remains in a puncture wound is called an embedded object. As with other puncture wounds, external bleeding is generally not severe. However, internal bleeding can be severe if the penetrating object damages major blood vessels or internal organs. Infection is also a potential risk.

After calling an ambulance, provide the following care:

1. Help the victim into the most comfortable position, often partly sitting up with the head and shoulders supported.

2. Control bleeding and care for wounds and burns.

3. Immobilise any fractures (see Chapter 14).

4. Continue to monitor the victim's condition closely and treat the victim for shock.

5. If the victim becomes unconscious, place the victim on the side and care for the airway, breathing and circulation following the Basic Life Support flow chart (page 35).

Crush Wounds

A crush wound occurs when something large and heavy strikes or falls on the victim (Figure 12-3). The victim may be struck by a car, for example, or hit by a falling girder. Crush injuries are often very serious because of injury to bones as well as extensive soft tissue damage. Even if the victim seems relatively uninjured immediately after being extricated from the crushing force, internal injury can soon lead to a life-threatening condition.

If the crushing force remains in place for more than an hour, the person's blood pressure may drop because of extensive bleeding into the injured area and severe shock may develop. Damaged muscle tissues may have released toxins that accumulate in the injured area. Releasing the victim from the pressure of the crushing

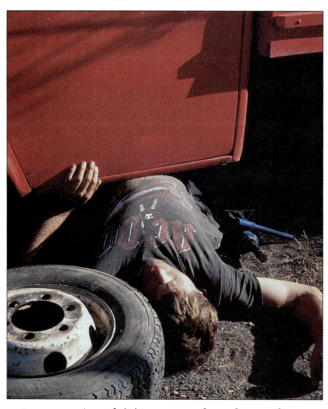

FIGURE 12-3 *A crush injury occurs when a large or heavy object falls on a person.*

object may allow these toxins to flood into other parts of the body, causing further damage such as kidney failure.

The symptoms and signs of a crush injury include numbness or tingling in the crushed limb or area, swelling and rigidity in the area, bruising, symptoms and signs of shock, and symptoms and signs of fractures (see Chapter 14).

Follow these guidelines of care for a crush injury:

1. Remove the crushing force **immediately** if possible. If the victim has been trapped longer than 60 minutes, call the emergency services but do not release the person.

2. Control the bleeding and call an ambulance.

3. Treat for shock.

4. Immobilise any fracture.

5. Monitor the victim's condition while waiting for the ambulance.

Lacerations, Incisions, Avulsions and Amputations

Lacerations, incisions, **avulsions** and **amputations** are similar in that the injury is caused by a shearing force from something sharp. Controlling the bleeding is the first goal. If the piece of skin or appendage is avulsed, such as a dangling skin flap, do not remove it. Return it to its original position before applying the pressure dressing and bandage. Do not wash the severed part, even if it is contaminated with foreign material.

If the victim has an amputation in which a body part has been completely severed (see Figure 12-4), follow these guidelines:

1. Control any bleeding.

2. Retrieve the severed body part and place it in a plastic bag. Gently inflate the bag by trapping surrounding air to protect the part. Seal the bag.

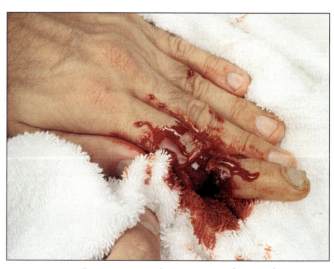

FIGURE 12-4 *In an amputation an appendage such as a finger is completely removed.*

3. If possible, keep the part cool by floating the bag in a container of water with a few ice cubes added (Figure 12-5). Avoid direct contact between the part and ice.

4. Mark the package with the victim's name and the time of the injury.

5. Make sure the part is transported to the medical facility with the victim.

Puncture Wounds, Embedded Objects and High Velocity Wounds

A puncture wound is often serious, even if bleeding is light. The victim needs immediate medical attention because of the risk of infection and possibility of injury to internal organs.

A small foreign body in a wound can be removed if you can wipe it off easily or rinse it off with cold water. If a larger embedded object is still in the wound, follow these additional guidelines:

1. *Do not* remove the object, because it may be plugging the wound and restricting bleeding.

2. Squeeze the edges of the wound together around the object to put pressure on the wound.

3. Use bulky dressings to stabilise the object. Any movement can result in further tissue damage (Figure 12-6A).

4. Control bleeding by bandaging the dressings in place around the object (Figure 12-6B).

A high velocity wound occurs when an object hits the body with great speed, such as a bullet from a firearm. In such cases be sure to look for an exit wound, which may be more serious than the wound where the bullet or object entered the body. Care for both wounds and, because there may also be serious internal bleeding and injury, call an ambulance immediately.

Why should an embedded object be left in the wound?

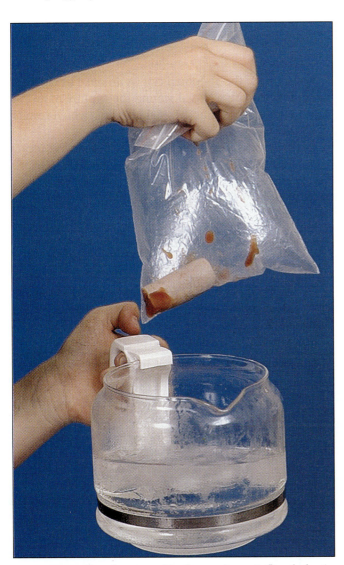

FIGURE 12-5 *Put the severed body part in an inflated plastic bag, and put the bag in ice water.*

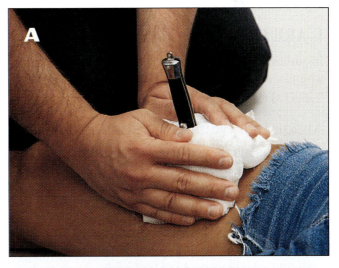

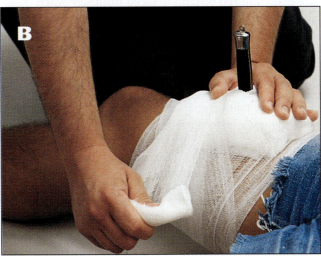

FIGURE 12-6 A *Use a bulky dressing to support an embedded object.* **B** *Use bandages over the dressing to control bleeding.*

FRONT VIEW   **BACK VIEW**

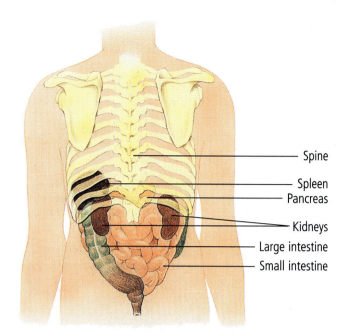

Liver
Stomach
Gallbladder
Large intestine
Small intestine

Spine
Spleen
Pancreas
Kidneys
Large intestine
Small intestine

FIGURE 12-7 *Unlike the organs of the chest or pelvis, organs in the abdominal cavity are relatively unprotected by bones.*

CARE OF SPECIAL WOUNDS

In addition to special care for different types of wounds, some wounds in certain areas of the body also require special attention.

Abdominal Wounds

The abdomen is the area immediately below the chest and above the pelvis. It is easily injured because there is no bony covering. The upper abdomen is partially protected in front by the lower ribs and at the back by the spine. The muscles of the back and abdomen also help protect the internal organs, many of which are vital (Figure 12-7). Most important are the organs that are easily injured or tend to bleed profusely when injured, such as the liver, spleen and stomach. Injuries to any of these organs can cause life-threatening internal or external bleeding and may lead to infection.

In addition to a visible abdominal wound, the symptoms and signs of a serious abdominal injury include:

- severe pain
- bruising
- external bleeding
- nausea and/or vomiting (sometimes containing blood)
- weakness
- symptoms and signs of shock
- pain, tenderness or a tight feeling in the abdomen

An injury to the abdomen can be an open or closed wound. Even with a closed wound the rupture of an organ can cause serious internal bleeding, which results in shock.

With a severe open injury, abdominal organs sometimes protrude through the wound (Figure 12-8A). To care for an open wound in the abdomen, follow these steps:

1. Carefully position the victim in a half sitting position with knees bent up, to prevent the wound from gaping open. Support the head and shoulders. Remove clothing from around the wound (Figure 12-8B).

2. *Do not* apply direct pressure on the wound, but control bleeding by carefully squeezing the edges of the wound together.

3. *Do not* try to push organs back into the abdomen.

4. Apply moist, bulky sterile dressings loosely over the wound to avoid damage to internal organs from drying out or sticking to the dressings (Figure 12-8C). (Warm tap water can be used.)

5. Secure the dressing with a broad bandage (Figure 12-8D).

6. Continue to monitor the victim's condition closely. Be prepared to treat the victim for shock.

7. If the victim becomes unconscious, place the person on the side and care for the airway, breathing and circulation following the Basic Life Support flow chart (see page 35).

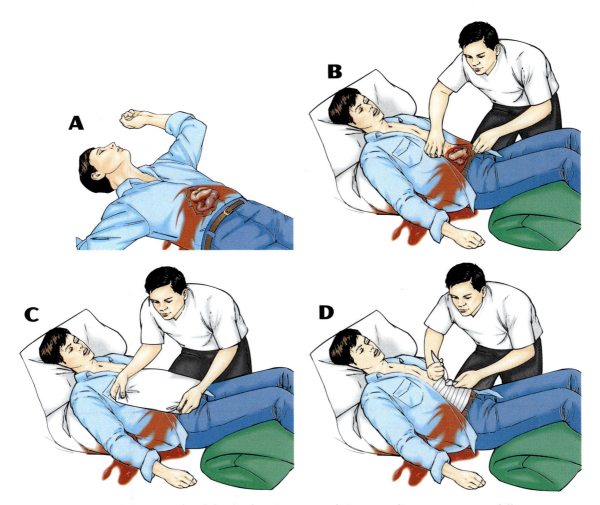

FIGURE 12-8 **A** *Severe open injuries to the abdominal cavity can result in protruding organs.* **B** *Carefully remove clothing from around the wound.* **C** *Apply a large, moist, sterile dressing loosely over the wound.* **D** *Secure the dressing with a broad bandage.*

Penetrating Chest and Back Wounds

Penetrating wounds to the chest or back range from minor to life-threatening. Stab and gunshot wounds are examples of penetrating wounds. A forceful puncture may penetrate the rib cage and allow air to enter the chest through the wound (Figure 12-9). This does not allow the lungs to function normally. The penetrating object can also injure any structure within the chest, including the lungs. Refer to Chapter 7 on the risk of pneumothorax.

*Why is it necessary to apply **moist** dressings to protruding abdominal organs?*

4

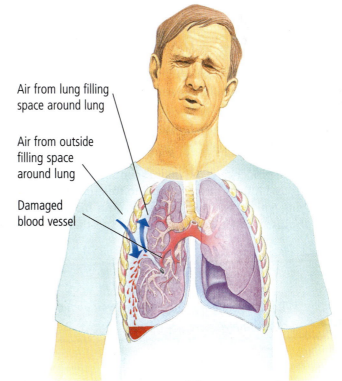

Air from lung filling space around lung

Air from outside filling space around lung

Damaged blood vessel

FIGURE 12-9 *A puncture wound that penetrates the lung, or the chest cavity surrounding the lung, allows air to go in and out of the cavity.*

INHALATION

EXHALATION

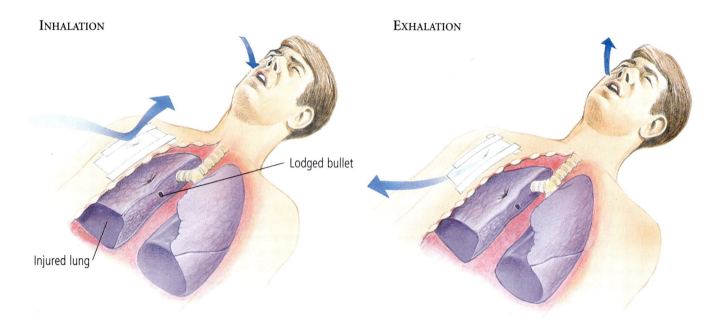

Lodged bullet

Injured lung

FIGURE 12-10 *A special dressing with the bottom unsealed keeps air from the wound during inhalation and allows air to escape during exhalation.*

Penetrating wounds cause varying degrees of internal or external bleeding. If the injury penetrates the rib cage, air can pass freely in and out of the chest cavity and the victim cannot breathe normally. With each breath the victim takes, you hear a sucking sound coming from the wound. This is the primary sign of a penetrating chest injury, called a sucking chest wound.

The symptoms and signs of a penetrating wound to the chest or back may include the following:

- pain in the chest or back
- difficulty breathing
- cyanosis seen around the mouth or in the nail beds
- frothy, blood-tinged liquid coughed up
- bloody liquid bubbling from the wound during breathing
- sucking sound with breathing
- symptoms and signs of shock

Without proper care, the victim's condition will worsen. The affected lung or lungs will fail to function and breathing will become more difficult. Your main concern in this situation is the problem of breathing.

Give the following care for penetrating chest and back wounds:

1. Assist the victim into the most comfortable position, often sitting up. Support the head and shoulders.

2. Cover the wound with a sterile dressing. For a sucking chest wound, cover the wound with a dressing that does not allow air to pass through it. If it is available, you can use aluminum foil folded several times and placed over the wound to make an effective dressing. Tape the dressing in place on three sides only. The lower edge should remain loose to keep air from entering the wound during inhalation but allowing it to escape during exhalation (Figure 12-10). If no occlusive dressing is available, use a folded cloth or, as a last resort, your hand.

3. Continue to monitor the victim's condition closely and treat the victim for shock.

4. If the victim becomes unconscious, place the person on the affected side and care for the airway, breathing and circulation following the Basic Life Support flow chart (see page 35).

What does coughing up blood tell you about a chest injury?

Why is it best to use a special dressing to care for a sucking chest wound?

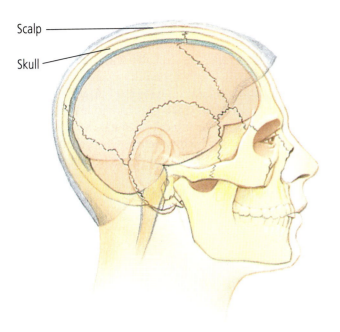

Scalp
Skull

FIGURE 12-11 *The head is easily injured because it lacks the padding of muscle and fat found in other areas of the body.*

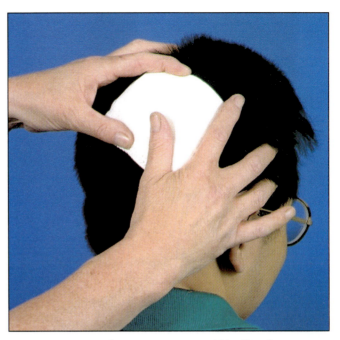

FIGURE 12-12 *Apply pressure to control bleeding from a scalp wound.*

Scalp Wounds

The head is easily injured because it lacks the padding of muscle and fat in other areas of the body. You can feel bone just beneath the surface of the skin over most of the head, including the chin, cheekbones and scalp (Figure 12-11). Bleeding from the scalp is a special concern because the skull beneath the scalp may also be injured. Because the skin is often stretched tightly over the skull, a scalp wound may gape open when the skin splits.

Scalp bleeding can be minor or severe. The bleeding is usually easily controlled with direct pressure but, because the skull may be fractured, be careful to press gently at first (Figure 12-12). If you feel a depression, a spongy area or bone fragments, do not put direct pressure on the wound. As with all head injuries, call an ambulance. If you suspect a fracture, control the bleeding with gentle pressure on the area around the wound. Examine the injured area carefully because the victim's hair may hide part of the wound.

If the victim has a scalp wound without a suspected fracture, give the following care:

1. Control the bleeding with firm direct pressure.

2. Apply a dressing and hold it in place with your hand.

3. Secure the dressing with a roller or triangular bandage (Figure 12-13).

4. Help the victim into a comfortable position lying down with head and shoulders raised.

5. Continue to monitor the victim's condition closely. Be prepared to treat the victim for shock.

6. If the victim becomes unconscious, place the person on the side and care for the airway, breathing and circulation following the Basic Life Support flow chart (see page 35).

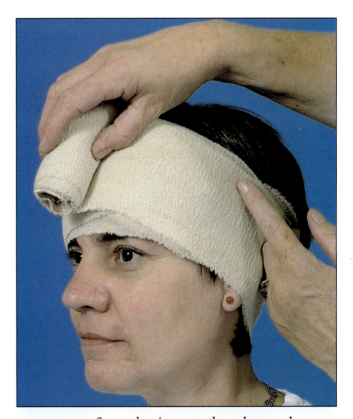

FIGURE 12-13 *Secure dressings onto the scalp wound with a bandage.*

Remember:

A victim who has sustained a blow severe enough to damage the scalp may suffer from concussion or other head injuries.

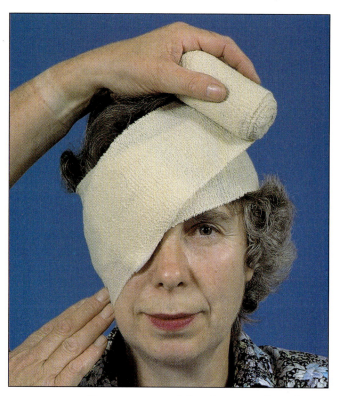

FIGURE 12-14 *For an eye wound, bandage a sterile pad over the eye.*

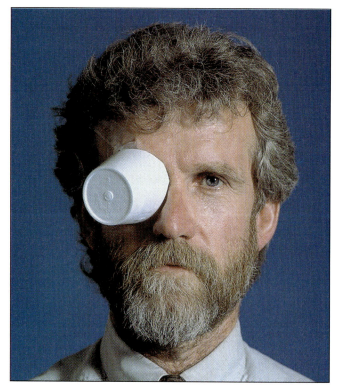

FIGURE 12-15 *For an object impaled in the eye, use a paper cup over the object to support it before bandaging.*

Eye Injuries

Injuries to the eye can involve the bone and soft tissue surrounding the eye, or the eyeball itself. Blunt objects like a fist or a baseball may injure the eye area, or a smaller object may penetrate the eyeball. Any eye injury might be serious as even small injuries can lead to scarring of the cornea or infection, which can later affect vision. Injuries which penetrate the eyeball or cause the eye to be removed from its socket are very serious and can cause blindness.

Symptoms and signs of an eye injury may include:

- impaired or total loss of vision in the injured eye
- pain in the eye
- copious tears in the eye
- spasm of the eyelids
- loss of blood or fluid from the eye

After calling an ambulance, follow these guidelines to help a victim with an eye injury:

1. Assist the victim to rest in the most comfortable position. Support the head and advise the victim to avoid movement.

2. If there is no object embedded in the eye, cover the injured eye with a sterile pad. Bandage the pad in place without putting any pressure on the eyeball (Figure 12-14).

3. Do not attempt to remove any object embedded in the eye. If an object is protruding from the eye, place a sterile dressing around the object and bandage it in place. Stabilise the embedded object in place as best you can. You can do this by taping a paper cup over the object to support it before applying a bandage (Figure 12-15).

4. Never put direct pressure on the eyeball.

5. Ask the victim to keep the unaffected eye closed to keep blood, fluid or dirt from entering it. Advise the victim to avoid moving the unaffected eye, because any movement will also involve movement of the injured eye.

Foreign bodies which get in the eye, such as dirt, sand or slivers of wood or metal, are irritating and can cause significant damage. The eye produces tears immediately in an attempt to flush out such objects. Pain from the irritation is often severe, and the victim may have difficulty opening the eye because light further irritates it.

First, try to remove the foreign body by telling the victim to blink several times, then try gently flushing the eye with water (see Figures 11-9 and 11-10 in Chapter 11). If the object remains, cover the eye with a pad held in place with tape and seek professional medical attention.

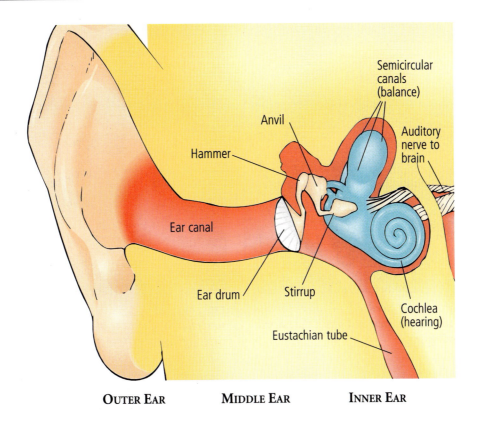

Semicircular
canals
(balance)

Anvil

Auditory
nerve to
brain

Hammer

Ear canal

Ear drum

Stirrup

Cochlea
(hearing)

Eustachian tube

OUTER EAR   **MIDDLE EAR**   **INNER EAR**

FIGURE 12-16 *A cross-section of the ear. The eardrum is easily injured by objects inserted in the ear.*

Ear Wounds

Ear injuries are common, with either the outer soft tissue of the ear or the eardrum within the ear itself being injured (Figure 12-16). Open wounds, such as lacerations or abrasions, can result from recreational injuries, such as being struck by a ball or falling off a bike. An avulsion of the ear may occur when a pierced earring catches on something and tears away from the ear. You can control bleeding from the soft tissues of the outer ear by applying direct pressure to the affected area.

If the victim has a serious head or spine injury, blood or other fluid may be in the ear canal or be draining from the ear. *Do not* attempt to stop this drainage with direct pressure.

The ear can also be injured internally. A direct blow to the head may rupture the eardrum. Sudden pressure changes, such as those caused by an explosion or a deep-water dive, can also injure the ear internally. The eardrum can be injured by an object being pushed into the ear or by falling while water skiing.

A foreign object, such as dirt or an insect, can become lodged in the ear canal. If you can easily see and grasp the object you can remove it, but do not try to remove any object by using a toothpick, cotton-tipped applicator or a sharp item of any sort. You could force the object farther into the canal or puncture the eardrum. Sometimes you can remove the object if you pull down on the earlobe and tilt the head to the affected side. If you cannot easily remove the object, seek professional medical assistance.

The symptoms and signs of a serious ear injury may include:

- pain
- deafness or impaired hearing
- bleeding from the ear
- signs related to injury within the skull: watery fluid mixed with blood from the ear, headache or an altered conscious state

After calling an ambulance, give the following first aid for a serious ear injury:

1. Assist the victim into a comfortable position, sitting up with the head tilted toward the side of the injury.

2. Loosely cover the ear with a sterile dressing, and bandage it lightly. Do not plug the ear with a dressing or try to stop the flow of blood or fluid from the ear.

3. Continue to monitor the victim's condition closely. Be prepared to treat the victim for shock.

4. If the victim becomes unconscious, place the person on the side and care for the airway, breathing and circulation following the Basic Life Support flow chart (see page 35).

Nose Wounds

Nose injuries are usually caused by a blow from a blunt object and often result in a nose bleed. High blood pressure or changes in altitude can also cause nose bleeds. Sneezing, picking the nose and blowing the

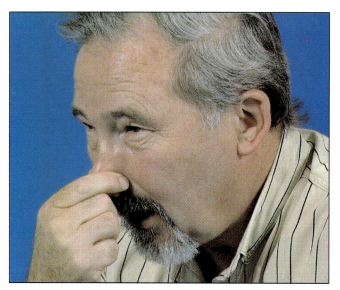

FIGURE 12-17 *To control a nose bleed, advise the victim to lean forward with the mouth open and pinch the nostrils together until the bleeding stops.*

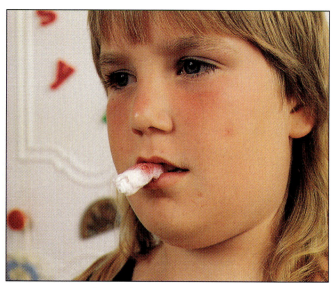

FIGURE 12-18 *If a tooth is knocked out and you are unable to replace it, cover the bleeding socket with a thick pad or dressing and ask the victim to bite on it.*

nose may also cause a nose bleed. Significant bleeding may lead to the victim inhaling or swallowing blood, which can cause a breathing problem or vomiting.

Give the following care for a nose bleed:

1. In most cases, bleeding can be controlled by asking the victim to sit with the head slightly forward while pinching the nostrils together (Figure 12-17). Instruct the victim to breathe through the mouth.

2. Ask the victim to spit out any blood in the mouth.

3. While the victim holds the nostrils closed, clean around the nose and mouth with a dressing moistened with water. Do not pack a dressing inside the nostrils.

4. When the bleeding stops, tell the victim to avoid rubbing, blowing or picking the nose, because this could restart the bleeding.

You should seek medical care if the nose bleed continues after 30 minutes, if bleeding recurs or if the person says the bleeding is the result of high blood pressure, or if a fracture of the nasal bones or skull is possible.

If you think a foreign object is in the nose, look into the nostril. If you see the object and can easily grasp it, then do so. However, do not probe the nostril with your finger. Doing so may push the object farther into the nose and cause bleeding or make it more difficult to remove later. If the object cannot be removed easily, the person should receive medical care.

Teeth and Mouth Wounds

Your primary concern for any injury to the mouth is to ensure an open airway, as mouth injuries may cause breathing problems if blood or loose teeth obstruct the airway. Swelling or a fracture may also obstruct breathing. Bleeding from mouth wounds can be extensive.

Give the following care for wounds inside the mouth:

1. If you do not suspect a serious head or spine injury, place the victim in a seated position with the head tilted slightly forward to allow any blood to drain. If the wound is on one side, tilt the head toward that side.

2. If the victim cannot sit up, place the victim on the side to allow blood to drain from the mouth.

3. Ask the victim to spit out any blood in the mouth to prevent swallowing it.

4. Put a dressing over the wound and apply pressure with the fingers. For injuries which penetrate the lip, place a rolled dressing between the lip and the gum. You can place another dressing on the outer surface of the lip. If the tongue is bleeding, apply direct pressure between thumb and forefinger over a dressing.

5. Do not rinse out the mouth because this could interfere with blood clotting. Tell the victim to drink cool or cold fluids for the rest of the day. Applying cold to the lips or tongue can also help reduce swelling and ease pain.

6. If the bleeding continues after 10 to 20 minutes, the victim should seek additional medical attention.

If one or more of the victim's teeth have been knocked out, replace the tooth if possible. If this is not possible due to other injuries, control the bleeding and save the tooth for replacement. To control the bleeding, cover the bleeding socket with a thick pad or dressing and ask the victim to bite on it and to hold it in place for 10 to 20 minutes (Figure 12-18). Do not put a dressing *into* the space left by the missing tooth. Ask the victim to spit out any blood. Follow the guidelines for mouth wounds and avoid rinsing the mouth or drinking warm fluids. Seek dental advice if the bleeding does not stop.

See the sidebar "Now Smile" (opposite page) on caring for dislodged teeth.

NOW SMILE

Knocked-out teeth no longer spell doom for pearly whites. Most dentists can successfully replace a knocked-out tooth if they can do so quickly, and if the tooth is properly cared for.

Replacing a tooth is similar to replanting a tree. On each tooth, tiny root fibres called periodontal fibres attach to the jawbone to hold the tooth in place. Inside the tooth, a canal filled with bundles of blood vessels and nerves runs from the tooth into the jawbone and surrounding tissues.

When these fibres and tissues are torn from the socket, it is important that they be replaced within 60 minutes. Generally, the sooner the tooth is replaced then the greater the chance it will survive. The knocked-out tooth must be handled carefully to protect the fragile tissues. Be careful to pick up the tooth by the chewing edge (crown) only; do not rub or handle the root part of the tooth. You may be able to replace the tooth in its socket while the victim is being transported. If not, it is best to preserve the tooth by placing it in the victim's own mouth, between the lip and gums. However, for a small child or a victim who is crying or who may swallow or aspirate the tooth, keep the tooth moistened with the victim's own saliva in a closed container until it reaches the dentist. If it is difficult to get enough saliva, use a small amount of milk. Never use water because this can damage the protective membrane and the tooth will die.

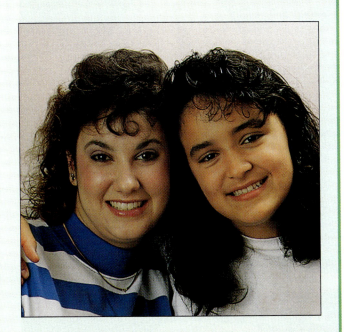

A dentist or doctor will clean the tooth, taking care not to damage the root fibres. The tooth will then be placed back into the socket and secured with a special splint. The splint keeps the tooth stable for two to three weeks while the fibres reattach to the jawbone. The bundles of blood vessels and nerves grow back within six weeks. ■

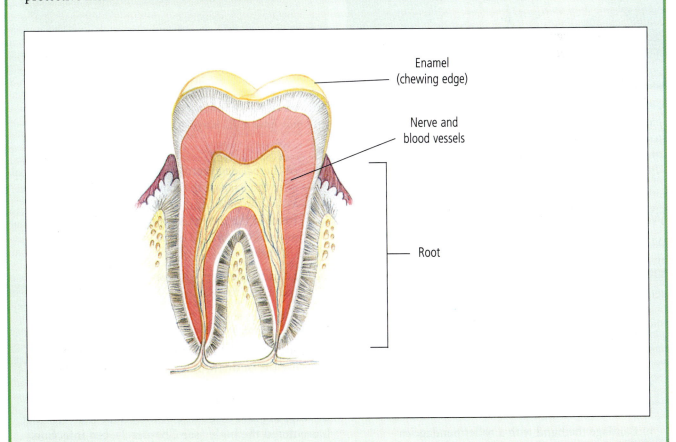

Enamel (chewing edge)

Nerve and blood vessels

Root

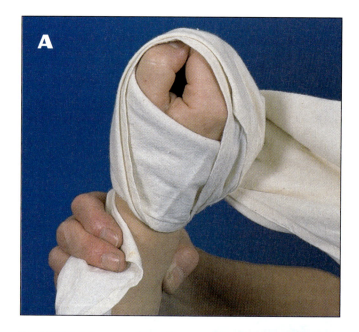

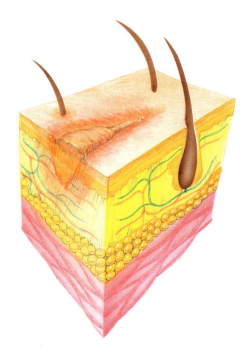

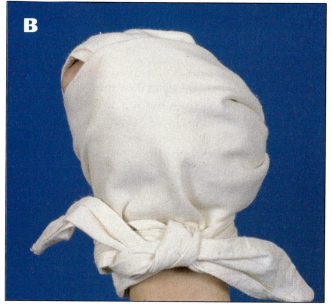

FIGURE 12-19 *Dressing and bandaging a wound in the palm of the hand.* **A** *Put a sterile dressing or pad over the wound and apply pressure.* **B** *Have the victim make a fist over the pad, and wrap a bandage as shown to hold the dressing in place.*

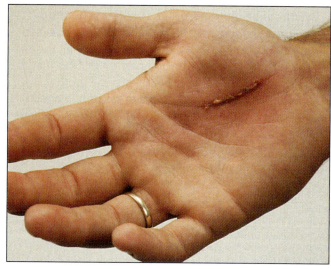

FIGURE 12-20 *An infected wound may become swollen and may have a discharge of pus.*

Wounds in the Palm of the Hand

Wounds to the palm of the hand may bleed seriously and may involve injuries to bones or nerves in the hand. Provide the following care until the victim can get medical attention:

1. Control bleeding with a sterile dressing or pad on the wound and apply pressure.

2. Help the victim to maintain pressure on the dressing by making a fist of the hand or grasping the fist of the injured hand with the other hand.

3. Elevate the extremity, with the elbow supported.

4. Bandage the hand with a roller bandage or triangular bandage (Figure 12-19). Wrap one end of the bandage across the front of the fist, then up over the back of the hand and down to the wrist. Wrap the other end of the bandage across the front of the fist in the opposite direction, and around the wrist. Tie the ends on the outside of the wrist.

5. Support the arm with an elevation sling (see Chapter 14).

Infected Wounds

Any wound can be infected by micro-organisms entering the body from the air or any object that touches the wound (Figure 12-20). The body's lymphatic system attempts to control the infection by trapping and disposing of infectious material that has entered the body (see Chapter 2), but infection can still occur.

A wound that has not begun to heal well after 2 days may be infected. Infections can spread through the body and become serious or even life-threatening.

The symptoms and signs of a infected wound may include:

- pain and soreness persisting in the wound
- swelling and redness of the wound and surrounding area
- warmth around the wound area
- pus oozing from the wound
- fever
- swelling and tenderness in lymph glands

More serious infections may cause a person to develop a fever and feel generally unwell. Anyone suspected of having an infected wound should seek medical attention as soon as possible.

CARE OF MINOR WOUNDS

Minor wounds are small, superficial wounds which usually do not need to be seen by a doctor or ambulance personnel. Consider a wound to be minor only if it meets all three of these criteria:

- The wound is shallow and damage to the skin is superficial.
- Bleeding is minimal and stops quickly.
- The wound is smaller than 2.5 centimetres.

A more extensive or deeper wound requires medical assessment and may need stitches.

The care for a minor wound includes covering the wound with a dressing to prevent infection.

Preventing Infection

Even with a minor wound, it is important to take steps to prevent infection, as micro-organisms can enter the body through even the smallest wound. Your goal is to prevent infection in both the victim and yourself and others who may come in contact with that person's blood or body fluids from the wound.

When caring for any wound, prevent infection by:

- washing your hands well
- avoiding direct contact with any wound
- wearing disposable latex gloves
- cleaning the wound carefully
- using only sterile dressings and supplies
- washing and disinfecting all used equipment
- disposing of used supplies correctly

A STITCH IN TIME...

It can be difficult to judge when a wound should be seen by a doctor for stitches. A general rule of thumb is that stitches are needed when the edges of skin do not fall together or when any wound is more than 2.5 centimetres long or on or near a joint. Stitches speed the healing process, lessen the chances of infection and reduce scarring. They should be placed within the first few hours after the injury, although it is never too late for medical treatment. The following major injuries often require stitches:

- Bleeding from an artery or uncontrollable bleeding.
- Deep cuts or avulsions that show the muscle or bone, gape widely or involve the hands or feet.
- Cuts where the wound edges may separate, such as over joints.
- Large or deep punctures.
- Large or deeply embedded objects.
- Human and animal bites.
- Wounds that, if left unattended, could leave a conspicuous scar, such as those which involve the face, especially the lip or eyebrow.

If you are caring for a wound and think it may need stitches, it probably does. Once applied, stitches are easily cared for by keeping the wound area protected and dry. If the wound gets red or swollen or if pus begins to form, notify your doctor.

Stitches in the face are often removed in less than a week. In other parts of the body, they may be left in place for 10 to 14 days. Some stitches dissolve naturally and do not require removal. ▪

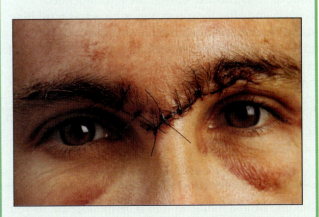

Wash your hands both before and after caring for a wound. Wash them thoroughly with soap and water (Figure 12-21). Use a sink in a rest room or utility area, not in a food preparation area. Also, wash any equipment used thoroughly before immersing any item in disinfectant solution (see next section of this chapter).

Always wear disposable latex gloves whenever there is a possibility of contacting blood or body fluids and whenever giving wound care (Figure 12-22). When wearing gloves, consider them contaminated and do not handle other objects such as a pen or comb. Do not attempt to clean or reuse disposable gloves. Remove them by peeling them off inside out, and dispose of them properly into a container reserved for contaminated waste.

See Chapter 13 for information about using sterile dressings.

Antiseptics and Disinfectants

An **antiseptic** is a substance which helps to limit the growth and spread of micro-organisms in and around a wound. In first aid, an antiseptic is usually in liquid form and may need to be diluted before use. When dilution is required, be sure to follow the manufacturer's instructions, and use accurate measuring containers. Some antiseptics are packaged for first aid use in the form of sterile swabs presoaked in the antiseptic solution. Alcohol should not be used on an open wound because it can cause pain and increase tissue damage.

In medical centres and hospitals, sterile dressings impregnated with antiseptic may be used, particularly where a wound infection would be a serious complication, such as with burns. In first aid, antiseptics are used only for cleaning minor wounds such as an abrasion and should not be used on a bleeding wound or for any injuries which will be seen by a doctor.

A **disinfectant** is a chemical used to destroy harmful micro-organisms. It is a stronger substance than an antiseptic and is not safe for use on human skin.

A disinfectant is used frequently in the sterilisation of instruments after they have been used for wound care. However, it is effective only at the recommended strength and after thorough prewashing and scrubbing of the instrument to remove blood and other body fluids. If an unwashed or dirty instrument is immersed in a disinfectant solution, harmful micro-organisms may survive, especially when an alcohol-based solution is used.

The recommended solution for chemical disinfection of instruments is 70 per cent alcoholic chlorhexidine (see Appendix B on page 364).

Cleaning a Minor Wound

Bleeding from a minor wound is easily stopped, so you can clean and care for the wound without first seeking medical attention (Fig 12-23). Follow the steps outlined in the practice guide at the end of the chapter.

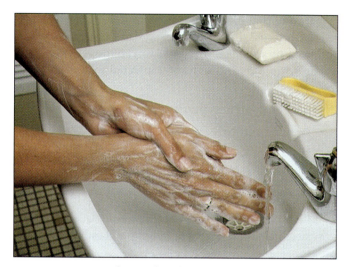

FIGURE 12-21 *Wash your hands before and after caring for a wound.*

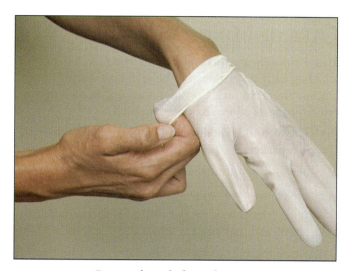

FIGURE 12-22 *Put on gloves before taking care of a wound. Fold back the cuff to avoid tearing the glove while sliding your hand in.*

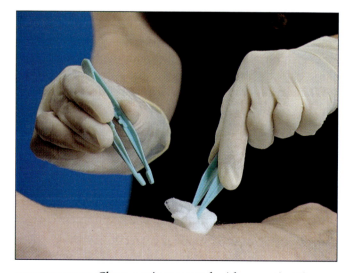

FIGURE 12-23 *Clean a minor wound with an antiseptic swab.*

Summary

- Types of wounds include contusions, abrasions, incisions, lacerations, avulsions, punctures, crush wounds and blast wounds.

- Consider all wounds to be major and in need of medical attention unless the damage is superficial, bleeding is minimal and the wound is smaller than 2.5 centimetres and does not involve a moving surface or joint.

- The care of all major wounds involves stopping the bleeding, covering the wound with a dressing and seeking medical help.

- Certain types of wounds require special treatment:
  —abdominal wounds
  —penetrating chest and back wounds
  —scalp wounds
  —eye wounds
  —ear wounds
  —nose wounds
  —teeth and mouth wounds
  —wounds in the palm of the hand
  —infected wounds
  —bites

- With all wounds take steps to prevent infection by, for example, washing hands, wearing disposable latex gloves and using sterile dressings.

- Care for minor wounds by cleaning the area, using an antiseptic and applying a sterile dressing.

Answers to Application Questions

1. Both open and closed wounds can cause injury to underlying tissue and bleeding. Open wounds can often be more serious, however, because the break in the skin surface provides an entry point for infection.

2. Tetanus is a serious infection by micro-organisms found in the soil and other outdoor locations. It can enter the body easily through any kind of open wound but is more common in puncture wounds. Everyone should keep their tetanus immunisation current to prevent the possibility of infection.

3. The embedded object may be plugging the wound and applying pressure on tissues which restricts bleeding. If the object is removed, severe bleeding may occur.

4. Moist dressings provide protection for the delicate internal organs which would otherwise be very easily damaged. The dressings should be moist to keep the organs from drying out and the dressings from sticking.

5. Coughing up blood is a sign of bleeding in the chest. This indicates that blood vessels, chest muscles and other tissues are damaged. For instance, a lung may be punctured. More importantly, coughing up blood indicates that blood is entering and to some degree obstructing the airway, which may make breathing more difficult. Coughing up blood is also a warning sign that, if the victim becomes unconscious, there is a high probability that blood will be aspirated into the lungs.

6. When air enters the chest through a wound, one or both lungs may fail to function. A special dressing, one that does not allow air to enter, prevents air from being sucked into the chest when the victim inhales, helping the victim to breathe more easily.

Study Questions

1. **Match each type of injury to its example.**

   a. Abrasion.

   b. Avulsion.

   c. Puncture.

   d. Bruise.

   _____ Torn earlobe.

   _____ Black eye.

   _____ Scraped knee.

   _____ Gunshot wound.

2. **Match each type of wound with the appropriate care.**

   a. A major open wound.

   b. A major open wound with an embedded object.

   c. A minor open wound.

   d. A severed body part.

   _____ Pack dressing around the object and then use a pressure bandage over the dressings.

   _____ Wash the wound thoroughly with soap and water.

   _____ Put in an inflated plastic bag and place into iced water.

   _____ Use bulky dressings to control bleeding.

3. **List four signs of infection.**

4. **To protect a minor open wound from infection:**

   a. wash the area with soap and water

   b. apply a clean dressing

   c. apply an antibiotic ointment.

   d. a and b.

   e. a, b and c.

5. **The differences that distinguish major open wounds from minor open wounds are:**

   a. the severity of bleeding

   b. the depth of tissue damage

   c. the amount of pain that the victim is experiencing.

   d. a and b.

   e. a, b and c.

6. *In caring for major open wounds, you should:*

  a. apply a dressing and control bleeding
  b. wash the wound
  c. recommend to the victim to get a tetanus booster shot, if necessary.
  d. a and c.
  e. a, b and c.

7. *When caring for an injury in which the body part has been completely severed, you should:*

  a. place the part directly on ice
  b. seek medical assistance and make sure the part is transported with the victim
  c. wash the body part thoroughly with soap and water
  d. place the part in sealed bag surrounded by iced water.
  e. b and d.

8. *When caring for an injury with an embedded object, you should:*

  a. remove the object
  b. allow the area to bleed freely
  c. stabilise the object in the position you find it.
  d. b and c.
  e. a, b and c.

9. *At the scene of a car crash, a victim has blood seeping from his ear. You should:*

  a. loosely cover the ear with a sterile dressing
  b. do nothing; this is a normal finding in a head injury
  c. collect the fluid in a sterile container for analysis
  d. pack the ear with sterile dressings to prevent further fluid loss

10. *Caring for an injury to the eyeball includes:*

  a. avoiding direct pressure on the eyeball
  b. removing an object penetrating the eye
  c. covering the unaffected eye.
  d. a and c.
  e. a, b and c.

11. *As you begin to apply direct pressure to control bleeding for a scalp injury, you notice a depression of the skull in the area of the bleeding. How should you alter care?*

Answers are in Appendix A (page 362).

Cleaning and Dressing a Wound

Prepare the area and the victim

- Choose an area that is clean, quiet and well lit. Ensure that the surface of the working area has been well cleaned. Assist the victim to assume a comfortable position with the wound accessible for cleaning.

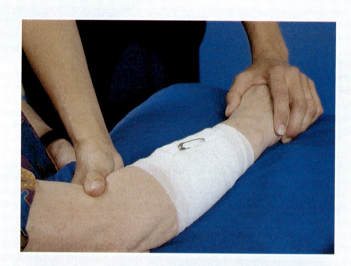

Prepare equipment

- Arrange the following equipment and supplies on a clean surface:
  - Sterile single-use dressing pack with tray, 3 forceps, drape, 3 gauze and 6 swabs.
  - Scissors.
  - Antiseptic.
  - Adhesive tape.
  - Appropriate wound dressings.
  - Disposable latex gloves.
  - Roller bandage.
  - Waste bag.
  - Clean work area.

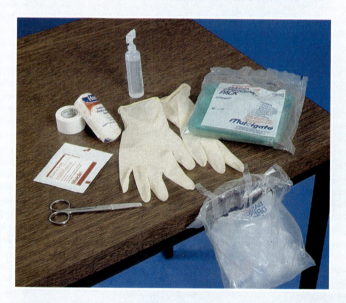

Prepare for aseptic technique

- Take off and discard into a waste bag any bandage and outer dressings from the wound (leave any dressings in direct contact with the wound).
- Wash and dry your hands.

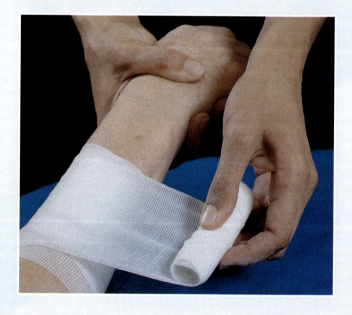

PRACTICE GUIDE

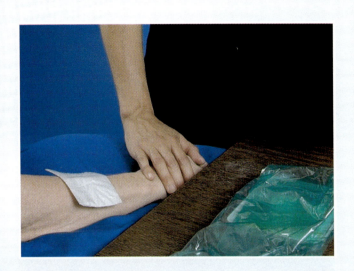

Open the dressing pack.

- Unwrap the cover of the tray, touching the corners only.

- Using the cover as a sterile field, pour antiseptic solution into the tray.

- Open the dressings to be used. Place them onto the sterile field without touching it.

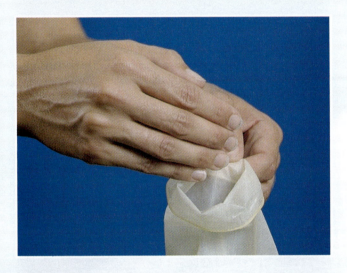

Put on gloves

- Wash your hands and dry them with a disposable towel.

- Touching only the inside of the glove, put on the gloves, allowing only the donned glove to touch the other glove.

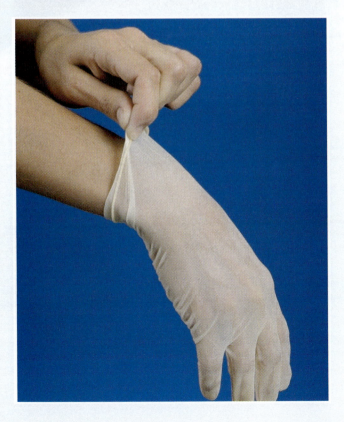

Cleaning and Dressing a Wound

Uncover the wound

- Using one pair of forceps in each hand, place the drape under the wound.

- Use the third pair of forceps to remove the remaining dressing from the wound and discard both the dressing and the forceps.

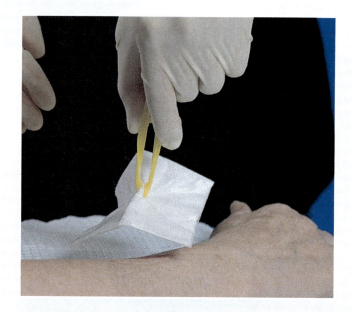

Clean the wound

- Using forceps in each hand, soak the swabs in the antiseptic and wring out.

- The forceps in your dominant hand are now considered "dirty" and the other set clean. Pick up a swab with the clean forceps and transfer it to the dirty forceps.

- With each swab and using the "dirty" forceps, wipe the wound only once, along the edge closest to the wound. Repeat with additional swabs to clean the whole wound, working from the inside to the outside edges of the wound.

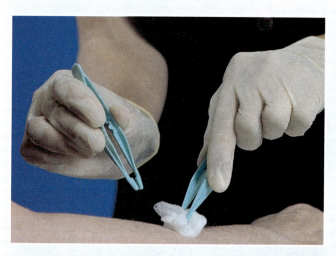

- Discard each swab into the bag after use.

- Dry the wound with gauze in the same manner.

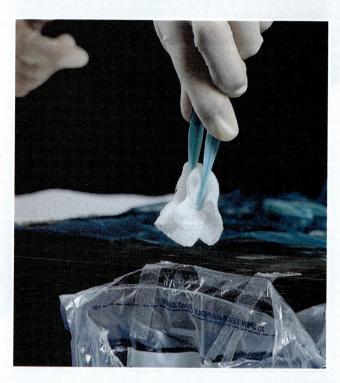

PRACTICE GUIDE

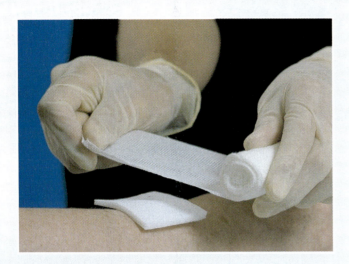

Cover the wound

- Cover the wound with a new dressing, and secure it with tape and a bandage.

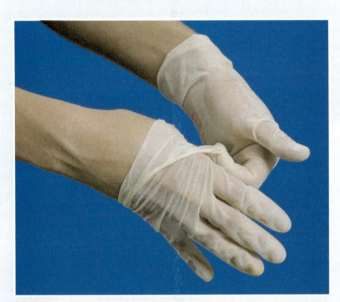

Complete the procedure

- Gather up all equipment into the sterile field.
- Remove one glove, touching the dirty side only. Slip this hand inside the other glove and remove it by turning it inside out.

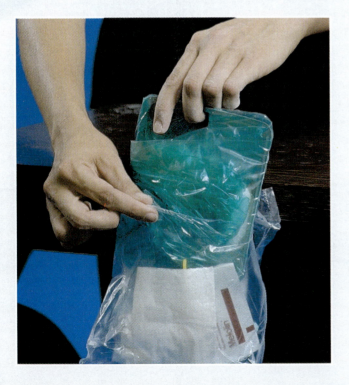

- Discard all used supplies into the bag and seal it for disposal.
- Clean the work surface.
- Wash your hands thoroughly.
- Record the procedure and your observations of the wound.
- Refer any redness, discharge or pain for medical advice.

Dressings and Bandages

IN **PREVIOUS CHAPTERS** you have learned that dressings and bandages are used in the care of bleeding and wounds. In situations with severe bleeding, the correct application of a dressing or bandage can save the victim's life. Each wound requires a dressing suitable for the area in which it occurs and the severity of the injury. Slings and splints are also used to support and immobilise an injured area.

This chapter outlines the different kinds of dressings and bandages, and how to use them for bleeding, wounds and other injuries.

For Review

A basic understanding of the circulatory system, skin and the inter-relationship of the body systems (Chapter 2), how to control bleeding (Chapter 5), treat shock (Chapter 6) and care for wounds (Chapter 12) will help your understanding of the chapter.

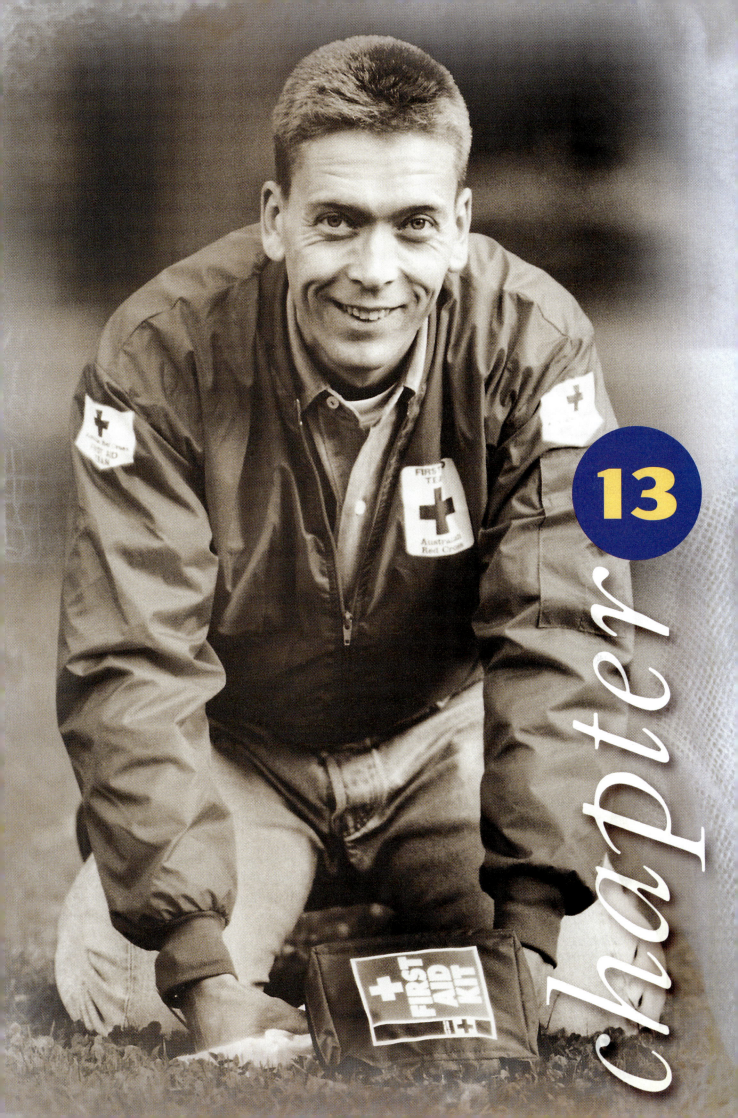

chapter

13

Key Terms

Bandage: Material used to wrap or cover a part of the body, commonly used to hold a dressing or splint in place.

BPC dressing: A machine-compressed sterile combine dressing stitched to a bandage, used for controlling bleeding in a large area; commonly used by defence personnel and also known as mines or field dressings. (BPC refers to British Pharmacopoeia Codex, an international published standard for drugs and bandages.)

Combine dressing: A dressing made up of layers of gauze and cotton wool, used when bulk is needed for controlling bleeding or for absorbing discharge from a wound.

Dressing: A pad placed directly on a wound to absorb blood and other body fluids and to provide a barrier against infection.

Sling: A bandage used to hold, support or immobilise a body part.

Splint: A commercial or improvised device used to immobilise an injured or fractured body part.

As discussed in Chapter 12, all open wounds need some type of covering to help control bleeding and prevent infection. These coverings are commonly referred to as **dressings** and **bandages**, of which there are many different types. The type you use and your method of applying it depend on the type of injury and the materials at hand.

DRESSINGS

Dressings are placed directly on the wound to absorb blood and other fluids and to provide a barrier against infection. To minimise the chance of infection, dressings should be sterile. Most dressings are porous, allowing air to circulate to the wound to promote healing. Absorbency is also important to allow sweat and other moisture around the wound to evaporate to keep the wound as dry as possible. Standard dressings are available in different types and varying sizes.

Another function of dressings is to help blood to clot and thus stop bleeding. Although blood sticking to the dressing sometimes makes it difficult to remove later, the benefits of a dressing are much more important than any damage which may occur when it is removed. Some dressings have non-adherent surfaces to prevent them from sticking to the wound.

General Principles for Applying Dressings

Regardless of the specific injury and type of dressing used, follow the general principles for cleaning a wound whenever applying a dressing (see also Chapter 12):

- Wash your hands before and after applying the dressing and bandage, and wear disposable latex gloves.
- Use a sterile dressing large enough for the wound and to extend about 2 centimetres beyond it on all sides. In an emergency, use any clean, non-fluffy material.

- In a minor wound where bleeding has stopped, clean the wound with an antiseptic solution before dressing it (see Chapter 12). With a large wound which will require medical attention, do not try to clean the wound; leave this to the medical professionals, who will provide care.

- Keep the dressing and wound as free from contamination as possible. Do not touch it with your hands unnecessarily, or breathe or cough over it.

Dressings for Major Wounds

For most larger wounds, use an unmedicated sterile dressing (Figure 13.1). This may be either a **combine dressing**, or for very large or deep wounds a **BPC dressing**. Do not use plain gauze unless that is the only dressing available in an emergency. Combine dressings are made up of layers of gauze and cotton wool, used when bulk is needed for controlling bleeding or for absorbing discharge from a wound. BPC dressings (sometimes called field, mines or wound dressings) are made of cotton wool and gauze layers already attached to a roller bandage for easier application. These dressings are compressed to only a fraction of their size, and come in individually sealed protective wrappers to maintain sterility. Follow the general principles for all dressings, using these specific steps to apply a BPC dressing:

1. Open the outer package and any inner wrapping from the dressing (Figure 13-2).

2. Hold one end of the bandage in each hand as you position the unfolded dressing over the wound. Lower the dressing into place on the wound.

3. Wrap the shorter end of the bandage around the extremity and dressing to hold it in place. Then wrap the other end around and over the dressing until it is covered.

4. Tie the ends of the bandage over the dressing site with a reef knot, as shown on page 237.

Non-Adherent Dressings

As dried blood and fluids may stick to dressings and make them difficult to remove later, non-adherent dressings have been developed which can be removed easily (Figure 13-3). Non-adherent dressings can be used on any wound as long as they cover the wound properly, but they are most useful for skin surface injuries such as abrasions and burns. Some non-adherent dressings have a perforated plastic layer on one side which lets blood pass through to the absorbent part of the dressing; with this type, always place the plastic film surface against the wound.

Special non-adherent dressings, called tulle gras dressings, have a film of sterile ointment or paraffin and are used for serious burns and extensive abrasions. Some of these dressings contain an antiseptic which helps prevent infection. An absorbent pad placed over these dressings will help to absorb fluids from the wound.

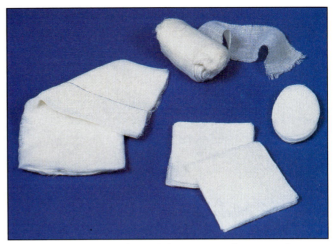

FIGURE 13-1 *Non-medicated dressings used to control bleeding or cover a large wound.*

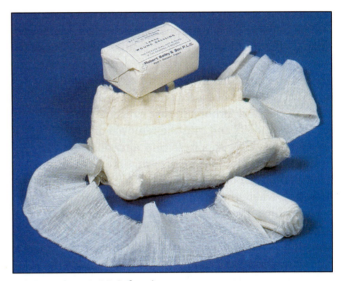

FIGURE 13-2 *A BPC dressing.*

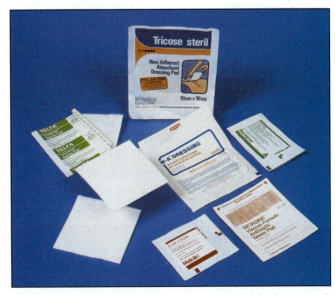

FIGURE 13-3 *Non-adherent dressings are used for burns and abrasions.*

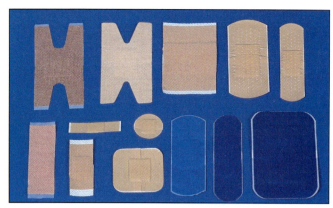

FIGURE 13-4 *Adhesive dressings for minor wounds.*

Adhesive Dressings for Minor Wounds

Adhesive dressings have an absorbent pad backed with an adhesive strip or backing which holds the dressing in place. These dressings are available in many sizes and shapes (Figure 13-4). Use the dressings, which are packaged individually in a closed sterile wrapping, rather than the continuous strip type where the edges are exposed and may become contaminated.

A special waterproof adhesive dressing should be used by food handlers and must be removed and replaced every few hours with a fresh one, after allowing the wound to "breathe". These dressings are blue coloured so that they can be easily detected if they fall off. In any situation where the wound may become wet, such as when fishing, the person should use waterproof adhesive dressings but must remember to remove the dressing at least once a day to let the wound dry out.

Follow these steps to apply an adhesive dressing:

1. Clean and dry the skin around the wound.

2. Take off the outer wrapper. Hold the dressing by the protective strips covering the adhesive sections.

3. Peel back the edge of the strips away from the dressing. Do not touch the dressing itself.

4. Place the dressing pad on the wound and pull the protective strips back and off the adhesive sections. Pat the adhesive sections firmly against the skin to make sure they stick in place securely.

5. With waterproof dressings or any wound covering which becomes wet or soiled, remove the dressing at least once a day, clean the wound area if necessary and apply a new adhesive dressing.

COLD COMPRESSES

The care of closed wounds such as bruises or musculoskeletal injuries (see Chapter 14) often includes the use of a cold compress or ice pack to reduce pain and swelling. A cold compress may be a towel or similar absorbent cloth soaked in cold or ice water and wrung out so that it is not dripping wet. An ice pack is a bag half filled with crushed or cube ice and sealed after the air is squeezed out. The bag is then wrapped in a damp cloth to prevent ice contacting the skin.

Place the cold pack on the injury for 10 minutes and then check the wound site. The wet cloth compress may need to be recooled with cold water and wrung out again. Remove an ice pack if the skin becomes painfully cold or red; increased redness indicates increased blood flow. (For further information on soft tissue injuries see pages 202-221.)

Where musculoskeletal injuries are likely, such as in sports, commercial ice packs are available which can be kept in a freezer. There is also a disposable cold pack which uses a chemical reaction to produce the cold for one application only. These are ideal for sports teams playing away from club rooms or in a remote facility.

BANDAGES

A bandage is any material used to wrap or cover any part of the body. Bandages are used to:

- hold dressings in place
- apply pressure to control bleeding
- protect a wound from dirt and infection
- prevent swelling
- restrict movement
- provide support to an injured limb or body part

Many different types of bandages made of many different materials are available commercially. The two primary types of bandages used for most wounds are roller bandages, which can be wrapped around a body part, and triangular bandages, which can be folded, wrapped and tied in different ways for different injuries.

General Principles for Applying Bandages

Regardless of the type of bandage used, follow these general principles:

- Assist the victim to sit or lie in a comfortable position. Support the injured extremity or part in the position in which it will be bandaged.

- Always use a reef knot (see page 237) to tie bandages. For pressure bandages to control bleeding, tie the knot over the wound. For bandages used for immobilisation, tie the knot on the opposite side to the wound.

- Apply the bandage securely and firmly enough to hold the dressing in place and apply the needed pressure or immobilisation, but not so tightly that it restricts circulation. When bandaging an extremity, leave the fingernails or toenails exposed so that you can check that the circulation is not impaired.

Checking Circulation in a Bandaged Extremity

Always check the victim's circulation beyond the bandage to make sure the bandage is not too tight. Check immediately after putting on the bandage and then 10 minutes later. Loosen, adjust or remove a bandage which impairs circulation.

Follow these steps to check circulation:

1. Press one of the fingernails or toenails beyond the bandage until the nail bed turns white.

2. Release the nail. It should quickly become pink again.

3. If the nail bed remains white or blue, the bandage is too tight and should be loosened. Other symptoms and signs of impaired circulation include the following:

   — The fingers or toes have a tingling sensation or a lack of feeling.

   — The victim feels pain in the extremity.

   — The fingers or toes feel cold to the touch.

   — The pulse is absent or weak in the extremity compared to the other side.

   — The victim cannot move the fingers or toes.

Types of Bandages

Either roller bandages or triangular bandages are used with most types of large or major wounds. A third type of bandage, the tubular gauze bandage, is used for fingers and toes.

Roller Bandages

Roller bandages may be used to:

- Apply pressure to control bleeding.
- Keep dressings in place.
- Support an injured part.

Roller bandages are made of various materials, including cotton, gauze, elastic and synthetic fibres (Figure 13-5). They are commercially available in different widths.

The appropriate width of the roller bandage depends on the wound. For a finger, use a width of 2.5 centimetres; for the hand or foot, 5 centimetres; for the arm, 5 or 6 centimetres; for the leg, 7.5 or 9 centimetres; and for the trunk, 10 or 15 centimetres.

Follow these steps to apply a roller bandage:

1. Support the extremity or area in the position in which it will be bandaged. Keep the bandage rolled with only a few centimetres loose in a "tail" at any time.

2. Keep the roll of the bandage uppermost, and apply the bandage from the inner side outward and from below the wound upward.

3. Place the tail of the bandage below the wound or injury and make one full turn around the extremity or trunk to hold the tail in place (Figure 13-6A).

4. Make spiral turns around the extremity or trunk, working upwards. Each turn should overlap two-thirds of the preceding turn (Figure 13-6B).

5. At the end of the roll, make a last turn so that it overlaps the previous turn and secure the end of the bandage with a bandage clip, safety pin or adhesive tape (Figure 13-6C).

6. Check the circulation below the bandage and adjust it if necessary.

Elastic roller bandages that stretch are usually used for sprains or other musculoskeletal injuries where even pressure is necessary to support the joint or prevent swelling. With elastic roller bandages there is a risk of stretching them too tightly and impairing circulation. Be sure to check the circulation frequently, and loosen the bandage if necessary. A new type of elastic roller

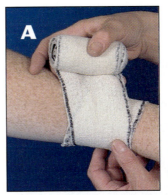
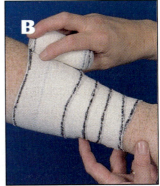
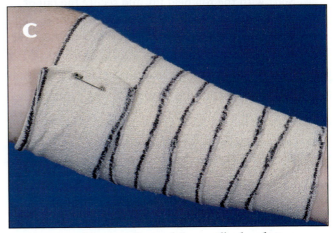

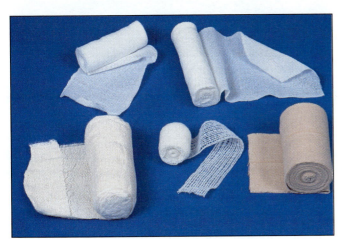

FIGURE 13-5 *Roller bandages are made of various materials, including cotton, gauze, elastic and synthetic fibres.*

FIGURE 13-6 *The steps for applying a roller bandage (see description above).*

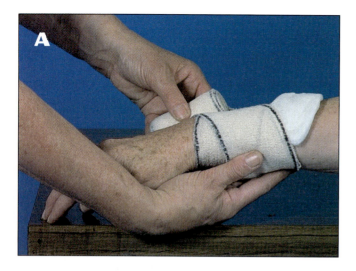

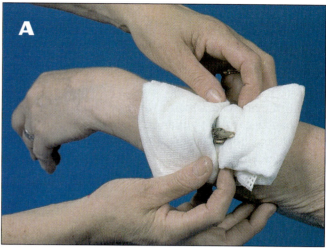

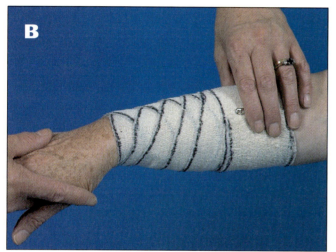

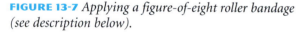

FIGURE 13-7 *Applying a figure-of-eight roller bandage (see description below).*

bandage is printed with small rectangles that become square shapes when the bandage is stretched the correct amount during application.

Figure-of-Eight Roller Bandaging

A roller bandage can be applied in a figure-of-eight pattern to provide even pressure on an arm or leg, as follows:

1. Start with the roll held up, and secure the tail of the bandage with one turn below the wound, working from the inside outward (Figure 13-7A).

2. Still working from inside outward, make a series of figures-of-eight up the extremity (Figure 13-7B).

3. Secure the end of the bandage with a bandage clip, safety pin or adhesive tape.

Bandaging Around an Embedded Object

Chapter 12 describes care of a wound in which a foreign object is embedded. Leave the object in the wound, as it may be helping to control the bleeding. Bandaging avoids putting pressure on the object.

1. Build up dressings around the foreign body to finish above the height of the object (Figure 13-8A).

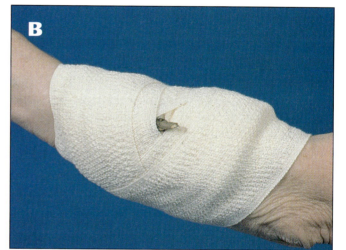

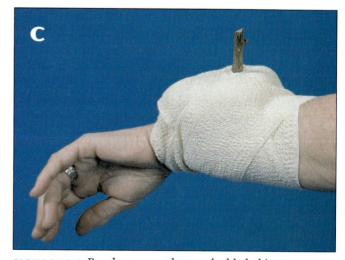

FIGURE 13-8 *Bandage around an embedded object to stabilise it in the wound (see description below).*

2. Secure the dressings in place by wrapping the roller bandage diagonally both above and below the wound (Figure 13-8B) before passing the bandage over the dressing and lightly over the object.

3. If the object is large and protruding above the dressings, bandage firmly on all sides of the object over the dressings and protect from further injury, but do not pass the bandage over the object (Figure 13-8C).

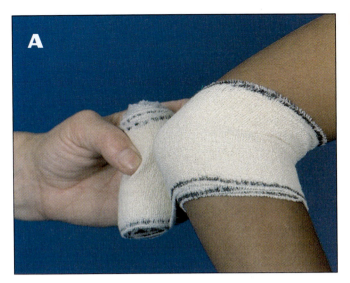

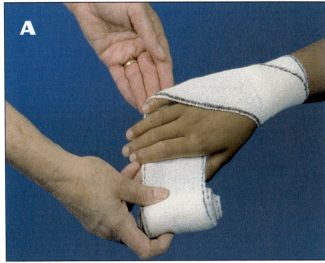

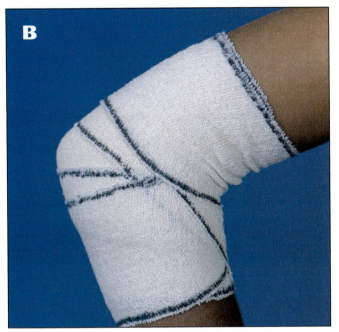

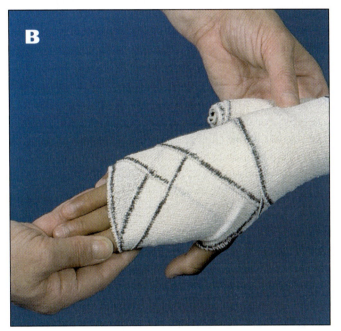

FIGURE 13-9 *Applying a roller bandage around an elbow or knee (see description below).*

FIGURE 13-10 *Bandaging the hand with a roller bandage (see description below).*

Bandaging the Elbow or Knee

To apply a roller bandage to an elbow or knee:

1. Ask the victim to support the limb in the most comfortable position, put the tail of the bandage inside the joint and make one full turn over the point of the elbow or knee to secure it, working from the inside outwards (Figure 13-9A).

2. Make the next turn above the joint, covering two-thirds of the first turn; then make a turn below the joint, overlapping the first turn by two-thirds (Figure 13-9B).

3. Make alternating turns above and below the joint, covering each previous turn by about two-thirds.

4. Make the last turn above the joint with a straight turn, and secure the end.

5. Check the circulation.

Bandaging the Hand or Foot

The following steps are for bandaging the hand with a roller bandage (for wounds to the palm of the hand, see Chapter 12). Use the same method for the foot.

1. With the victim supporting the arm with the palm down, start by securing the tail of the bandage with one turn around the wrist.

2. Bandage diagonally across the back of the hand to the base of the little finger, around the palm and diagonally across the back of the hand to the wrist in a figure-of-eight (Figure 13-10A).

3. Use additional figures-of-eight to cover the hand, leaving the fingertips exposed (Figure 13-10B). Finally, make a straight turn at the wrist and secure the end.

4. Check the circulation and adjust the bandage if necessary.

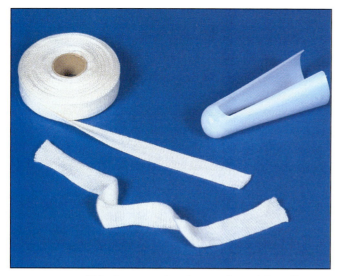

FIGURE 13-11 *Tubular gauze bandage and special applicator used to bandage fingers and toes.*

Tubular Gauze Bandages

Tubular gauze bandage is a commercial bandage made of a roll of seamless stretch gauze tubing used to bandage fingers and toes. A special applicator is used with the tubular gauze (Figure 13-11). For wounds to fingers or toes this bandage is easier and faster to apply than a roller bandage and often holds in place better.

The directions for using tubular bandage with the applicator are printed on the package. The following is a summary of these steps.

1. Cut a piece of bandage at least three times as long as the finger.

2. Push the gauze tube entirely onto the applicator.

3. Push the applicator over the finger. Hold the end of the tubular bandage at the base of the finger and, with the other end of the gauze still on the applicator, pull the applicator back off the finger (Figure 13-12A).

4. Rotate the applicator at the end of the finger to twist the gauze once or twice around. Then push the applicator back onto the finger using a rotary action to roll down a second layer on the finger (Figure 13-12B).

5. Use adhesive tape to secure the end of the bandage.

> ## Remember:
> *Rotate the tubular gauze applicator to apply the second layer so that it conforms to the dressing and the finger.*

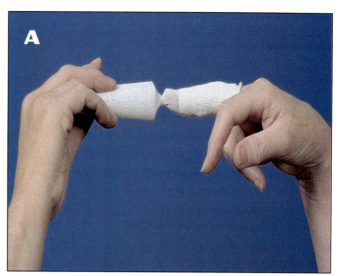

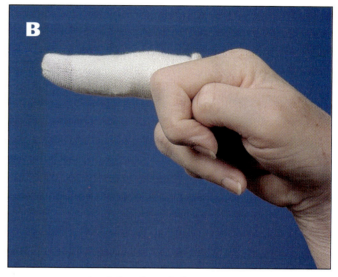

FIGURE 13-12 *Applying the tubular gauze bandage with an applicator (see text description opposite).*

Triangular Bandages

Triangular bandages are large triangular pieces of cloth which can be folded in different ways for different uses as bandages or slings. Triangular bandages are commercially available or can be made by cutting a piece of cloth at least 1 metre square diagonally in half. Fold the triangular bandage into a broad or narrow bandage as needed.

Broad triangular bandages are used for securing splints or immobilising an extremity during transport. The fold for a triangular bandage is as follows:

1. Fold the point to the base (Figure 13-13A).

2. Fold the bandage in half in the same direction (Figure 13-13B).

Narrow triangular bandages can be used to secure a dressing at a joint or around an extremity if a roller bandage is not available, and to make a collar and cuff sling.

To make a narrow triangular bandage, first follow the steps for making a broad bandage and then fold it in half again in the same direction (Figure 13-13C).

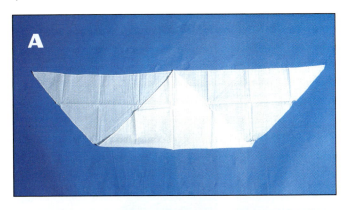

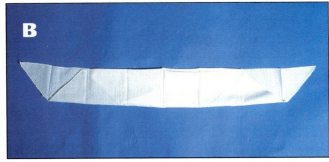

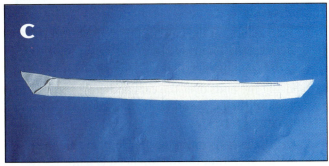

FIGURE 13-13 *Making a broad or narrow triangular bandage (see description on previous page).*

Reef Knot for Triangular Bandages

Use a reef knot to tie bandages because they do not slip, they untie easily and are flat and comfortable. The procedure is as follows:

1. Pass the left end over and then under the right (Figure 13-14A) and then bring both ends back.

2. Reverse the procedure by passing the right end over and then under the left (Figure 13-14B).

3. Pull the knot tight and tuck in the ends or fasten them to the bandage (Figure 13-14C).

4. If the position of the knot causes discomfort for the victim, put padding under it. Check that the knot does not press against a bone or the back of the neck when used with a sling.

5. To untie the knot, grasp a pair of parallel ends as they protrude from the knot and pull them smoothly apart. Slip the knot off the remaining ends (Figure 13-14D).

6. Alternatively, hold the bandage firmly with one hand and grasp one of the ends. Pull gently across the knot with a steady movement, then slip the knot apart.

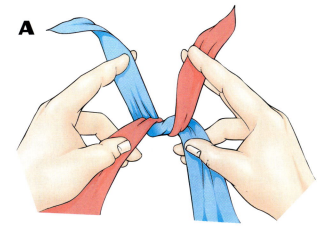

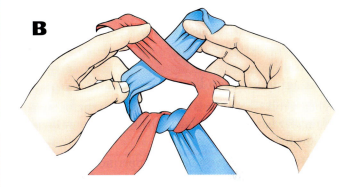

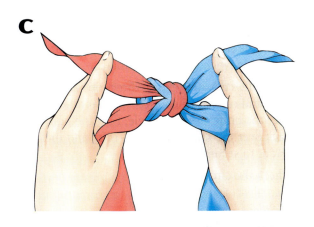

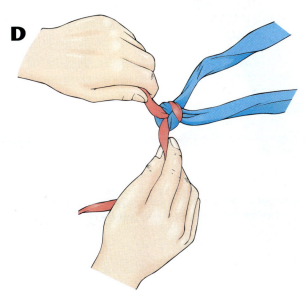

FIGURE 13-14 A, B AND C *Tying and* **D** *untying a reef knot.*

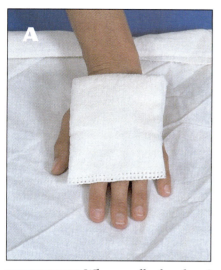
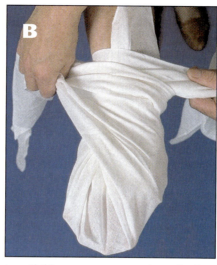
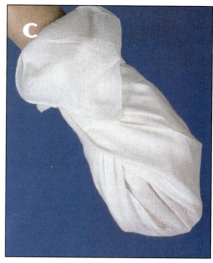

FIGURE 13-15 *When a roller bandage is not available, you can use a triangular bandage for the hand (see description below).*

Bandaging the Hand or Foot

When a roller bandage is unavailable, you can use a triangular bandage to bandage the hand, foot or knee. Follow these steps:

1. Keeping the dressed injury uppermost, place the hand or foot onto the triangular bandage with the fingers or toes towards the point (Figure 13-15A). Fold a hem along the base if necessary for a small hand or foot.

2. Bring the point of the bandage up over the hand or foot to reach the wrist or ankle.

3. Cross the ends in opposite directions around the hand or foot (Figure 13-15B), and tie them over the point of the triangle. Fold the point back over the knot (Figure 13-15C) and tuck it under to secure it.

4. Check the circulation.

Bandaging the Scalp

A triangular bandage can be used to hold a dressing in place on the scalp but should not be used in an attempt to control bleeding.

1. Fold a hem on the base of the triangle and put the hem on the forehead above the eyebrows with the point hanging down at the back of the neck.

2. Bring the ends over the ears and cross them at the back of the head and at the base of the skull (Figure 13-16A).

3. Bring the ends round to the front and tie them with a reef knot on the forehead (Figure 13-16B).

4. Support the head with one hand, and use the other hand to pull down the point of the bandage at the back to tighten the bandage over the scalp. Then fold the point upwards and fasten it to the bandage on top of the head with a safety pin.

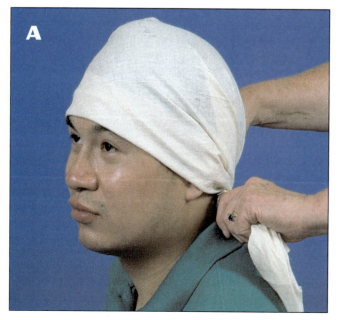
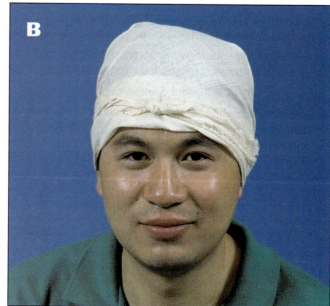

FIGURE 13-16 *Bandaging the scalp.*

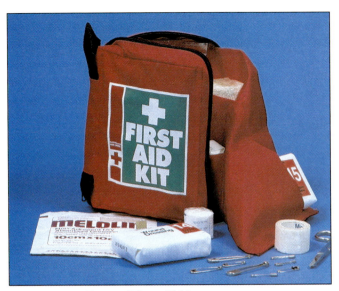

FIGURE 13-17 *Personal first aid kit.*

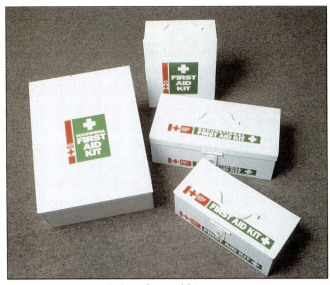

FIGURE 13-18 *Workplace first aid kits.*

FIRST AID KITS

Although you can improvise dressings and bandages in an emergency, using proper sterile supplies is safer. Keep a variety of dressings and bandages in your first aid kit in an airtight container. Do not keep the kit in a damp place such as a bathroom.

Family First Aid Kit

Keep a personal first aid kit in a convenient place in your home (Figure 13-17). The following contents are what Australian Standard 2675 "Portable First Aid Kits for Use by Consumers" requires as the minimum standard.

- 3 packets of gauze swabs (3 or 5 to a pack)
- 3 individual hand towels or tissues in a pocket-sized pack
- 5 adhesive dressing strips (assorted widths)
- 1 roll of adhesive tape (at least 25 millimetre wide and 2.5 metres long)
- 2 sterile non-adherent dry dressings (10 x 10 centimetres)
- 1 no. 14 BPC wound dressing
- 1 x 5 centimetres stretch bandage
- 1 x 7.5 centimetres stretch bandage
- 1 triangular bandage
- 5 safety pins
- 1 pair of blunt/sharp scissors
- 1 pair of splinter forceps
- pencil and note pad
- 3 plastic bags

Optional inclusions:

- 3 antiseptic swabs
- 1 combine dressing (9 x 20 centimetres)

In addition, latex disposable gloves are recommended.

Workplace First Aid Kits

The contents of first aid kits in the workplace are stipulated by regulations which vary in each State and Territory. If you are responsible for maintaining the first aid kit in your workplace, check it periodically to ensure all equipment and supplies are present and in good condition (Figure 13-18).

SPLINTS

A splint is a commercial or improvised device used to immobilise an injured or fractured body part, particularly when a victim is being moved or transported.

Commercial splints are available, but improvised splints can be made of many different materials. Another body part can also be used as a splint. For example, an injured leg can be splinted to the uninjured leg with bandages around both. Padded boards, fence palings, rolled newspapers and sticks can be used to splint an arm or leg. A pillow or rolled blanket can be used to splint the lower leg or ankle. Any rigid material which is long and wide enough to support the injured extremity can work as a splint.

Select a splint which is long enough to extend past the joints both above and below the injury. Ensure the splint is padded, with extra padding where the bones contact the splint, such as at the elbow, knee, wrist or ankle. Natural hollows such as behind the knee also should be padded.

Chapter 14 gives detailed steps on how to apply splints.

Remember:

Before applying a splint to an injured limb, note which position is chosen by the victim for comfort and pain relief.

Slings

A sling is a bandage used to hold, support and immobilise an upper extremity when it or the chest is injured. Slings are usually made from triangular bandages, but in an emergency any improvised material can be used. An injury is best supported in the position which the victim adopts, with one of the following slings.

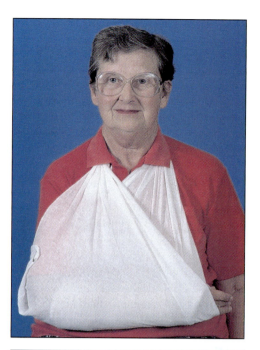

Arm Sling

An arm sling is used to hold the forearm across the chest in cases of injuries to the arm or hand. It is also used for some chest injuries. The Practice Guide at the end of this chapter details the steps for applying an arm sling.

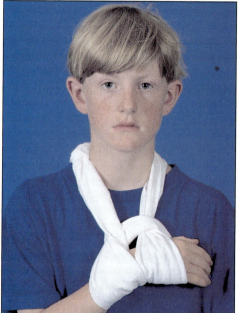

Collar and Cuff Sling

The collar and cuff sling is used to support the upper arm in an injury when pressure should not be put on the elbow. A clove hitch must be used so that the loops do not slip and cut off the circulation. The Practice Guide at the end of the chapter details the steps for the collar and cuff sling.

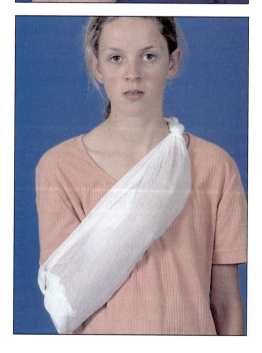

Elevation Sling

An elevation sling supports the hand and forearm in a higher position than the arm sling. This is used when there is bleeding from the hand or there are chest or shoulder injuries. It should not be used for injuries of the elbow. The Practice Guide at the end of the chapter details the steps for applying the elevation sling.

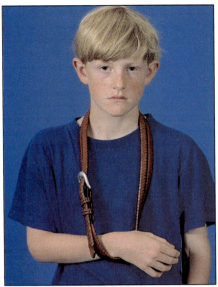

Improvised Slings

If no bandages are available, the person's clothing can be used to provide support. For example, turn up the bottom of the shirt or top, use a tie or belt or place the hand inside the shirt or jacket.

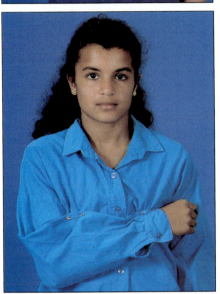

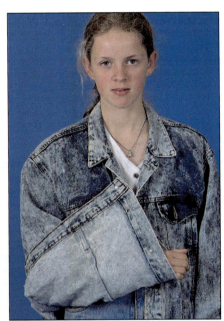

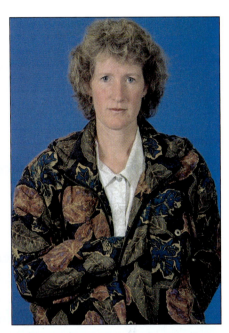

Summary

- Dressings are used to absorb blood and other fluids and to prevent infection.
- With all dressings, wash hands before and after application, wear latex gloves, use a dressing large enough to extend beyond the wound and use only sterile dressings if they are readily available in an emergency.
- Types of dressings include major wound dressings, non-adherent dressings and adhesive dressings.
- Cold compresses are used for some closed wounds and musculoskeletal injuries to reduce pain and swelling.
- Bandages are used to hold dressings in place, to apply pressure to control bleeding, to help protect a wound from dirt and infection, to prevent swelling and to support and immobilise an injured body part.
- Apply bandages with the body part in a comfortable position, with padding at bony areas, and with enough firmness to apply pressure when needed without restricting circulation.

- Always check the circulation after bandaging an extremity.
- Types of bandages include roller bandages, triangular bandages, tubular gauze bandages, slings and splints.
- Keep first aid kits well stocked with dressings and bandages.

Remember:

If no regular dressings are available in an emergency, think of the following improvised articles:

- *Clean cotton laundry, especially recently ironed sheets, t-shirts, pillowcases, etc.*
- *Laundry on a washing line, preferably of non-fluffy cloth.*
- *Clean material which has been exposed to strong sunlight.*

Study Questions

1. **List two purposes of dressings.**

2. **A dressing of the correct size will:**
   a. cover the shape and size of the wound exactly
   b. wrap all the way around the extremity
   c. apply pressure only in the centre of the wound
   d. extend past the edges of the wound in all directions

3. **If a dressing slips off the wound before you bandage it in place, what should you do?**
   a. Start again with a new dressing.
   b. Slide the dressing back onto the wound from one side.
   c. Put the same dressing back on.
   d. Use the same dressing again but turn it over to the other side.

4. **How often should you check the skin under an ice compress?**
   a. Every minute.
   b. At least every 10 minutes.
   c. Every hour.
   d. When the victim says the skin feels cold.
   e. b and d.

5. **List two purposes of bandaging.**

6. **When applying a bandage:**
   a. cover the dressing completely
   b. cover fingers or toes
   c. remove any blood-soaked bandages and apply new ones.
   d. a and c.

7. **When you press and release the victim's fingernail to check circulation, you should consider circulation to be restricted if:**
   a. the victim feels pain
   b. the victim feels anxious
   c. the nail bed stays white
   d. the nail bed becomes pink

8. **Each turn of a roller bandage around an extremity should cover the previous turn by:**

    a. one-quarter
    b. one-half
    c. one-third
    d. two-thirds

9. **A reef knot is used to tie triangular bandages because:**

    a. it does not slip
    b. it unties easily
    c. it lies flat
    d. all of the above

10. **The purpose of the collar and cuff sling is to:**

    a. avoid putting pressure on the collar bone as other types of slings do
    b. support the upper arm without putting pressure on the elbow
    c. prevent the forearm from pressing on a broken rib.
    d. All of the above.

Answers are in Appendix A (page 362).

Arm Sling

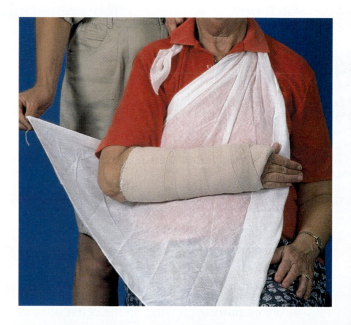

Position the victim

- Ask the seated victim to support the forearm with the hand slightly higher than the elbow.

Position the bandage

- Prepare the bandage by holding it with the longest side (base) held vertically beside the body, with the right angled point over the elbow on the injured side.

- Slip one end of the triangular bandage between the chest and forearm at the hollow between the elbow and chest.

- Bring the upper end up to the shoulder on the uninjured side and around the back of the neck to near the collar bone on the injured side.

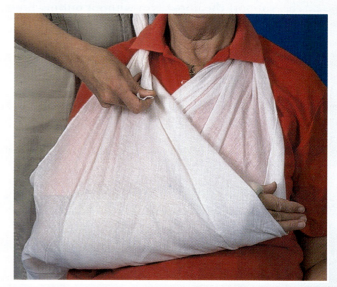

Tie the bandage

- Bring up the lower end of the bandage to tie it to the first end at the hollow of the collar bone.

- Use a reef knot.

- Use the collar of the shirt, dress or T-shirt to keep the knot padded and off the skin.

- Ensure that the finished position of the sling keeps the hand slightly higher than the elbow.

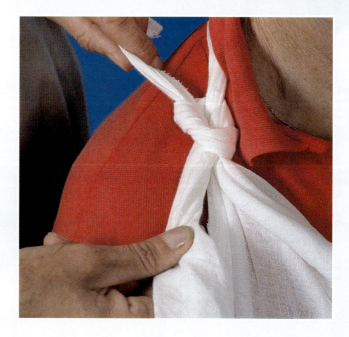

PRACTICE GUIDE

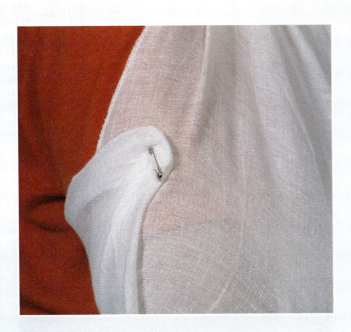

Complete the bandage

■ Bring the point of the triangle forward from behind the elbow and pin it to the front of the bandage with pin head pointing downwards.

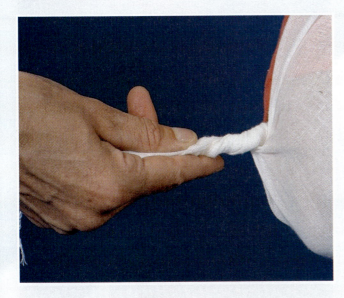

■ Alternatively, twist the end of the bandage and tuck it inside the sling.

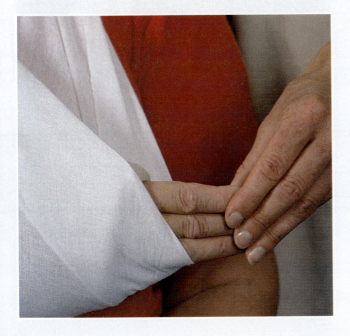

Check circulation

■ Check the circulation and adjust the bandage if necessary.

Elevation Sling

Position the victim

- Ask the victim to sit and hold the injured arm in a raised position with fingertips reaching almost to the opposite shoulder.

Position the bandage

- Open the triangular bandage with the point over the elbow and the longest side (base) vertically along the body. Place the upper end over the hand which is close to the shoulder on the uninjured side.

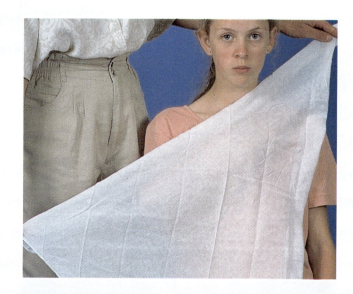

- Ease the base of the bandage under the hand, forearm and elbow.
- Bring the lower end around to the back and up to meet the other end across the uninjured shoulder.

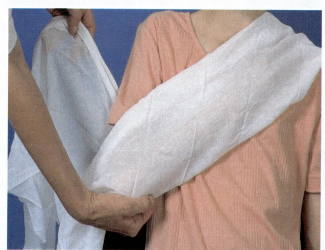

Adjust sling

- Adjust the height of the sling.
- Twist the bandage gently to hold the hand in place, and tie the ends on the uninjured side above the collar bone.

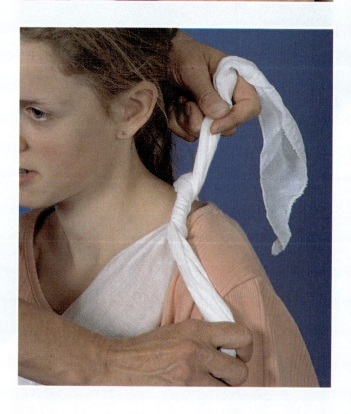

PRACTICE GUIDE

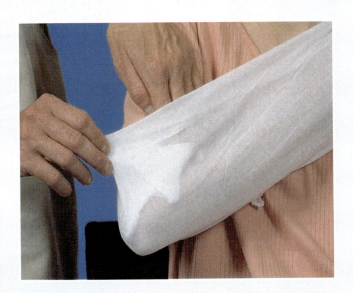

Complete the sling

- Tuck in the point of the triangle over the elbow and take it behind the elbow.

- Secure the fold with a safety pin with the point downward.

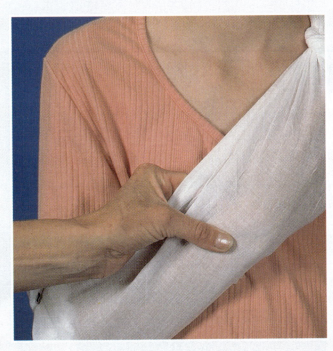

Check circulation

- Check the circulation and adjust the sling if necessary.

Collar and Cuff Sling

Position the victim

- Ask the victim to sit and hold the injured arm supported with the fingers pointing toward the opposite shoulder.

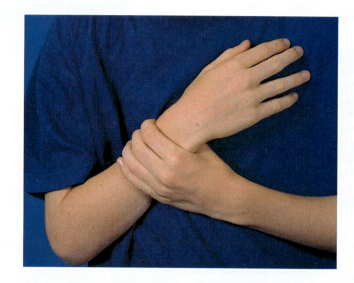

Prepare the sling

- Use a narrow triangular bandage, tie or belt at least 1 metre long. Fold it with two loops over the centre of the bandage, each pointing in opposite directions.
- Bring the loops together with the ends trapped between the loops.

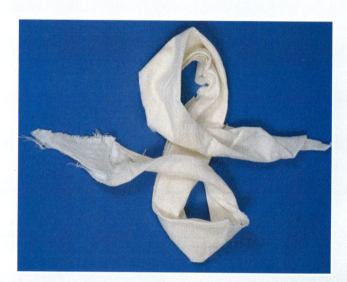

Position the sling

- Slip the loops over the victim's hand and position them at the wrist.

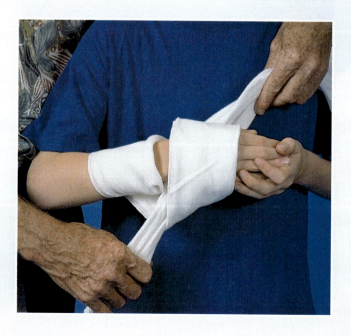

PRACTICE GUIDE

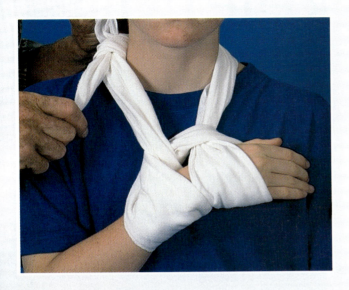

- Adjust the height of the sling so that it is comfortable to the victim.
- Tie the ends around the neck, with the reef knot over the hollow of the collar bone on either side in the most comfortable position.

Check circulation

- Check the circulation and adjust the sling as needed.

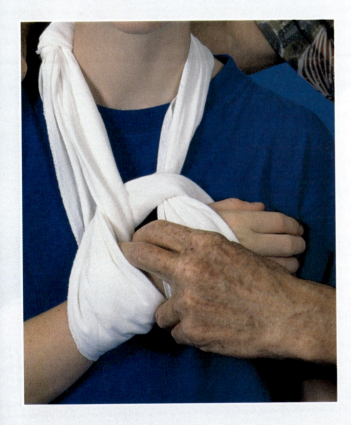

Musculoskeletal Injuries

IN PREVIOUS CHAPTERS you have learned how to care for injuries to the body's soft tissues. Injuries can also occur to the bones, as well as to the muscles and the ligaments and tendons. These musculoskeletal injuries can be minor and cause only pain and temporary disability, or they can be very serious and life-threatening if they are fractures that cause heavy bleeding or damage to other organs.

This chapter outlines how to recognise different musculoskeletal injuries and how to care for them.

For Review

Before reading this chapter, a review of the anatomy and function of the musculoskeletal system (Chapter 2) will assist your understanding of the chapter. A knowledge of how the musculoskeletal system interacts with the nervous system, how to perform a secondary survey (Chapter 3) and how to manage bleeding (Chapter 5) and shock (Chapter 6) will also be of benefit.

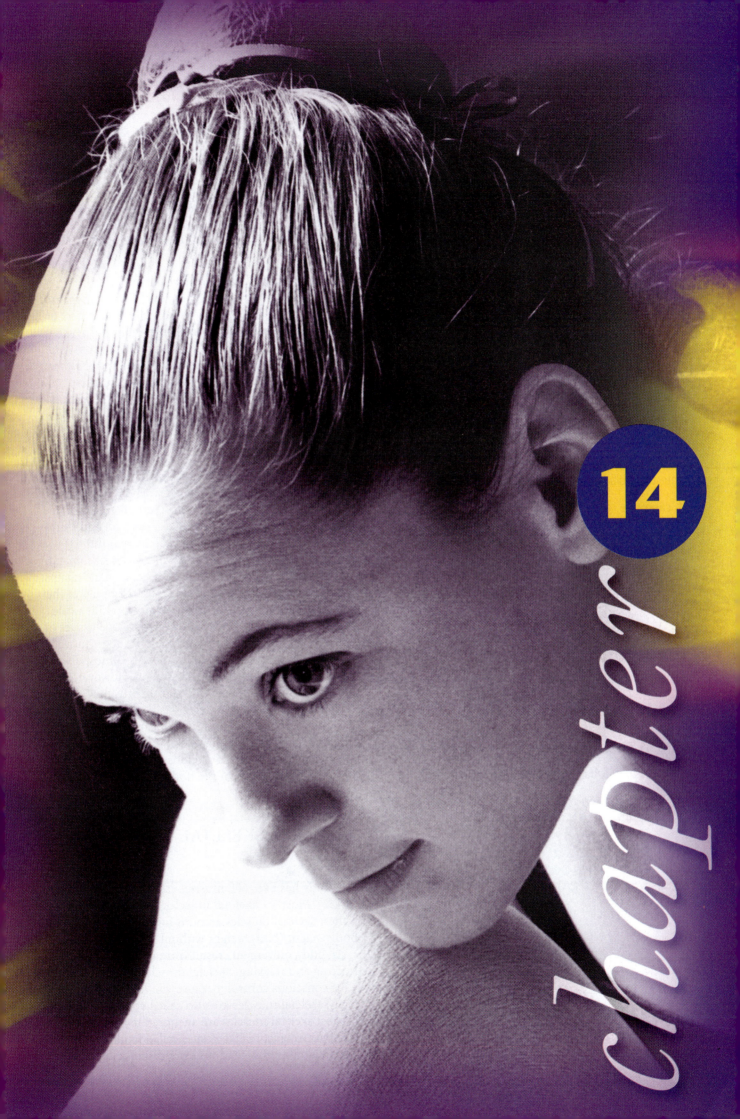

14

chapter

Key Terms

Body splinting: Using a sound body part to support an injured one, for example, using an uninjured leg to support an injured one.

Bone: A dense, hard tissue that forms the skeleton.

Dislocation: The displacement of a bone from its normal position at a joint.

Extremities: The arms and legs, hands and feet.

Fracture: A break or disruption in bone tissue.

Immobilisation: The use of a splint or other method to keep an injured body part from moving.

Joint: A structure where two or more bones are joined.

Ligament: A fibrous band that holds bones together at a joint.

Muscle: A tissue that lengthens and shortens to create movement.

Pelvis: The lower part of the trunk containing the intestines, bladder and reproductive organs.

Rib cage: The cage of bones formed by the 12 pairs of ribs, the sternum and the spine.

Skeletal muscles: Muscles that attach to bones.

Spinal column: The column of vertebrae extending from the base of the skull to the tip of the tailbone (coccyx).

Spinal cord: A bundle of nerves extending from the base of the skull to the lower back, protected by the spinal column.

Splint: A device used to immobilise body parts.

Sprain: The stretching and tearing of ligaments and other soft tissue structures at a joint.

Strain: The stretching and tearing of muscles and tendons.

Tendon: A fibrous band that attaches muscle to bone.

Vertebrae *(ver-te-bray)*: The 33 bones of the spinal column.

It is the summer holidays at the beach. High school and university students are having fun in the sun. The weather is great, the water refreshing. The day is perfect for playing cricket on the sand.

Later in the day the tide has come in, and three young men are playing near the surf. Two of them run into the surf chasing a long hit, and dive head first to reach for the ball. As they strike the water a wave crashes over them, forcing them underwater and into a sandbar. Both strike their heads on the sandy bottom. The result? Both are pulled from the surf by their friends. One is lucky and escapes with only a concussion. The other, not so lucky, suffers a broken neck and spinal cord damage.

Injuries to the musculoskeletal system are common. Thousands of people at home, at work or at play injure their **muscles, bones, ligaments, tendons** or **joints.** No age group is immune. A person may fall and bruise the muscles of the hip, making walking painful. Heavy machinery may fall on a worker and break ribs, making breathing difficult. A person who braces a hand against a dashboard in a car crash may injure the bones at the shoulder, disabling the arm. A person who falls while skiing may twist a leg, tearing the supportive tissues of the knee and making it impossible to stand or move.

Although musculoskeletal injuries are almost always painful, they are rarely life-threatening. However, when not recognised and taken care of properly, they can have serious consequences and even result in permanent disability. In this chapter, you will learn how to recognise and care for musculoskeletal injuries. These injuries are arranged in different sections in the chapter based on the different areas of the body: head and spine, chest, pelvis and extremities.

MUSCULOSKELETAL SYSTEM

Muscles

The body has over 600 muscles (see Chapter 2, pages 21–22). Most are **skeletal muscles** which attach to the bones. Skeletal muscles account for most of your lean body weight (body weight without excess fat).

All body movements result from skeletal muscles contracting and relaxing. Skeletal muscle actions are under your conscious control; because you move them voluntarily, skeletal muscles are also called voluntary muscles.

Most skeletal muscles are anchored to bone at each end by strong, cord-like tissues called tendons. Muscles and their adjoining tendons extend across joints.

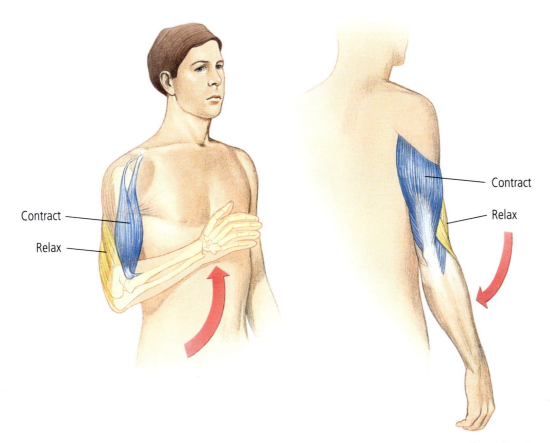

FIGURE 14-1 *Movement occurs when one group of muscles contracts and an opposing group of muscles relaxes.*

When the brain sends a command to move, electrical impulses travel through the spinal cord and nerve pathways to the individual muscles and stimulate the muscle fibres to contract. When a muscle contracts the muscle fibres shorten, pulling the ends of the muscle closer together. The muscles pull the bones, causing motion at the joint.

Motion is usually caused by a group of muscles close together pulling at the same time. For instance, the hamstring muscles are a group of muscles at the back of the thigh. When the hamstrings contract, the leg bends at the knee. The biceps are a group of muscles at the front of the arm. When the biceps contract, the arm bends at the elbow. Generally, when one group of muscles contracts, another group of muscles on the opposite side of the body part relaxes (Figure 14-1). Even simple tasks, such as bending to pick up an object from the floor, involve a complex series of movements in which different muscle groups contract and relax.

Injuries to the brain, the spinal cord or the nerves can affect muscle control. A loss of muscle control is called paralysis. Less serious or isolated muscle injuries may only affect strength because adjacent muscles can often assume the function of the injured muscle (Figure 14-2).

Skeleton

As described in Chapter 2, the skeleton is formed by bones of various sizes and shapes. It protects vital organs

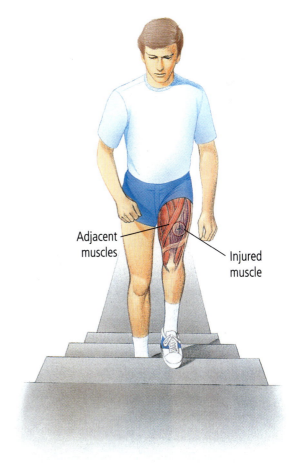

FIGURE 14-2 *Adjacent muscles can often assume the function of an injured muscle.*

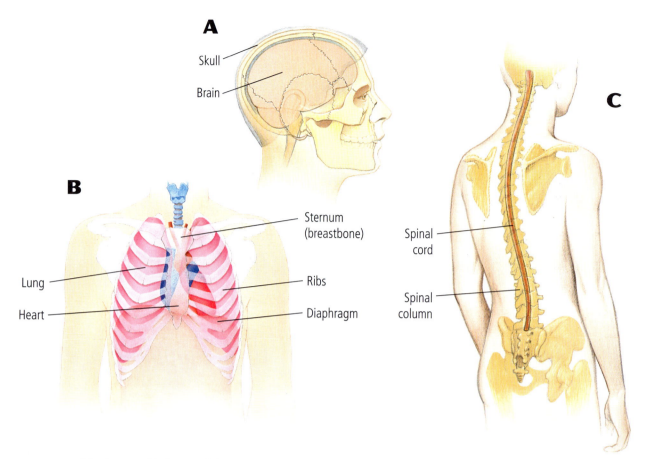

FIGURE 14-3 A *The immovable bones of the skull protect the brain.* **B** *The rib cage protects the lungs and heart.* **C** *The spinal cord is protected by the vertebrae.*

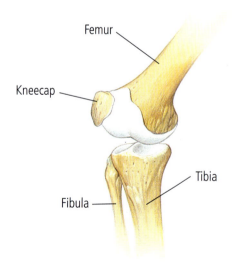

FIGURE 14-4 *Bone surfaces at the joints are smooth.*

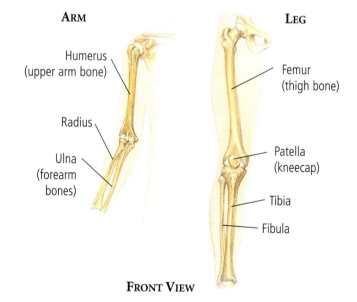

FRONT VIEW

FIGURE 14-5 *Leg bones are larger and stronger than arm bones because they carry the body's weight.*

and other soft tissues (see Figure 2-14 on page 21). For example, the skull protects the brain (Figure 14-3A); the ribs protect the heart and lungs (Figure 14-3B); the spinal cord is protected by the canal formed by the bones that form the spinal column (Figure 14-3C).

Bones

Bones are hard, dense tissues with a strong, rigid structure which helps them to withstand stresses that cause injuries. The shape of bones depends on what the bones

do and the stresses on them. For instance, the surfaces of bones at the joints are smooth (Figure 14-4). Although similar to the bones of the arm, the bones of the legs are much larger and stronger because they carry the body's weight (Figure 14-5).

Bones have a rich supply of blood and nerves. Some bones store and manufacture red blood cells and supply

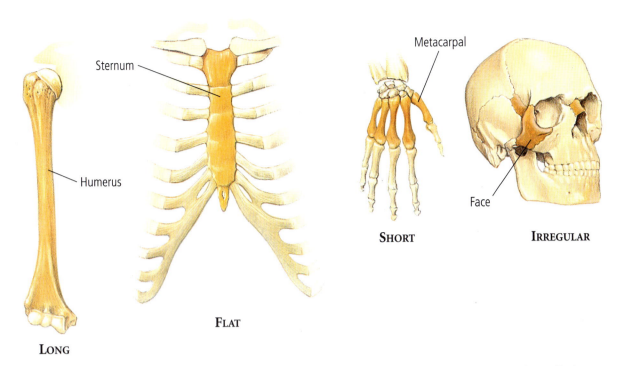

FIGURE 14-6 *Bones vary in shape and size. They are weakest at the points where they change shape and usually fracture at these points.*

them to the circulating blood. Bone injuries can bleed and are usually painful; the bleeding can become life-threatening if not properly cared for. Bones heal by forming new bone cells; they are the only body tissue that can regenerate in this way.

Bones weaken with age. In young children, bones are more flexible and are therefore less likely to break. In contrast, elderly people have more brittle bones that are more likely to give way to even everyday stresses, which can cause significant injuries. For instance, an elderly person pivoting with the weight on one leg can break the strongest bone in the body, the thigh bone. This gradual weakening of bone is called osteoporosis (see page 257).

Bones are classified as long, short, flat or irregular (Figure 14-6). Long bones are longer than they are wide; they include the bones of the upper arm (humerus), the forearm (radius, ulna), the thigh (femur) and the lower leg (tibia, fibula). Short bones are about as wide as they are long; they include the small bones of the hand (metacarpals) and feet (metatarsals). Flat bones have a relatively thin, flat shape; they include the breastbone (sternum), the ribs, the shoulder blade (scapula) and some of the bones that make up the skull. Bones that do not fit into the other categories are called irregular bones; they include the vertebrae and the bones of the face. Bones are weakest at the points where they change shape and usually fracture at these points.

Joints

A joint is a structure formed by the ends of two or more bones coming together. Most joints allow motion, but the bone ends at some joints are fused together, which restricts motion. Fused bones form solid structures that protect their contents (Figure 14-7).

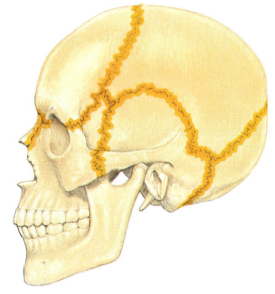

FIGURE 14-7 *Fused bones, such as the bones of the skull, form solid structures that protect their contents.*

Joints are held together by ligaments. Ligaments resist joint movement. Joints surrounded by ligaments have restricted movement, with joints that have few ligaments moving more freely. For instance, the shoulder joint, with few ligaments, allows greater motion than the hip joint, although their structure is similar. Joint motion also depends on the bone structure.

Joints that move more freely have less natural support and are therefore more prone to injury. However, all joints have a normal range of movement. When a joint is forced beyond its normal range, ligaments stretch and tear. Stretched and torn ligaments permit too much motion, and consequently make the joint unstable.

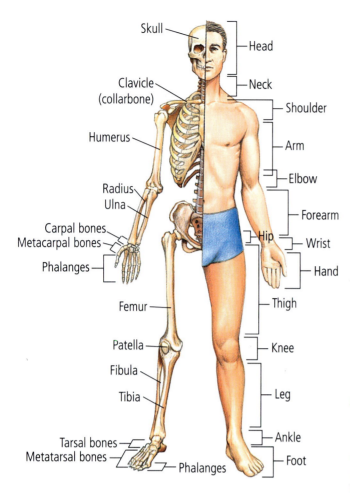

FIGURE 14-8 *Bones that can be seen and felt beneath the skin provide landmarks for locating parts of the body.*

Unstable joints can be disabling, particularly when they are weight-bearing, such as the knee or ankle. Unstable joints are prone to re-injury and often develop arthritis in later years.

Parts of the Skeleton

The bony structures that form the skeleton define the parts of the body. For example, the head is defined by the bones that form the skull and face, and the chest is defined by the bones that form the rib cage, sternum and spinal column. Prominent bones, which can be seen or felt beneath the skin, provide landmarks for locating parts of the body, as illustrated in Figure 14-8.

INJURIES TO THE MUSCULOSKELETAL SYSTEM

Injuries to the musculoskeletal system occur in a variety of ways, and are more commonly caused by physical force.

Types of Musculoskeletal Injuries

The four basic types of musculoskeletal injuries are **fracture, dislocation, sprain** and **strain**. Injuries to the musculoskeletal system can be classified according to the body structures that are damaged. Some injuries

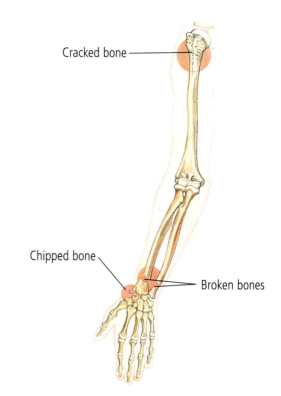

FIGURE 14-9 *Fractures include chipped or cracked bones and bones broken all the way through.*

may involve more than one type of injury; for example, a direct blow to the knee may injure both ligaments and bones. Injuries are also classified by the nature and extent of the damage.

Fractures

Fractures are breaks or disruptions in bone tissue. They include chipped or cracked bones, as well as bones that are broken all the way through (Figure 14-9). Fractures are commonly caused by direct and indirect forces. However, if strong enough, twisting forces and strong muscle contractions can also cause a fracture.

Fractures are classified as open or closed. An open fracture involves an open wound. Open fractures often occur when the limb is severely bent, causing bone ends to tear the skin and surrounding soft tissues, or when an object penetrates the skin and breaks the bone. Bone ends do not have to be visible for a fracture to be classified as open. Closed fractures leave the skin unbroken and are more common than open fractures. Open fractures are more serious because of the risks of infection and severe blood loss. Both open and closed fractures may be "complicated", however, when there is an associated injury to a major nerve, organ or other structure caused by the broken bone ends. Although fractures are rarely an immediate threat to life, any fracture involving a large bone can cause severe shock because bones and soft tissue may bleed heavily internally or externally.

Fractures are not always obvious unless there is a sign such as pain, deformity or an open wound with protruding bone ends. The way in which the injury occurred is often enough to suggest a fracture.

THE BREAKING POINT

Osteoporosis, a metabolic bone disorder usually discovered after the age of 60, affects 30 per cent of people over the age of 65. It will affect one out of four Australian women and occurs less frequently in men. Fair-skinned women with ancestors from northern Europe, the British Isles, Japan or China are genetically predisposed to osteoporosis. Inactive people are more susceptible to osteoporosis. Other risk factors include smoking, alcohol excess, regular use of certain medications including glucocorticoids, and poor dietary calcium intake.

Osteoporosis occurs when there is a decrease in the calcium content of bones. Normally, bones are hard, dense tissues which endure tremendous stresses. Bone-building cells constantly repair damage that occurs as a result of everyday stresses, keeping bones strong. Calcium is a key to bone growth, development and repair. When the calcium content of bones decreases, bones become frail, less dense and less able to repair the normal damage they incur.

This loss of density and strength leaves bones more susceptible to fractures. Where once tremendous force was necessary, fractures may now occur with little or no stress to the part, especially to hips, vertebrae and wrists. Spontaneous fractures are those that occur without trauma. The victim may be taking a walk or washing dishes when the fracture occurs. Some hip fractures thought to be caused by falls are actually spontaneous fractures which caused the victim to fall.

Peak bone mass is achieved around the ages of 17 to 20, and then subsequently falls. The amount of calcium absorbed from the diet naturally declines with age, making calcium intake increasingly important.

When calcium in the diet is inadequate, calcium in bones is withdrawn and used by the body to meet its other needs, leaving bones weakened.

Building strong bones before the age of 35 is the key to preventing osteoporosis. Calcium and exercise are necessary to bone building. The Australian Institute of Health and Welfare (AIHW) recommends an intake of 800 milligrams of calcium each day for adults. Many physicians recommend an intake of 1000 milligrams for women aged 19 and over. Three to four daily servings of low-fat dairy products should provide adequate calcium. Vitamin D is also necessary because it aids in the absorption of calcium. Exposure to sunshine enables the body to make vitamin D. Fifteen minutes of sunshine on the hands and face of a young, light-skinned individual are enough to supply the recommended daily allowance of 5 to 10 micrograms of vitamin D per day. Dark-skinned and elderly people need more sun exposure. People who do not receive adequate sun exposure need to consume vitamin D. The best sources are vitamin-fortified milk and fatty fish such as tuna, salmon and eel.

Calcium supplements combined with vitamin D are available for those who do not take in adequate calcium. However, before taking a calcium supplement you should consult a doctor. Many highly advertised calcium supplements are ineffective because they do not dissolve in the body.

Exercise seems to increase bone density and the activity of bone-building cells. Regular exercise may reduce the rate of bone loss by promoting new bone formation and also stimulate the skeletal system to repair itself. An effective exercise program, such as aerobics, jogging or walking, uses the weight-bearing muscles of the legs. ■

Dislocation

A dislocation is a displacement or separation of a bone from its normal position at a joint (Figure 14-10). Dislocations are usually caused by severe forces. Some joints, such as the shoulder or fingers, dislocate easily because their bones and ligaments do not provide adequate protection. Others, such as the elbow or the joints of the spine, are well protected and therefore dislocate less easily.

A force violent enough to cause a dislocation can also cause a fracture and can damage nearby nerves and blood vessels.

Dislocations are generally more obvious than fractures because the joint appears deformed. The displaced bone end often causes an abnormal lump, ridge or depression, sometimes making dislocations easier to identify than other musculoskeletal injuries.

Sprains

A sprain is the partial or complete tearing of ligaments and other tissues at a joint. A sprain usually results when the bones that form a joint are forced beyond

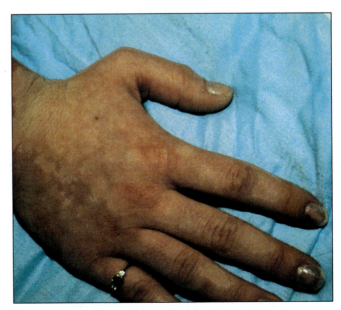

FIGURE 14-10 *Because of deformity, dislocations are generally more obvious than fractures.*

their normal range of motion (Figure 14-11). The more ligaments torn, the more severe the injury. The sudden, violent forcing of a joint beyond its limit can completely rupture ligaments and dislocate the bones. Severe sprains may involve a fracture of the bones that form the joint, or ligaments may pull a bone away at the point of attachment.

Mild sprains, which only stretch ligament fibres, generally heal quickly. The victim may have only a brief period of pain and quickly return to activity with little or no discomfort. For this reason, people often neglect sprains and the joint is often re-injured. Severe sprains that involve a fracture usually cause pain when the joint is moved or used. The weight-bearing joints of the ankle and knee and the joints of the fingers and wrist are sprained most often.

Strains

A strain is a stretching and tearing of muscle or tendon fibres. It is sometimes called a muscle pull or tear. Because tendons are tougher and stronger than muscles, tears usually occur in the muscle itself or where the muscle attaches to the tendon. Strains are often the result of over-exertion, such as lifting something too heavy or working a muscle too hard. They can also result from sudden or unco-ordinated movement.

Strains sometimes recur chronically, especially to the muscles of the neck, lower back and the back of the thigh. Neck and back problems are two of the leading causes of absenteeism from work, accounting for many compensation claims and much lost productivity.

Which do you think is more severe, a strain or sprain? Why?

Symptoms and Signs of Musculoskeletal Injuries

Common symptoms and signs associated with musculoskeletal injuries include:

- pain
- swelling
- deformity
- discolouration of the skin
- inability to use the affected part normally
- feeling of grating of broken bone ends, or the sound of a snap or pop at the time of injury
- symptoms and signs of shock (Chapter 6)

Pain, swelling and discolouration of the skin commonly occur with any significant injury. Irritation to nerve endings that supply the injured area causes pain, which is the body's indicator that something is wrong. The injured area may be painful to touch and to move. Swelling is caused by bleeding from damaged blood vessels and tissues in the injured area. However, swelling is often deceptive: it may appear rapidly at the site of injury, may develop gradually, or may not appear at all. Swelling by itself is not a reliable indicator of the severity of an injury or of the structures involved. Bleeding may discolour the skin in surrounding tissues. At first, the skin may only look red then, as blood seeps to the skin's surface, the area begins to look bruised.

Deformity is also a sign of significant injury. Swelling, abnormal lumps, ridges, depressions or unusual bends or angles in body parts are types of deformities. Marked deformity is often a sign of fracture or dislocation (Figure 14-12). Comparing the injured part to an uninjured part on the opposite side of the body may help you detect deformity.

A victim's inability to move or use an injured part may indicate a significant injury. The victim may tell you that movement is impossible, or that it is simply too painful to move. Moving or using injured parts can disturb tissues, further irritating nerve endings, which causes or increases pain. Often, the muscles of an affected area contract and pull the bone pieces out of alignment. This may cause pain, contracture of a limb and deformity of a part.

Similarly, a victim often supports the injury in the most comfortable position. To manage musculoskeletal injuries, try to avoid any motion or use of an injured body part that causes pain.

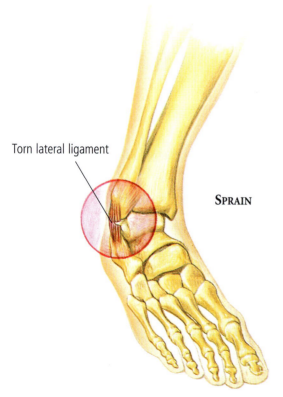

Torn lateral ligament

SPRAIN

FIGURE 14-11 *A sprain results when bones that form a joint are forced beyond their normal range of motion.*

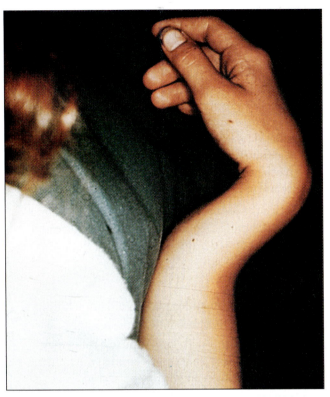

FIGURE 14-12 *Marked deformity is often a sign of fracture or dislocation.*

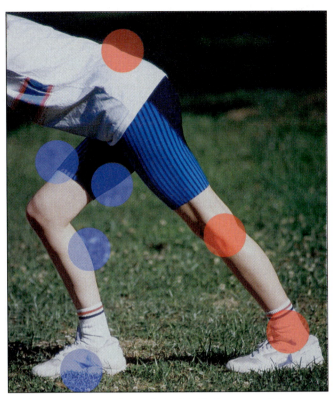

FIGURE 14-13 *A sprain involves the soft tissues at a joint (indicated in red). Strains involve the soft tissue structures that, for the most part, stretch between joints (indicated in blue).*

Symptoms and Signs of Specific Musculoskeletal Injuries

In the secondary survey, you may notice certain telltale symptoms and signs that help you determine the type of injury. Often, what the victim feels or can recall from the moment of injury provides important clues.

Sprains or strains are fairly easy to tell apart. Because a sprain involves the soft tissues at a joint, pain, swelling and deformity are generally confined to the joint area. Strains involve the soft tissue structures that, for the most part, stretch between joints. In most strains, pain, swelling and any deformity are generally in the areas between the joints (Figure 14-13). Sprains and strains are sometimes referred to as soft tissue injuries and may involve damage to muscles, ligaments, tendons, veins, arteries and nerves.

However, it is not always easy to determine if an injury involves a fracture or dislocation. Sometimes, the only reliable way to determine whether the injury is a sprain, strain, fracture or dislocation is by x-ray. Always treat such an injury as a fracture if you are uncertain of its severity.

Assessment of Musculoskeletal Injuries

You identify and care for injuries to the musculoskeletal system during the secondary survey. Because they appear similar, it may be difficult for you to determine exactly what type of injury has occurred. One method of assessment of such injuries is the use of the acronym SALTAPS, described by Dr Russell Gibbs in his book *Sports Injuries* (Sun Books, Melbourne, 1977):

Stop, Ask, Look, Touch, Active movement, Passive movement, Stand.

1. *Stop* the victim from further activity and movement.

2. *Ask* the victim about what happened, where it hurts, and so on.

3. *Look* at the injured area for swelling, bruising, and deformity, comparing one side of the body to the other for any differences.

4. *Touch* the area involved gently to assess for pain or tenderness, warmth or muscle spasms.

5. If the first four steps do not reveal significant injury, ask the victim to try *Active movement* of the injured area. If the victim cannot move the body part, seek immediate medical advice.

6. If the victim can freely move the area actively, then use *Passive movement* to assess the range of movement of the part by asking the victim with an injured upper extremity to squeeze your hands or, with a lower extremity injury, to push the feet against the resistance of your hands. A loss of power or co-ordination may indicate a more serious injury and medical advice is needed.

7. Check whether the victim can *Stand* up and move unassisted. If the victim cannot do this without support or is in significant pain, seek medical advice before any further movement is attempted.

COLD COMPRESSES FOR SPRAINS AND STRAINS

Sprains and strains are common injuries in many sports and part of the specialty treatment area of sports medicine. In addition to other care given for sprains and strains, cold compresses are often used as soon as any bleeding has been controlled.

How cold helps initially

When a person twists an ankle or knee, the tissues underneath the skin are injured. Blood and fluids seep out from the torn blood vessels and cause swelling to occur at the site of the injury. Once bleeding has been controlled, cold can be applied to make the broken blood vessels constrict, thus limiting further blood and fluid loss.

Cold has been widely used as a first response to a sprain or strain, but recent research has shown that cold is best used only after any internal bleeding has been controlled, as cold inhibits clotting initially. For example, a likely ankle sprain, requires initial first aid for the damage to internal blood vessels and muscle fibres, and cold can then be used in the second stage of treatment as an aid to recovery.

Applying a Cold Compress

1. Soak a cloth or other suitable material in cold or iced water. Squeeze out any excess water so that the cloth is damp but not dripping, and place it over the area of injury.

2. Replace the compress regularly or drip more cold water onto the old one to ensure that the cooling is maintained. Cool the injury for 10 minutes, then check the skin temperature and colour, and remove the compress if reddening occurs.

3. If necessary, hold the compress in position with an open-weave bandage.

Applying an Ice Pack

1. Fill a plastic bag or ice bag half to two-thirds full of crushed or cubed ice. Exclude all air, seal the bag and wrap it in a damp cloth. The ice pack should be large enough to cover the entire area of the injury. (A packet of frozen peas wrapped in a cloth can be used as this easily moulds to the shape of the injured body part.)

2. Place the ice pack over the injury for a maximum of 10 minutes. Check the skin temperature and colour regularly, and remove the ice pack if reddening occurs.

Notes:

- *Always* wrap an ice pack in a damp cloth to avoid burning the skin.

- Elite athletes with larger muscle mass may need to have an ice pack applied for longer periods under medical supervision.

How heat helps later on

A sports physician often advises applying ice to the injury after the initial first aid has been given. Ice packs may be applied for 10 minutes at a time and continued periodically for up to 72 hours or until the tissues are no longer hot to the touch. After that, heat applications may be prescribed. Heat speeds up the chemical reactions needed to repair tissue. White blood cells move in to rid the body of infections, and other cells begin the repair process. Even though heat has a later role in treatment of an injury, always apply cold before heat and consult your doctor for clearance to start.

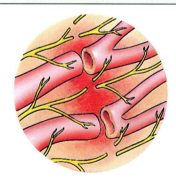 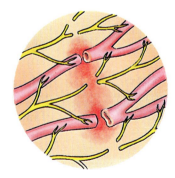 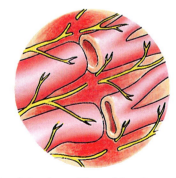

An injury damages blood vessels, causing bleeding in the injured area. Injury irritates nerve endings, and thus causes pain.

Applying ice or a cold pack constricts blood vessels, slowing bleeding that causes the injury to swell. Cold deadens nerve endings and thus relieves pain.

Applying heat dilates blood vessels, increasing blood flow to the injured area. Nerve endings become more sensitive.

Care for Musculoskeletal Injuries

Some musculoskeletal injuries are obvious because they involve severe deformities such as protruding bones or bleeding. Also, the victim may be in much pain. Do not be distracted by pain as such injuries are rarely life-threatening. Complete the primary survey and care first for any life-threatening conditions. Then complete the secondary survey and care for any other injuries. Call for an ambulance, especially if:

- the injury involves the head, neck or back
- the injury impairs walking or breathing
- you see or suspect multiple musculoskeletal injuries

If an ambulance is on the way, do not move the victim unnecessarily. Control any bleeding and take steps to minimise shock. Monitor the ABC.

Remember:

Sometimes it is difficult to tell whether an injury is a fracture, dislocation, sprain or strain. When in doubt, always treat such an injury as a fracture.

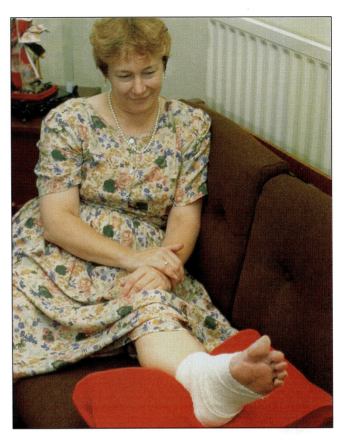

FIGURE 14-14 *General care for all musculoskeletal injuries is similar. Remember compression, elevation and rest.*

Soft Tissue Injuries

Injuries to muscles, ligaments and other soft tissues can occur with or without a fracture. If you do not suspect a fracture, control bleeding with compression, elevation and rest (Figure 14-14). Apply ice after bleeding is controlled.

Compression

Apply a firm supporting bandage to give an even pressure over the injured area. Use light padding under the bandage if the pain is severe.

Elevation

Elevating the injured area helps slow the flow of blood and reduces swelling. If possible, raise the injured area above the level of the heart. Remember, *do not* attempt to elevate a part you suspect is fractured until it has been splinted or fully immobilised.

Rest

Avoid any movements or activities which cause pain. Help the victim into the most comfortable position. If you suspect head, neck or back injuries, leave the victim lying flat.

Ice

Once any bleeding has been controlled, apply a wrapped ice pack or cold compress (see opposite page). Cold helps reduce swelling and eases pain and discomfort.

Fractures

The main aim of treatment for any fracture is to prevent movement at the injury site. If you suspect a fracture, you must support or immobilise the injured part.

The purposes of support and **immobilisation** for an injury are to:

- lessen pain
- prevent further damage to soft tissues
- reduce the risk of serious bleeding
- reduce the possibility of loss of circulation to the injured part
- prevent a closed fracture from becoming an open fracture

You can *support* an injured part by leaving it as found and packing available material around it to give support. This allows the victim to relax the muscles surrounding the area and helps relieve pain.

You can *immobilise* an injured part by applying a **splint**, sling or bandages to keep the injured body part from moving. A splint is a device that maintains an injured part in place. If necessary, a sound leg can be used to support an injured one by tying bandages around both limbs. This is a type of **body splinting**. A Practice Guide at the end of this chapter gives the detailed steps for using the body as a splint for the lower leg. If body splinting is not possible or greater support is needed, such as to transport the victim a long way, then a more rigid splint is required. An effective splint must extend

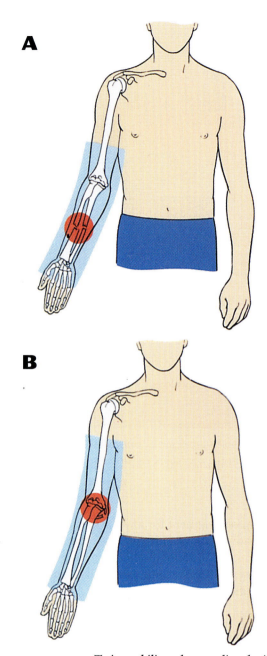

A

B

FIGURE 14-15 A *To immobilise a bone, splint the joints above and below the fracture.* **B** *To immobilise a joint, splint the bones above and below the injured joint.*

above and below the injury site (Figures 14-15A and B). For instance, to immobilise a fractured bone, the splint must include the joints above and below the fracture. Practice Guides 2 and 3 at the end of this chapter detail the steps for applying both soft and rigid splints.

When using a splint, follow these four basic principles:

- Splint only if necessary, and if you can do it without causing more pain and discomfort to the victim.

- Splint an injury in the position you find it.

- Splint the injured area and the joints above and below the injury site.

- Check the circulation before and after splinting.

In general, you don't need to apply a splint if you are in a metropolitan area and ambulance assistance is

readily available. In this instance you should support the injury in the position in which you find it and not move the victim unnecessarily.

Injuries to Head and Spine

Recognising Serious Head and Spine Injuries

Injuries to the head or spine often damage both bone and soft tissue, including brain tissue and the **spinal cord**. It is difficult to determine the extent of damage in head and spine injuries. In most cases, the only way to assess the damage is by x-ray. You may not know the severity of an injury, so always provide initial care as if the injury is serious.

The Spine

The spine is a strong, flexible column that supports the head and the trunk and encases and protects the spinal cord. The spine consists of small bones called **vertebrae**, which have circular openings. The vertebrae are separated from each other by cushions of cartilage called discs (Figure 14-16A). This cartilage acts as a shock absorber when a person is walking, running or jumping. The spinal cord, a bundle of nerves, runs through the hollow part of the vertebrae. Nerve branches extend to various parts of the body through openings on both sides of the vertebrae.

The spine is divided into five regions: the cervical or neck region, the thoracic or midback region, the lumbar or lower back region, the sacrum and the coccyx, the small triangular bone at the lower end of the spinal column (Figure 14-16B).

Injuries to the spine often fracture the vertebrae and sprain the ligaments. These injuries usually heal without problems. With severe injuries, however, the vertebrae may shift and compress or sever the spinal cord. This can cause temporary or permanent paralysis, even death. The extent of the paralysis depends on which area of the spinal cord is damaged (Figure 14-16B).

Causes of Head and Spinal Injury

Consider the cause of the injury to help you determine when a head or spinal injury may be serious. The cause is often the best initial measure of severity. Survey the scene and think about the forces involved in the injury. Strong forces are likely to cause severe injury to the head and spine. For example, a driver whose head breaks a car windscreen in a crash may have a potentially serious head and spine injury. Similarly, divers

2 *How may compression or severing of the spinal cord cause death?*

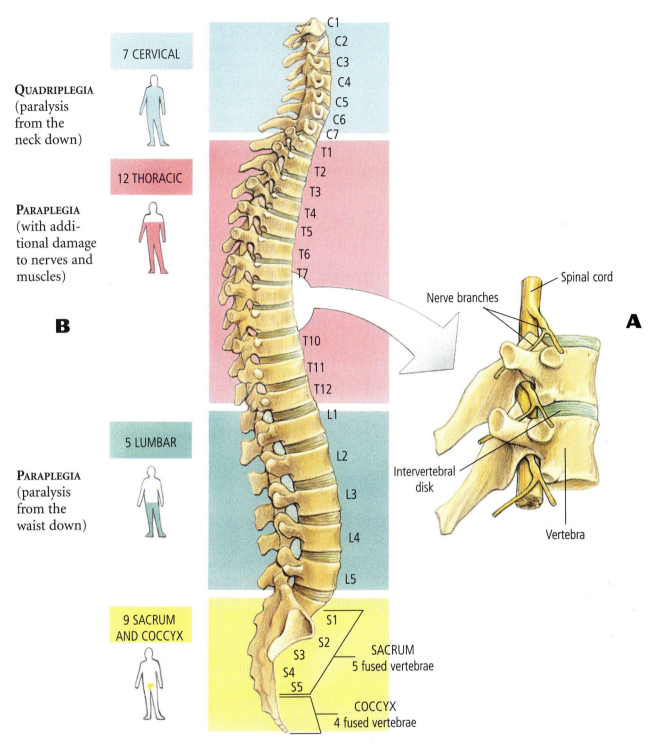

QUADRIPLEGIA (paralysis from the neck down)

7 CERVICAL

PARAPLEGIA (with additional damage to nerves and muscles)

12 THORACIC

B

5 LUMBAR

PARAPLEGIA (paralysis from the waist down)

9 SACRUM AND COCCYX

C1
C2
C3
C4
C5
C6
C7
T1
T2
T3
T4
T5
T6
T7
T10
T11
T12
L1
L2
L3
L4
L5
S1
S2
S3
S4
S5

Spinal cord

Nerve branches

A

Intervertebral disk

Vertebra

SACRUM
5 fused vertebrae

COCCYX
4 fused vertebrae

FIGURE 14-16 A *Vertebrae are separated by cushions of cartilage called discs.* **B** *The spine is divided into five regions. Traumatic injury to a region of the spine can paralyse specific body areas.*

who hit their heads on the bottom of a swimming pool may also have serious injuries.

Consider the possibility of a serious head and/or spine injury in several situations. These include:

- A fall from a height greater than the victim's height.
- A fall where the victim lands heavily on the head, back, feet or base of the spine.
- Any blow to the face, because an underlying injury may have occurred.

- Any diving mishap such as diving into shallow or murky water.
- Any injury involving a severe blunt force to the head or trunk, such as from a car or other vehicle.
- Any injury that penetrates the head or trunk, such as a gunshot wound.
- A motor vehicle collision involving a driver or passengers, especially when not wearing seat belts.

- Any situation where a person is thrown from a motor vehicle.
- Any injury in which a victim's helmet is broken, including a motorcycle, football or industrial helmet.
- Any incident involving a lightning strike.

Symptoms and Signs of Head and Spine Injuries

You may also notice the following symptoms and signs which indicate a serious head or spine injury. These may be obvious at first or may develop later:

- Changes in the conscious state (see Chapter 9).
- Severe pain or pressure in the head, neck or back.
- Tingling or loss of sensation in the extremities.
- Blood or other fluids in the ears or nose.
- Profuse external bleeding of the head, neck or back.
- Seizures.
- Impaired breathing or vision as a result of injury.
- Nausea or vomiting.
- Persistent headache.
- Loss of balance.
- Bruising of the head, especially around the eyes and behind the ears.
- Partial or complete loss of movement of any body part.
- Unusual bumps or depressions on the head or spine.

These symptoms and signs alone do not always suggest a serious head or spine injury, but they may do when combined with the cause of the injury. Regardless of the situation, always call an ambulance when you suspect a serious head or spine injury.

General Care for Head and Spine Injuries

Head and spine injuries can become life-threatening emergencies, as a serious injury can cause a victim to stop breathing. Providing care for serious head and spine injuries involves supporting the respiratory, circulatory and nervous systems. Always give the following care while waiting for ambulance personnel to arrive:

1. Maintain an open airway.
2. If unconscious, turn the victim carefully on the side.
3. Minimise movement of the head and spine.
4. Monitor the conscious state.
5. Ensure the victim is breathing.
6. Control any external bleeding.
7. Maintain normal body temperature.

Chapter 7 describes the care for victims of spinal injury in water (page 114).

Injuries to the Pelvis

The **pelvis** is the lower part of the trunk and contains the bladder, reproductive organs and part of the large intestine, including the rectum. Major arteries and nerves pass through the pelvis. The organs within the pelvis are well protected on the sides and back but not in front. Injuries to the pelvis may include fractures to the pelvic bones and damage to structures within, especially the bladder, urethra or bowel.

Symptoms and Signs of Pelvic Injury

Symptoms and signs of injury to the pelvis are the same as those for an abdominal injury (page 290). Certain pelvic injuries may also cause a loss of sensation in the legs or an inability to move them.

Care for Pelvic Injuries

Care for pelvic injuries is the same as that for abdominal injuries and serious musculoskeletal injuries. Give the following care while waiting for the ambulance:

1. Do not move the victim unless necessary. If you suspect a spinal injury, do not move the victim except in a life-threatening situation.
2. Control any external bleeding and cover any protruding organs.
3. Take steps to minimise shock.
4. If possible, try to keep the victim lying flat. If not, help the victim become comfortable.

An injury to the pelvis sometimes involves the genitals, the external reproductive organs. Genital injuries are either closed wounds, such as a bruise, or open wounds, such as an avulsion or laceration. Any injury to the genitals is extremely painful. Care for a closed wound as you would for any closed wound. If the injury is an open wound, apply a sterile dressing and direct pressure with your or the victim's hand. If any parts are avulsed, wrap them appropriately and make sure they are transported with the victim. Injuries to the genital area can be embarrassing for both the victim and the first aider. Explain briefly what you are going to do, and then do it. Do not act in a timid or hesitant manner. This will only make the situation more difficult for you and the victim.

Rib Fractures

A serious chest injury is a fracture of the **rib cage**, which is usually caused by direct force to the chest. Although painful, a simple rib fracture is rarely life-threatening (Figure 14-17). A victim with a fractured rib generally remains calm and takes shallow breaths because normal or deep breathing is painful. The victim will usually attempt to ease the pain by supporting the injured area with a hand or arm.

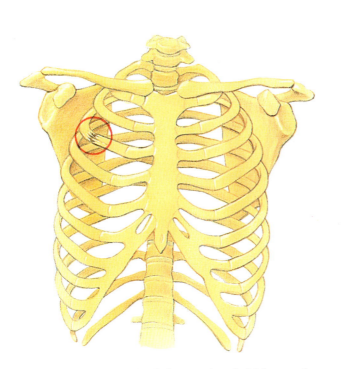

FIGURE 14-17 *A simple rib fracture is painful but rarely life-threatening.*

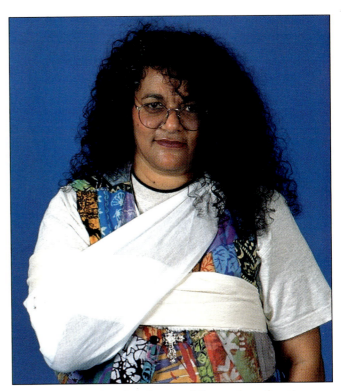

FIGURE 14-18 *Use a bandage, padding and an elevation sling for a rib fracture.*

Therefore, shallow breathing and holding the area are both signs of possible rib fracture. If you suspect a fractured rib, give the general care for musculoskeletal injuries together with this specific care:

1. Help the victim to rest in the position that makes breathing easiest.

2. If ambulance transport is delayed, binding the victim's arm to the chest over padding on the injured side will help support the injured area and make breathing more comfortable. Apply an elevation sling for extra support (Figure 14-18).

Injuries to the Limbs

Injuries to the **limbs**—the arms and legs, hands and feet—are quite common. They range from a simple bruise to a critical injury with severe bleeding, such as a fracture of the thigh bone. With any injury to the extremities, the prompt care you give can help prevent further pain and damage.

To care for musculoskeletal injuries involving the extremities follow these principles of general care for an injury:

1. If you suspect a serious injury, call an ambulance and until it arrives, continue to monitor the ABC.

2. Control bleeding.

3. Minimise shock.

4. Rest the injured body part.

5. Elevate the area if possible, if you do not suspect a fracture.

Upper Limb Injuries

The upper extremities are the arms and hands. The bones of each upper extremity include the collar bone (clavicle), shoulder blade (scapula), bones of the upper arm (humerus) and forearm (radius and ulna), and bones of the hand (carpals and metacarpals) and fingers (phalanges). Figure 14-19 (page 266) shows the major structures of the upper extremities.

The upper extremities are the most commonly injured area of the body. These injuries may occur in many different ways, the most frequent cause being a fall on an outstretched hand. Abrasions occur easily because the hands are rarely protected. Because a falling person instinctively tries to break the fall by extending the arms and hands, these areas receive the force of the body's weight. This can cause a serious injury, such as a severe sprain or dislocation of the wrist, the shoulder, elbow or a fracture of the arm between these joints.

When caring for upper extremity injuries, minimise any movement of the injured part. If an injured person is holding the arm securely against the chest, do not change the position. Holding the arm against the chest is an effective method of body splinting. Instead, help the person support the arm by binding it to the chest over padding. Caring for a victim with an upper extremity injury does not require special equipment.

FRONT VIEW   BACK VIEW

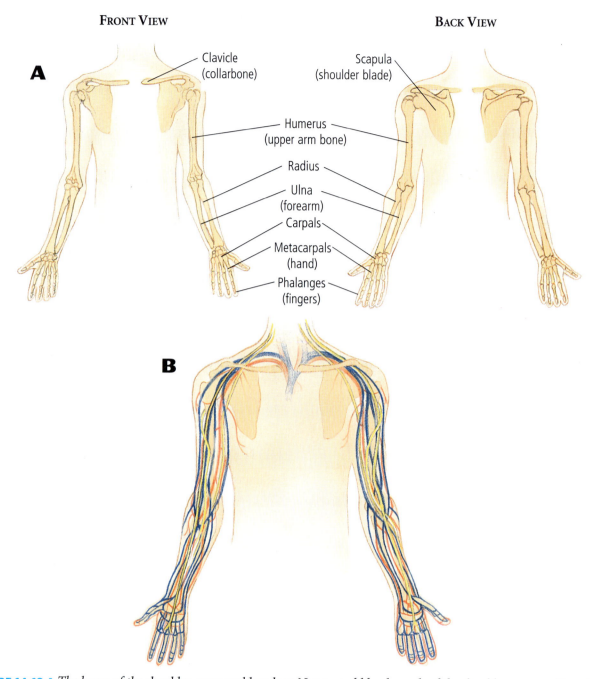

A

Clavicle
(collarbone)

Scapula
(shoulder blade)

Humerus
(upper arm bone)

Radius

Ulna
(forearm)

Carpals

Metacarpals
(hand)

Phalanges
(fingers)

B

FIGURE 14-19 A *The bones of the shoulder, arms and hands.* **B** *Nerves and blood vessels of the shoulder, arm and hands.*

Shoulder Injuries

The shoulder consists of three bones that meet to form the shoulder joint. These bones are the scapula, clavicle, and humerus. Injuries to the shoulder may involve a dislocation or fracture of one or more of these bones.

A dislocation is a common type of shoulder injury. Like fractures, dislocations often result from falls, when a person attempts to break a fall with an outstretched arm or lands on the point of the shoulder. The impact can force the arm against the joint formed by the scapula and clavicle (Figure 14-20). This can result in ligaments tearing, causing bones to displace and sometimes fracture.

Shoulder dislocations are painful and can often be identified by the deformity present. As with other

> **Remember:**
>
> *Never attempt to replace a dislocated shoulder because of the possibility of an associated fracture and the risk of damage to the nerves and blood vessels close to the joint.*

shoulder injuries, the victim often tries to minimise the pain by supporting the weight of the arm in the most comfortable position.

Scapula fractures are not common. A fracture of the scapula typically results from violent force. The symptoms and signs of a fractured scapula are the same as

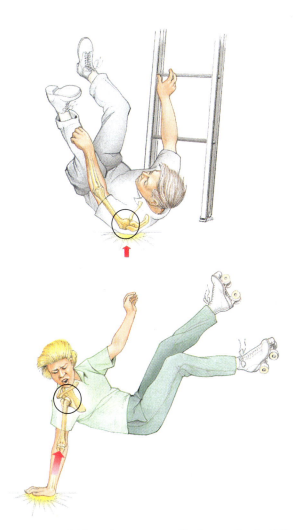

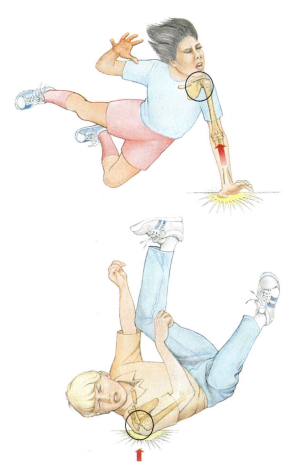

FIGURE 14-21 *A collar bone fracture is commonly caused by a fall.*

FIGURE 14-20 *Dislocations are usually the result of a fall.*

for any other extremity fracture, although you are less likely to see deformity of the scapula. The most significant symptom is the inability to move the arm.

Because it takes great force to break the scapula, consider that the force may have been great enough also to injure the chest wall. If the chest wall is injured, the victim with a fractured scapula may have difficulty breathing.

The most frequently injured bone of the shoulder is the clavicle, which is more commonly injured in children than it is in adults. Typically, the clavicle is fractured as a result of a fall (Figure 14-21). The victim usually feels pain in and around the shoulder area. A person with a fractured clavicle usually attempts to ease the pain by supporting the weight of the arm. As the clavicle lies directly over major blood vessels and nerves to the arm, it is important to minimise movement of the injured area to prevent injury to these structures if the victim must be moved.

The largest bone in the upper arm is the humerus. This bone can be fractured at any point, although it is usually fractured at the upper end near the shoulder or in the middle of the bone. The upper end of the humerus often fractures in the elderly or in young children as a result of a fall. Breaks in the middle of the bone mostly occur in young adults.

When the humerus is fractured, there is danger of damage to the blood vessels and nerves supplying the entire arm. Most humerus fractures are very painful and will not permit the victim to use the arm. A fracture can also cause considerable arm deformity.

Care for Shoulder and Upper Arm Injuries

There is a serious risk of damage to the nerves and blood vessels of the surrounding area if injuries to the shoulder or upper arm are moved unnecessarily. The aim of care is to assist the victim to support the injury in the most comfortable position and to obtain ambulance assistance.

In summary, this is the care you should provide for shoulder injuries:

1. Control any external bleeding.

2. Allow the victim to continue to support the arm in the most comfortable position.

3. If the victim is holding the arm away from the body, use a pillow, rolled blanket or similar object to fill the gap between the arm and chest to provide support for the injured area.

4. Remember, most victims feel more comfortable supporting their own injury (Figure 14-22, page 268).

Elbow Injuries

Injuries to the elbow can cause permanent disability, because all the nerves and blood vessels to the forearm and hand go through the elbow. Therefore, take elbow injuries seriously because of the serious risk of damage to the blood supply to the area. Like other joints, the elbow can be sprained, fractured or dislocated. Injuries to a joint like the elbow can be made worse by movement. If the victim says that the elbow cannot be moved, *do not* try to move it. Support the arm and immobilise it in the position in which you find it. Call an ambulance immediately.

In addition, provide the following specific care:

1. Control any external bleeding.

2. Support the arm from the shoulder to the wrist in the best way possible. This can be done by packing available material around the injury and encouraging the victim to relax the muscles surrounding the area (Figure 14-22).

3. If the elbow is straight, use body splinting and secure the arm at the wrist and upper arm with narrow or broad bandages.

4. In all cases of fractures involving the elbow or forearm, treat the injury gently and *do not move the limb from the position the victim has adopted.*

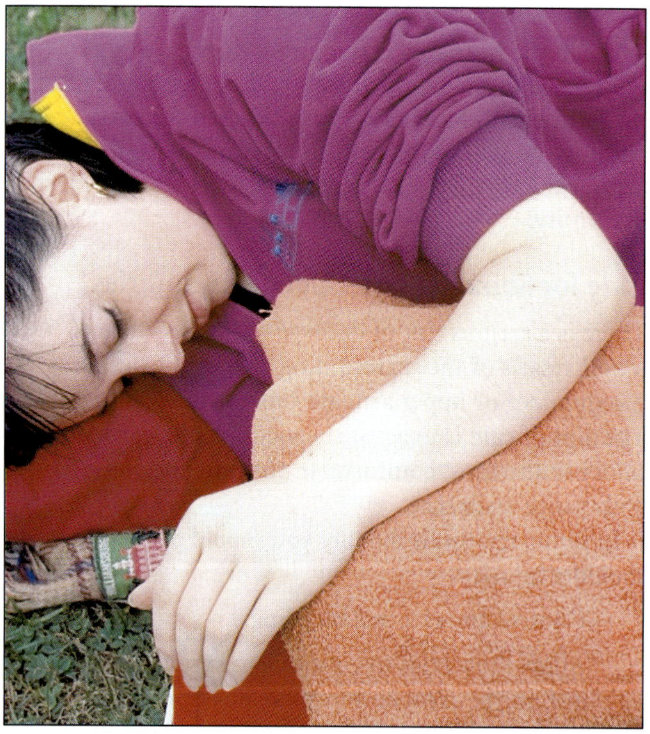

Forearm, Wrist and Hand Injuries

Fractures of the two forearm bones, the radius and ulna, are more common in children than they are in adults. If a person falls on an outstretched arm both bones may break, but not always in the same place. With forearm fractures, there may be an obvious deformity (Figure 14-23). Because the radial artery and nerve are near the bones, a fracture may cause severe bleeding or a loss of movement in the wrist and hand.

The wrist is a common site of sprains and fractures. It is often difficult to tell the extent of the injury. Therefore, care for wrist injuries in the same way as forearm injuries.

Because the hands are used in so many daily activities, they are very susceptible to injury. Most injuries to the hands and fingers involve only minor soft tissue damage. Home, recreational and industrial mishaps often produce lacerations, avulsions, burns and fractures of the hands.

With a suspected finger or thumb dislocation, *do not* attempt to put the bones back into place, as it is difficult to tell whether there may be an associated fracture.

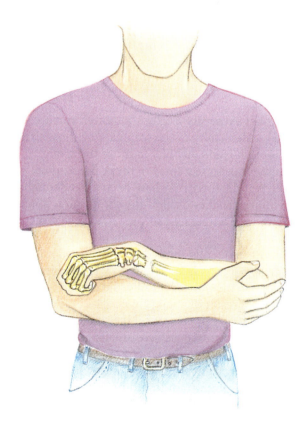

FIGURE 14-22 *Support the arm from the shoulder to the wrist in the best way possible.*

FIGURE 14-23 *Fractures of both forearm bones at the wrist often cause a characteristic S-shaped deformity.*

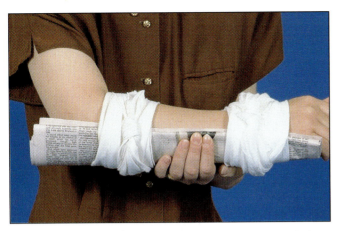

FIGURE 14-24 *Splinting a forearm fracture with a rolled newspaper or magazine.*

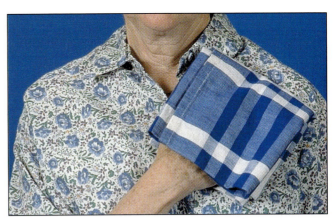

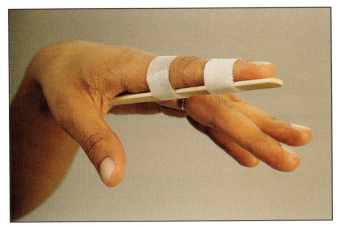

FIGURE 14-25 *An ice cream stick can be used to splint a finger injury.*

To care for forearm, wrist and hand injuries, first control any external bleeding. These injuries are generally not life-threatening, and therefore an ambulance may not be required.

If an ambulance is not being used, immobilise and support the injured part with a splint (Figure 14-24). Practice Guide 3 at the end of the chapter describes the detailed steps for application of a rigid splint which can be used for forearm and wrist injuries.

A finger injury can be splinted with a small, straight splint improvised from an ice cream stick (Figure 14-25).

For hand fractures, protect the injured hand with a fold of soft padding over the front and back of the hand. Use an elevation sling to support the limb (see Chapter 13). The limb can be further supported by applying a broad bandage around the trunk and arm over the sling, tied in front on the non-injured side (Figure 14-26).

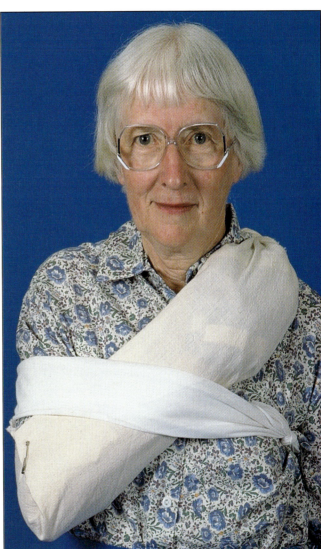

FIGURE 14-26 *Bandage and sling for a hand fracture (see text description below).*

Improvised Slings

If you do not have a triangular bandage available for making a sling, you can improvise one in several different ways (see page 241).

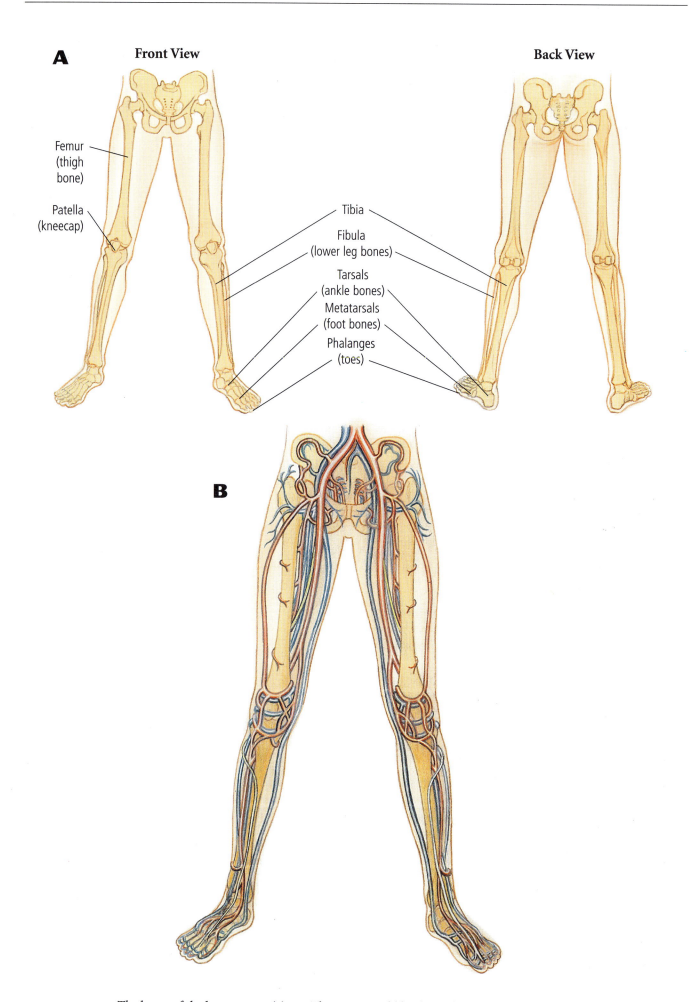

A Front View   Back View

Femur
(thigh
bone)

Patella
(kneecap)

Tibia

Fibula
(lower leg bones)

Tarsals
(ankle bones)

Metatarsals
(foot bones)

Phalanges
(toes)

B

FIGURE 14-27 A *The bones of the lower extremities.* **B** *The nerves and blood vessels of the lower extremities.*

Thigh and Lower Leg Injuries

The femur is the largest bone in the body. Because it bears most of the weight of the body, it is most important in walking and running. Thigh injuries range from bruises and torn muscles to severe injuries such as fractures and dislocations. The upper end of the femur meets the pelvis at the hip joint (Figure 14-28). Femur fractures involving the upper end of the bone are called fractures of the neck of the femur; these are more common in older adults. Even though the hip joint itself is not involved, such injuries are often called hip fractures.

A fracture of the femur usually produces a characteristic deformity. When the fracture occurs, the thigh muscles contract. Because the thigh muscles are so strong, they pull the broken bone ends together, causing them to overlap. This may cause the injured leg to be noticeably shorter than the other leg. The injured leg may also be turned outward (Figure 14-30). Other symptoms of a fractured femur include severe pain and inability to move the leg.

A fracture of the lower leg may involve one or both bones; often, both are fractured simultaneously. However, a blow to the outside of the lower leg can cause an isolated fracture of the smaller bone (fibula). Because these two bones lie just beneath the skin, open fractures are common (Figure 14-29). Lower leg fractures may cause a severe deformity in which the lower leg is bent at an unusual angle (angulated), as well as pain and inability to move the leg.

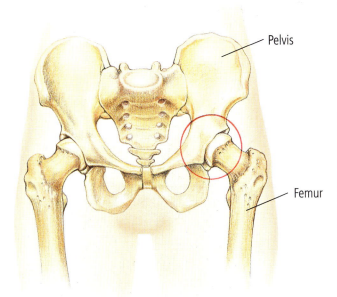

FIGURE 14-28 *The upper end of the femur meets the pelvis at the hip joint.*

Pelvis

Femur

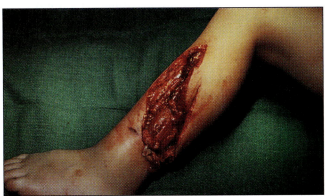

FIGURE 14-29 *A fracture of the lower leg can be an open fracture.*

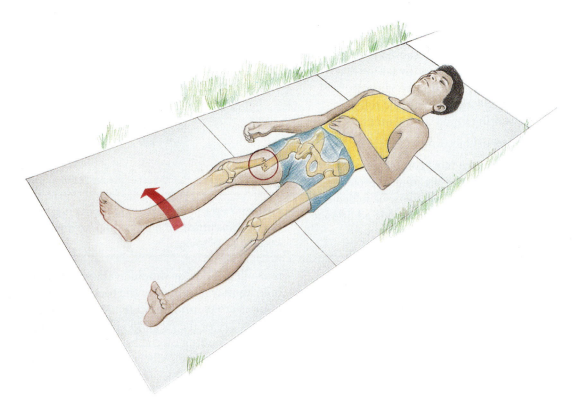

FIGURE 14-30 *A fractured femur often produces a characteristic deformity. The injured leg is shorter than the uninjured leg and may be turned outward.*

For the victim with a serious injury to the thigh or lower leg, provide the following specific care:

1. Control external bleeding. Call ambulance personnel immediately; they are much better prepared to care for a victim with a serious leg injury.

2. Support the injured area and help the victim rest in the most comfortable position. The ground itself acts as an excellent splint. If the victim's leg is supported by the ground, do not move it.

3. If ambulance assistance is delayed, you can use the uninjured leg as a splint in lower leg fractures (see page 279).

A fractured femur can cause serious bleeding, and the likelihood of shock is great. Keep the person lying down and minimise shock. Maintain normal body temperature, and ensure an ambulance has been called. Monitor the ABC and watch for changes in the victim's conscious state. *Do not attempt to splint a fractured femur because any movement risks serious complications.*

Knee Injuries

The knee joint is very vulnerable to injury. The knee involves the lower end of the femur, the upper ends of the tibia and fibula, and the patella (kneecap). The kneecap is a free-floating bone that moves on the lower front surface of the thigh bone. Knee injuries range from cuts and bruises to sprains, fractures and dislocations. Deep lacerations in the area of the knee can cause severe joint infections. Sprains, fractures and dislocations of the knee are common in athletic activities that involve quick movements or exert unusual force on the knee.

The kneecap is unprotected in that it lies directly beneath the skin. This part of the knee is vulnerable to bruises, lacerations and dislocations. Violent forces to the front of the knee, such as those caused by hitting the dashboard of a motor vehicle or by falling and landing on bent knees, can fracture the kneecap.

To care for an injured knee, provide the following specific care while waiting for an ambulance:

1. Control any external bleeding.

2. Support the knee in the most comfortable position. Place soft padding around the joint to protect it and provide comfort. A small pillow or folded coat or blanket under the knee may provide additional support and comfort (Figure 14-31).

Ankle and Foot Injuries

Ankle and foot injuries are commonly caused by twisting forces. Injuries range from minor sprains with little swelling and pain that heal with a few days' rest, to fractures and dislocations. As with other joint injuries, you cannot always distinguish between minor and severe injuries. You should initially care for all ankle and foot injuries as if they are serious. As with other lower extremity injuries, if the ankle or foot is painful to move, if it cannot bear weight or if the foot or ankle

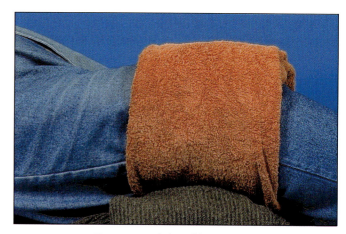

FIGURE 14-31 *Support an injured knee in the most comfortable position.*

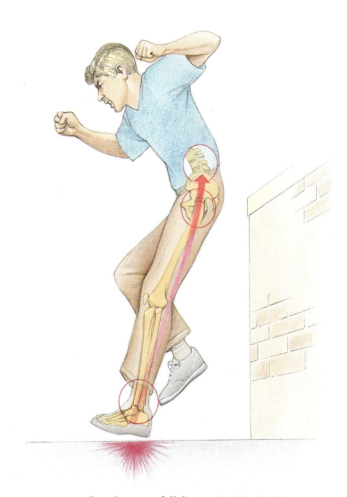

FIGURE 14-32 *In a jump or fall from a height, the impact can be transmitted up the legs, causing injuries to the ankles, knees, hips or spine.*

is swollen, a doctor should evaluate the injury. Foot injuries may also involve the toes. Although these injuries are painful, they are rarely serious.

Fractures of the feet and ankles can occur from forcefully landing on the heel. With any great force, such as falling from a height and landing on the feet, fractures are possible. The force of the impact may also be transmitted up the legs. This can result in an injury elsewhere in the body such as the thigh, pelvis or spine (Figure 14-32).

QUICK RECOVERY

The train track scars which once criss-crossed the injured knees of skiers, football players and arthritis sufferers have almost disappeared. Both the scars and the trauma of knee surgery have been diminished with the advent of a new medical technique: arthroscopy.

Arthroscopy has aided thousands of athletes cursed with "bad knees". Fifteen years ago, knee surgery meant a five-day hospital stay, a plaster cast and three to four months of rehabilitation. With arthroscopic surgery, many athletes leave the hospital the same day and begin rehabilitation within days of the procedure.

The most agile of joints, the knee, is also the most vulnerable. It joins the two longest bones of the body. Four ligaments attach to the bones and hold the knee together. Two cartilage discs serve as shock absorbers on the ends of the bones. Repeated and excessive shocks to the knee will splinter the cartilage pads and stretch or fray ligaments.

The arthroscope, a thin, steel, 25 centimetre telescope, allows orthopaedic surgeons to perform delicate joint surgery without cutting muscles and ligaments and lifting the kneecap to get to the injured area. After injecting a saline solution to distend the knee joint, the surgeon inserts the arthroscope through small puncture wounds into the space of the knee joint. By projecting magnified images inside the knee on to a screen, the arthroscope allows orthopaedic surgeons to use microsurgical instruments to smooth

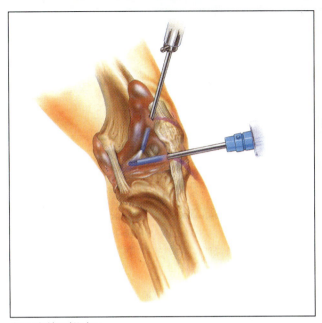

Source: Smith and Nephew

arthritic surfaces, remove chipped bones and cartilage and sew up torn ligaments.

The procedure is not limited to knees. Arthroscopes, some less than 1.7 millimetres in diameter, are being used to repair shoulders, ankles, wrists and even jaws. Not all joint problems can be repaired with arthroscopy, but most surgeons would agree that such advances in surgical procedures have had a profound impact on the lives of people who might otherwise be incapacitated. ■

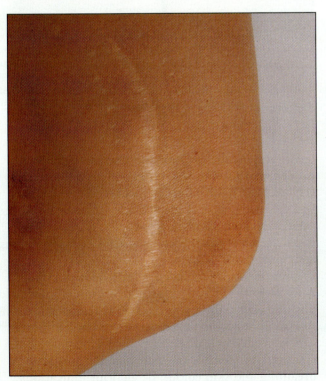

Traditional surgery.

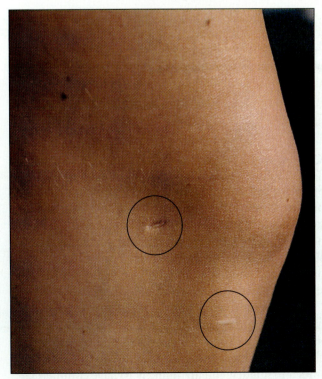

Arthroscopic surgery.

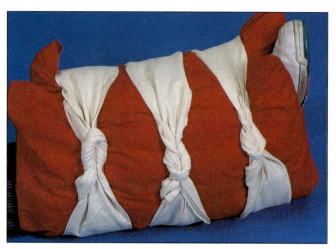

FIGURE 14-33 *An injured ankle can be immobilised with a pillow or rolled blanket secured with two or three bandages.*

Manage ankle and foot injuries by giving the following specific care:

1. Control external bleeding.

2. Immobilise the ankle and foot by using a soft splint such as a pillow or rolled blanket (Figure 14-33). See Practice Guide at the end of this chapter.

3. Elevate the injured ankle or foot to help reduce the swelling.

4. Suspect that any victim who has fallen or jumped from a height also may have injuries elsewhere. Call an ambulance and keep the victim from moving until it arrives.

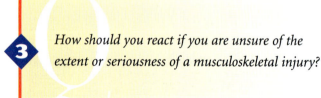

3   *How should you react if you are unsure of the extent or seriousness of a musculoskeletal injury?*

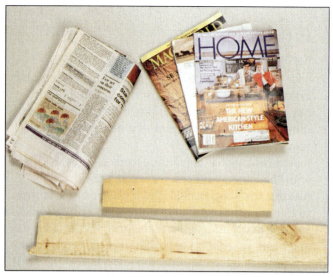

FIGURE 14-34 *Rigid splints include boards, metal strips, and folded magazines or newspapers.*

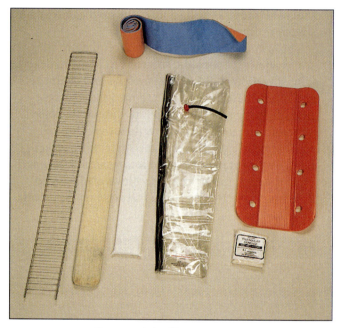

FIGURE 14-35 *Commercial splints.*

SPLINTS

Splints, whether commercially made or improvised, are of three types: soft, rigid and body splints. Soft splints include folded blankets, towels, pillows and a sling or narrow bandage. A sling is a triangular bandage tied to support an arm, wrist or hand (see Chapter 13). A wad of cloth and bandages can serve as effective splints for small body parts such as the hand or fingers.

Rigid splints include boards, metal strips and folded magazines or newspapers (Figure 14-34). Body splints use the body as a splint, securing an injured arm to the chest or an injured leg to the uninjured leg.

As a first aider, you are unlikely to have commercial splints immediately available to you. If they are available you should become familiar with their function

before you use them. Commercial splints include padded board splints, air splints and flexible splints (Figure 14-35). Air splints are not recommended for first aid use because of the difficulty of determining the correct inflation pressure. If the splint is overinflated, the increased pressure may restrict circulation and cause additional tissue damage.

After the injury has been splinted, recheck the ABC. Help the victim to rest in the most comfortable position and maintain normal body temperature. Reassure the victim and determine what additional care is needed and whether to call for an ambulance. Continue to monitor the victim's conscious state, breathing and skin colour. Be alert for indications that the victim's condition is worsening, e.g. symptoms and signs of shock.

TRANSPORTING A VICTIM

Some musculoskeletal injuries are obviously minor and do not require professional medical care. Others are obviously more serious and require you to call emergency personnel. If you discover a life-threatening emergency or think it likely one might develop, call an ambulance and wait for help. Always call an ambulance for any injury involving severe bleeding, injuries to the head, neck or back, and possible broken bones that may be difficult to transport properly, such as the hip and legs. Fractures of large bones are likely to cause serious bleeding and shock. You should also call an ambulance if the victim is distressed or in severe pain, as unnecessary movement will increase the degree of shock.

The advantages of using an ambulance include:

- the presence of trained personnel who can deal with any ongoing problems

- greater comfort for the injured person

- the availability of equipment such as oxygen, defibrillators, drugs, etc

- more rapid assessment in the Emergency Department of a hospital

Some injuries are not serious enough for you to call emergency personnel but still require professional medical care. If you decide to transport the victim yourself to a medical facility, you should immobilise the injury before moving the victim. Ask someone to drive so you can continue to provide care.

4 *Why are air splints not recommended for first-aid?*

Summary

- It is sometimes difficult to tell whether an injury is a fracture, dislocation, sprain or strain. When in doubt, treat it as a serious injury.

- Musculoskeletal injuries can have permanent, disabling effects on the body and can be life-threatening.

- Care for musculoskeletal injuries by providing the following care which focuses on minimising pain, shock and further damage to the injured area:
  - Manage airway or breathing problems.
  - Control external bleeding.
  - Minimise shock.
  - Support the injured area of the body.
  - Limit movement of the victim.
  - Seek advanced medical care.
  - If necessary, immobilise the injured area.
  - Elevate the area if possible.

- To decide whether a head or spine injury may be serious, consider its cause.

- If you suspect that the victim may have a fracture of the skull or spine, minimise movement of the injured area when providing care.

- An injury of the pelvis can be very serious because of bleeding or injury to abdominal organs; keep the victim from moving, call an ambulance and take steps to minimise shock.

- Care for injuries to the extremities includes the general care for all musculoskeletal injuries together with padding, bandaging and splinting the injured area for support and immobilisation.

Answers to Application Questions

1. Neither injury is always more severe than the other. Both injuries can range from mild, with slight stretching of the muscle, tendon or ligament, to severe, involving torn muscles or ligaments that require surgery. Both injuries can be disabling.

2. Compression or severing of the spinal cord may affect the nerves which control breathing, therefore causing breathing to stop.

3. It is often difficult to determine the seriousness of a musculoskeletal injury. It is important that at all times you direct care towards preventing further injury, which means that if you are unsure, you should treat the injury as serious.

4. Air splints are not recommended for first aid use as it is difficult to determine the correct inflation pressure. If the splint is over-inflated, additional serious injury can result.

Study Questions

1. **Match each term with the correct definition.**

   a. Bone.
   b. Dislocation.
   c. Fracture.
   d. Joint.
   e. Ligaments.
   f. Muscle.
   g. Skeletal muscles.
   h. Splint.
   i. Sprain.
   j. Strain.
   k. Tendon.

   _____ Device used to keep body parts from moving.
   _____ Displacement of a bone from its normal position at a joint.
   _____ Tissue that lengthens and shortens to create movement.
   _____ Broken bone.
   _____ Dense, hard tissue that forms the skeleton.
   _____ Injury that stretches and tears ligaments and other soft tissues at joints.
   _____ Fibrous band attaching muscle to bone.
   _____ Structure formed where two or more bones meet.
   _____ Injury that stretches and tears muscles and tendons.
   _____ Muscles that attach to bones.
   _____ Fibrous bands holding bones together at joints.

2. **List four principles of splinting.**

3. **List at least five situations that might result in serious head and/or spine injuries.**

4. **List at least six symptoms and signs of head or spine injuries.**

5. When caring for an injured joint, you should:

a. control external bleeding

b. straighten the fracture or dislocation before splinting

c. immobilise and support the fracture or dislocation in the position found.

d. a and c.

e. a, b and c.

6. You would suspect a fracture or dislocation if:

a. you saw severe swelling and discolouration

b. the area was significantly deformed

c. the victim heard a snap at the time of the injury.

d. All of the above.

7. You find a person lying at the foot of a steep cliff. Her right leg is twisted at an unusual angle and you can see protruding bones and blood. What do you do first?

a. Straighten the leg.

b. Do a primary survey.

c. Use direct pressure to stop the bleeding.

d. Look for material to use as a splint.

8. Immobilising a musculoskeletal injury helps to:

a. prevent further soft tissue damage

b. lessen pain

c. lessen the danger of infection.

d. a and c.

e. a and b.

9. When assessing the possibility of a head or spine injury, you should consider:

a. the cause of the injury

b. the symptoms and signs present

c. what bystanders who saw the injury occur can tell you.

d. a, b and c.

10. List three steps of general care for injuries to the extremities.

11. List two specific symptoms and signs of a fractured femur.

Answers are in Appendix A (pages 362–63).

Use of a Body Splint

You are out bushwalking and one of your party falls off a ledge. You are performing a secondary survey and suspect that the victim may have a lower leg injury. There is no deformity, so you decide to use the uninjured leg as a splint because the nearest ambulance is some distance away.

Control bleeding

- Control any external bleeding.
- Apply dressings and bandages over a wound as appropriate.

Help position the victim

- Help the victim into a position of comfort.
- Prepare to splint the injured leg to the uninjured leg.

Secure the injured limb to the uninjured limb

- Place padding between the knees and ankles.
- Gently slide the uninjured leg next to the injured leg.

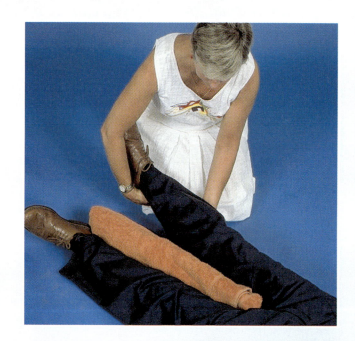

- Use a figure of eight narrow bandage around the ankles.

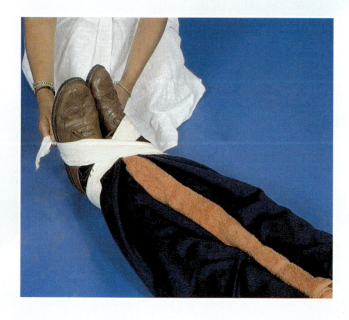

PRACTICE GUIDE

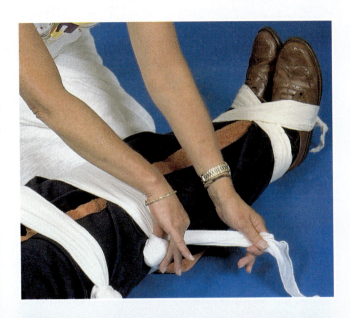

- Place a broad bandage around the knees.
- Place a broad bandage around the thighs.

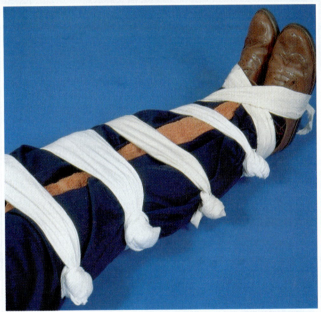

Stabilise the injured part

- Place a narrow bandage above and below the injury site.
- Tie the bandages on the uninjured side.

Prepare to transport

- Check frequently to see that the bandages are not too tight.
- If the victim complains of increasing localised pain from one or more bandages, loosen the bandages concerned.
- If more than one finger fits easily under the bandages, tighten them gently but firmly.

Using a Soft Splint

You are performing a secondary survey and suspect that the victim may have an ankle injury. You decide to use a soft splint to immobilise the injured area, as the nearest ambulance is some distance away.

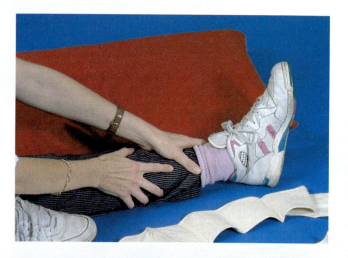

Control bleeding

- Control any external bleeding.
- Apply dressings and bandages over a wound as appropriate.

Help position the victim

- Help the victim into a position of comfort.
- Gently position the wounded ankle so that you can apply a soft splint.
- Leave the shoe and sock in place unless there is an open wound or severe swelling.
- Place three folded triangular bandages, one under the leg at the heel, one under the ankle and one under the lower leg.

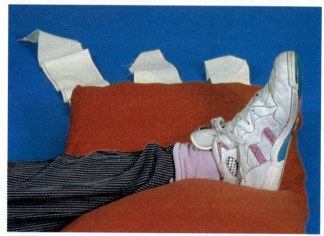

Position and secure the splint

- Fold or wrap a blanket or pillow gently around the ankle.
- Tie the first two bandages to secure the blanket or pillow around the ankle and lower leg.
- Tie the third bandage around the foot, from the heel to the front of the ankle.
- If more than one finger fits under the bandages, tighten them.

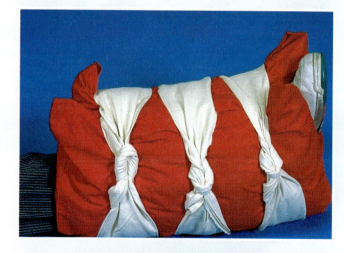

Elevate the injured part

- Check the circulation.
- If no fracture is suspected, elevate the foot.

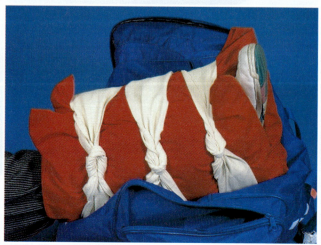

PRACTICE GUIDE

Using a Rigid Splint

You are performing a secondary survey and suspect that the victim may have a serious arm injury. You decide to support and immobilise the area of injury.

Control bleeding

- Control any external bleeding.
- Apply dressings and bandages over a wound as appropriate.

Help position the victim

- Help the victim into a position of comfort.

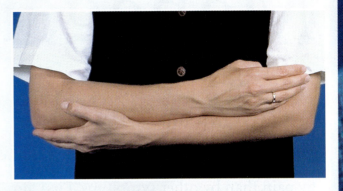

Immobilise and support the injured part with a splint

- Use a splint made of rolled up newspaper or magazine, or a flat board.
- If using newspaper or a magazine, roll it around the arm to fit closely at the elbow and hand. Otherwise, position the arm on a board which extends from the elbow to the fingers.
- Secure the splint with bandages or tape.

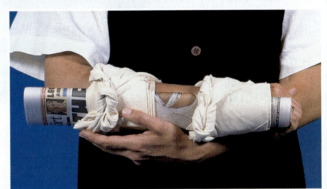

Check the circulation

- Check the circulation every 10 minutes by checking the fingers and radial pulse.

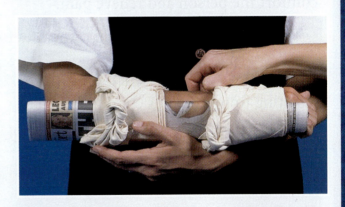

Support the arm

- Support the arm with an arm sling (see Chapter 13—Practice Guide for an arm sling).

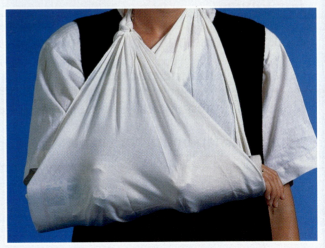

Pain Management

MOST INJURIES and many illnesses cause pain. Often the victim is more disturbed by pain than by other symptoms. First aid always initially addresses the cause of the pain, as pain is only a symptom of a condition requiring care rather than being the condition itself. Once you have cared for the injury or illness, you can take measures to comfort the person and relieve pain.

This chapter outlines general principles for managing pain, and how to identify pain resulting from a serious condition which requires medical attention. The chapter also describes care of common aches and pain.

For Review

A basic understanding of the body systems (Chapter 2) and the emergency action principles for all emergencies (Chapter 3) will help your understanding of the chapter.

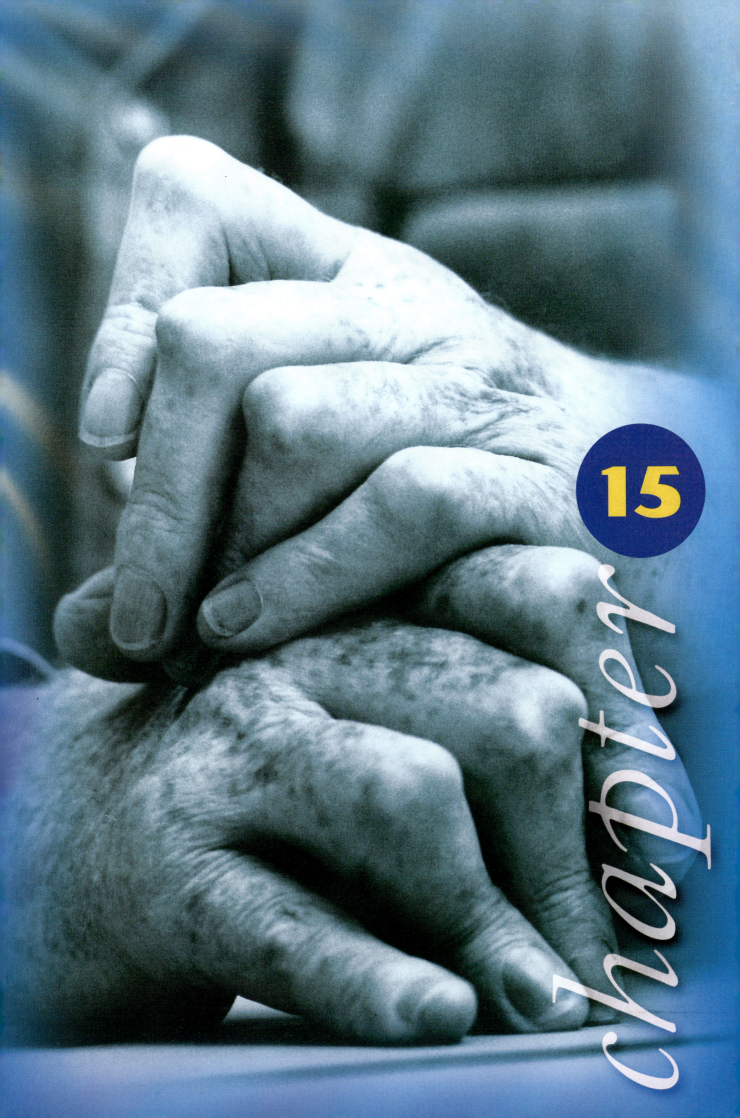

15

chapter

Key Terms

Abscess *(ab-sess)*: A collection of pus in a cavity which results from infection or injury to the tissues.

Analgesics *(an-al-gee-ziks)*: Drugs used for the relief of pain.

Appendicitis: An inflammation of the appendix causing abdominal pain.

Arthritis: An inflammatory condition of the joints causing pain and swelling.

Meningitis *(men-in-jy-tis)*: Infection or inflammation of the membranes covering the brain or spinal cord.

Migraine: A recurring, usually severe type of headache which may last for hours or days.

Pain: An unpleasant sensation caused by noxious stimulation of sensory nerve endings, often occurring as a symptom of infection, injury or other disorders.

Reassurance: The process of assuring a victim that help is on the way and that you will not leave the person alone; reassurance can help alleviate pain.

Ulcer: A usually painful crater-like sore in the stomach or other tissue resulting from an infection or other harmful condition.

Dianne was driving alone on the Pacific Highway, rushing to get home after a long day of babysitting her sister's children in a nearby town. Suddenly a kangaroo appeared at the edge of the road, and thinking it was about to bound out in front of her car, she turned the wheel too hard and lost control of the car. It went off the road and slammed into a tree. Dianne blacked out.

The only thing she knew when she regained consciousness was the pain—both legs in excruciating pain, filling her head and blotting out everything else. She closed her eyes tight against it. She vaguely knew someone was there, and realised that she must have had a car crash. She felt something being done to her body, but she couldn't think about anything except the pain. She wanted to scream and never stop screaming but her teeth were clenched tight…

Gradually she became aware of a voice saying something over and over. "You'll be okay," the voice was saying, "The ambulance is here, they're taking care of you now, you'll be okay." The voice was soothing, going on and on, a man talking, now describing the blue sky and clouds drifting by, telling her she was okay, she wasn't alone, maybe just a broken leg but she'd be swimming again soon, talking about boats out on the ocean, the voice going on and on. Slowly she felt a little better. When the ambulance crew told her they were going to lift her onto the stretcher she was ready, calmer now, and she understood what was happening. She'd be okay now. The pain was bad but it was manageable. She even opened her eyes in the bright sunlight as they rolled the stretcher to the ambulance—and saw that the voice came from a young man in jeans and T-shirt, not one of the ambulance crew. He smiled and pointed at the clouds drifting by, and said, "See—they are beautiful, aren't they?"

Later, arriving at hospital, the ambulance crew told her how the young man had stayed with her after calling for the ambulance, how he had covered her with a blanket from his car and held her hand and kept talking to her while they splinted her legs and dressed her wounds. "He talked about everything under the sun," one ambulance officer said with a laugh. She didn't remember most of it, but she did remember how soothing his voice had been and how much better she felt when she knew she wasn't alone.

Pain is one of the ways our body communicates with us, and therefore, serves as an important function. Pain forces us to pay attention to something that has happened or is happening inside our bodies. Not every illness or injury produces pain, but the presence or absence of pain is helpful in assessing a victim's condition.

Sometimes pain is obvious; for example, if you cut your finger on something sharp, you usually feel a sharp pain localised in the area of the cut. At other times pain is less localised and more difficult to interpret. For example, a pain running down the leg may be a symptom of a muscle strain or ruptured disc in the back, and a pain in the chest may seem like indigestion or heartburn but may actually be a heart attack.

What is important is to realise that when pain does exist, it may be a symptom of some illness, condition or injury. Neither the location nor severity of the pain automatically reveals the nature of the underlying problem, but it does suggest there is a problem, whether minor or serious. Therefore, you should always take seriously any complaints of pain by a victim. In some cases pain indicates a serious condition requiring medical attention, while in other situations the pain itself is the primary problem requiring care. When caring for a victim who is in pain, the most important priority is to care for whatever may be causing the pain, including seeking medical care if needed, and then care for the pain itself.

This chapter discusses general principles of pain management, techniques for lessening or alleviating pain and common aches and pains.

PRINCIPLES OF PAIN MANAGEMENT

Regardless of the type of pain or where it occurs in the body, you should follow these general principles of pain management:

1. *Address pain in the secondary survey, not the primary survey.* Remember that pain itself is not a life-threatening problem, although unrelieved pain will cause an increase in the output of certain hormones which can lead to cardiac and circulatory problems. Even if a victim is expressing great pain, your first concern must always be for any life-threatening conditions you find. Generally, a victim who is able to express pain is breathing and has a pulse, but this victim may have serious bleeding which requires immediate attention or may be going into shock. Until you are certain there are no serious or life-threatening conditions requiring immediate care, do not be distracted by the victim's communication of pain. This may mean, for example, quickly checking a crying child for bleeding or a possible fracture before giving a hug for comfort, or first stopping bleeding from an adult's leg wound before bandaging a broken arm, even if the victim is screaming in pain from the injury. Once you

have taken care of any serious problems, begin the secondary survey with an assessment based on the victim's complaint of pain.

2. *Pain should lead you to look for more serious problems.* Never ignore pain or assume it is caused by something minor. Look for other symptoms and signs, and consider what could be the cause of the pain. Persistent chest pain, for example, is the primary symptom of heart attack. Consider also the cause of an injury. For example, if a person in a serious car crash complains of neck pain, the neck may be seriously injured or fractured. Even a lesser pain, when associated with other symptoms or signs, may reveal a serious problem. Later sections in this chapter describe such kinds of pain, which are accompanied by other symptoms.

3. *Help manage pain while waiting for the ambulance.* With a serious injury or illness requiring medical attention, you can give care for the pain after you have done all you can for the injury or illness itself. Techniques of pain management are described in the next section.

4. *The severity of the victim's pain response does not indicate the severity of the condition.* In some cases you may have to pay less attention to the victim's response than to the injury itself. For example, a child who stubs a toe may scream and cry excessively even though the injury may be minor. The opposite is also true: a person may dismiss chest pain as mere indigestion when the pain is actually a heart attack occurring.

5. *Cultural and individual factors influence how a victim expresses pain.* Do not assess pain merely by what the person says. For example, a stoic person may feel great pain but not admit it. In some cases you may observe that the person's behaviour or facial expression reveals more about the pain than what the person says. For example, the person with a chest injury may grimace when moving a limb or take very shallow breaths to avoid pain.

6. *Assess the victim's pain repeatedly while waiting for medical aid.* Even if the person seems to be getting better, the condition may not be improving or it may be getting worse. Increasing pain should be noted and watched carefully because it *may* indicate a worsening condition.

GENERAL TECHNIQUES OF PAIN MANAGEMENT

Remember, always care for any conditions needing first aid before turning your attention to managing the pain itself. In many cases, managing the condition will help minimise the pain. Often your assistance will be required only for the short time it takes for the ambulance to arrive or the victim to reach medical assistance.

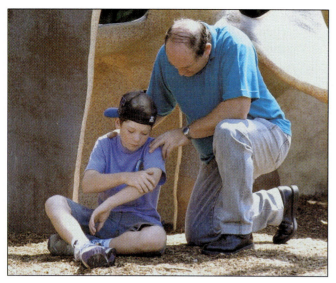

FIGURE 15-1 *Reassuring a victim can ease anxiety and help reduce the pain.*

In some other cases of minor pain resulting from a condition which does not require medical assistance, you may use pain management techniques to help the person get through the pain and return to activity.

Specific pains in certain body areas require specific care (see later sections). Following here are general techniques of pain management which may help with many kinds of pain.

Reassurance

When pain or fear is experienced, adrenaline is released within the body to stimulate a response. If you soothe and reassure the victim, the level of adrenaline will drop, the heart will slow down and the victim will begin to relax. Reassuring a victim that medical help is on the way and that you will stay there and continue helping them can ease their anxiety and help reduce the pain (Figure 15-1). You can also reassure a victim whose condition is not life-threatening that they'll be okay. However, with very severe injuries, do not offer false reassurance in cases where the victim may recognise the seriousness of the injury, because the person then may not believe you and the resulting lack of trust may worsen the situation.

It is reassuring to a victim to feel able to trust you and the first aid you are providing. Show the victim respect by first asking permission to help. Ask for and use the victim's name while giving care. These actions promote a positive relationship between you and the victim, which has psychological benefits.

Many victims also find touch reassuring. Be sure to ask first, because the person may feel your touch is a violation of personal space. Lightly touching the person's shoulder or holding the victim's hand can be reassuring. Using a cool cloth to gently stroke the person's forehead or face to remove perspiration can also be soothing.

If the victim is agitated by concern for other victims or other responsibilities or happenings, try to relieve that anxiety.

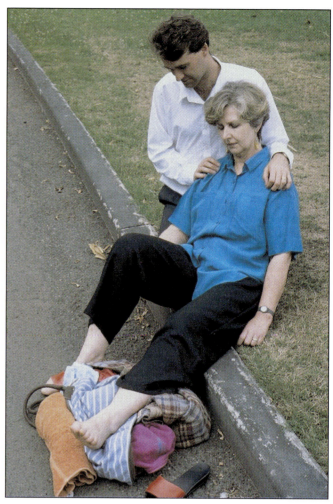

FIGURE 15-2 *Immobilise and support an injured area in the position of greatest comfort to help minimise pain which would result from movement.*

Positioning

Pain can be often alleviated by repositioning the person generally and supporting the injured body part. Often the victim naturally seeks out the position of greatest comfort, but you can help the person settle into that position if necessary. You can also use pillows or blankets to help support the person in the most comfortable position. Encourage the victim not to move around too much while waiting for the ambulance, because movement can often aggravate an injury and increase the pain.

Immobilisation of an injured body part follows the same principle. For example, fractures are immobilised with bandages and slings to minimise pain as well as to prevent further injury. Chapters 13 and 14 describe the use of various bandages and slings for immobilisation. Before bandaging, always observe how the victim positions the injured limb or body area, because the person usually seeks out the least painful position. It may not be possible or necessary to splint or immobilise a fracture, but simply helping to support the injury in the most comfortable position while waiting for the ambulance will help the victim to relax and so help relieve the pain (Figure 15-2).

Controlling the Environment

While waiting for the ambulance, you can also help manage the environment to reduce factors that might otherwise add to the victim's discomfort. Follow these guidelines if you can improve environmental conditions without leaving the victim or interrupting care:

1. Try to control other people at the scene. Keep onlookers well away from the victim, and try to keep nearby bystanders quiet. Bystanders may become very emotional at the sight of blood or injuries, or because of the condition of a victim, and their behaviour and words can be disturbing. If necessary, politely but firmly ask them to move away or be quiet.

2. Control the temperature of the environment if possible, such as by opening or closing doors and windows or adjusting heating or cooling controls. Outdoors, if the victim cannot be moved, take steps to help maintain normal body temperature (see Chapter 11). If it is raining, move the victim indoors if possible, or cover the person to prevent them from getting wet. If possible, remove any wet clothing from the victim.

3. Make the environment as pleasant as possible by controlling lighting and noise levels. A quiet, darkened room is more soothing than a bright room with a television or radio blaring in the background.

Maintaining Privacy and Dignity

Take steps to help the victim maintain personal privacy and dignity. In addition to keeping strangers back, cover any exposed body parts. If the victim is upset by soiled clothing, incontinence or aspects of personal appearance, you can help clean up the person as long as this does not interfere with care or cause movement which may result in additional injury or pain.

Distraction and Relaxation Techniques

A victim who is focused only on the pain will feel it most acutely. On the other hand, if the victim's thoughts can be turned to other things, the awareness of pain may diminish. Talking to the victim can be an effective distraction. Try to be natural in your tone of voice, and try to engage the person in conversation. With a child in pain, you may provide distraction by pointing out interesting things to look at in the environment, by telling a story or even by singing or humming in a soothing way. Do what seems natural and comfortable in the situation to try to distract the victim from dwelling on the pain. Watch for cues that the distraction may be working, and do not persist if your attempt seems to irritate the person.

Helping the person to relax physically will also minimise pain. Encourage the person to relax and to let the body go limp. Sometimes victims try to fight pain by clenching muscles in a way which actually increases the pain, for example, tensing muscles around a fracture. So, relaxing the body may help. Encouraging the victim to breathe slowly and rhythmically may help with relaxation. A light touch or rhythmic massage of the body in a non-injured location can work both by distracting the person's attention from pain and by helping to relax the muscles.

Minimising Shock

Remember that a victim in severe pain may go into shock. Therefore, be prepared to provide care to reduce the effects of shock (see Chapter 6).

Analgesics

As a general principle, first aiders should not give medication to victims, although you can assist a person to take a medication which is prescribed or which the person chooses to take independently. In some cases, if a person with minor pain has pain-killing tablets, you can assist by offering a glass of water or by helping to ensure the right dosage is taken.

In the workplace, follow the established guidelines for use of pain-relieving medication. For a child with minor pain, be sure to have permission from the parent or adult guardian. Remember that aspirin is not recommended for children.

MANAGEMENT OF SPECIFIC PAINS

In addition to the general pain management techniques described above, aches and pains in specific areas of the body may be given specific care.

Headache

A headache may be caused by many conditions, ranging from the common cold or sinus infection to stress, tension, eye strain, or lack of food or sleep. Headache may also be caused by more serious conditions such as internal pressure within the skull resulting from a head injury.

The pain of a headache may be continuous or throbbing and may remain steady or come and go. Headache which occurs together with other symptoms or signs may indicate a more serious condition. Complete the secondary survey and ask the person about other symptoms, then give the following care:

1. Seek immediate medical aid if the victim has any of the following symptoms:

   - fever
   - stiff neck
   - head injury
   - visual difficulties
   - slurring of speech
   - difficulty moving arms or legs
   - altered conscious state

2. Encourage the person to seek medical attention as soon as possible for headache with any of the following symptoms:

   • headache persisting over several days

   • headache which is worse in the morning

3. Put either a cold compress or hot water bottle wrapped in cloth on the victim's forehead. Use whichever one of these the victim prefers or is more convenient.

4. Encourage the person to lie down in a quiet, darkened room.

5. Victims may take their own pain-killing medication.

Sinus headache is a specific type of headache associated with inflammation of the sinuses caused by infection, a cold, asthma or hay fever. Typically this headache occurs together with a tenderness over the cheekbone on the affected side, a feeling of heaviness behind the nose and eyes, and possibly nasal discharge and fever. Consult a doctor if the symptoms persist or seem worse than those of a common cold.

Migraine

Migraine is a particular type of headache. Although this term is sometimes used loosely by people to describe a bad headache, migraine is a separate condition which can only be diagnosed by a doctor. The person with true migraine headaches, therefore, typically knows the diagnosis and often has been told by a doctor what to do when one occurs.

The symptoms of migraine are usually more severe than a common headache and may be incapacitating. Typically the headache is intense and throbbing and occurs on one side of the head only. The victim may look very pale. Sometimes migraines are triggered by stress or environmental conditions. They may be accompanied by nausea and vomiting and visual disturbances.

Care for a migraine is the same as for common headache. Take care to minimise noise and light because the victim is especially sensitive to these. The person may have medication prescribed by a doctor.

Earache

Ear pain can be caused by an injury or an infection which causes a build-up of fluid and/or pressure behind the eardrum. A change in altitude, such as in a descending aeroplane, can cause a painful pressure build-up. The ear is a sensitive organ, and even a small injury or swelling in the ear can produce much pain.

An earache may be accompanied by other symptoms and signs. An ear infection in a child or infant may also cause fever, crying, irritability and pulling at the affected ear.

Follow these guidelines to care for earache:

1. Seek immediate medical aid if the person has any of the following symptoms or signs:

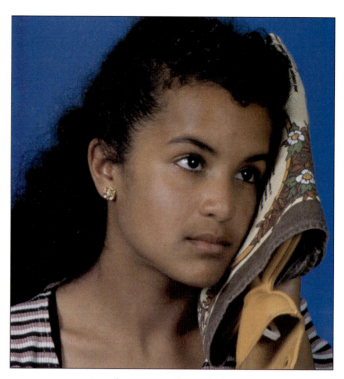

FIGURE 15-3 *Care for an earache includes use of a hot water bottle.*

   • injury to the ear

   • high fever

   • bleeding or discharge from the ear

2. Encourage the person to seek medical attention as soon as possible with any of the following symptoms:

   • fever or irritability in a child

   • persistent pain

   • deafness

   A child with an earache should always see a doctor because of the risk of an infection, which can lead to permanent damage to hearing.

3. Treat minor earache with a hot water bottle wrapped in cloth or a heating pad held against the ear (Figure 15-3).

4. Victims may take their own pain-killing medication.

5. To relieve ear pain resulting from pressure changes such as in an aeroplane's descent, encourage the person to swallow, drink water or yawn. Another effective way is to blow the nose while pinching the nostrils shut and keeping the mouth closed.

Eye Pain

Eye pain is rare but could be a symptom of a serious problem. Pain may be caused by an injury, infection or medical condition. A person with any eye pain should seek medical advice as soon as possible, because the condition causing the pain may threaten vision.

Symptoms other than pain are more common.

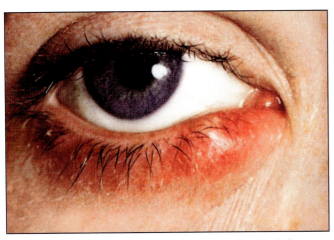

FIGURE 15-4 *A sty (a localised infection on the eyelid) can be painful.*

Burning or itching of the eye usually results from irritation caused by an infection, allergy or some environmental substance, such as smoke, dust or chlorine in swimming pool water. This burning or itching may not need treatment if it does not persist or recur. However, burning or itching accompanied by a discharge of pus often indicates an infection, and the person should seek medical attention. If vision is affected, the person should see a doctor as soon as possible.

A sty or obstructed tear duct may cause pain or tenderness near the eye. A sty is a localised infection which causes a red bump on the eyelid (Figure 15-4). Care for a sty with warm moist compresses several times a day for 15 minutes at a time. A sty which drains will usually heal by itself, but if it persists a doctor should be consulted. A blocked tear duct requires medical attention.

Care for a foreign body in the eye is described in Chapter 12, and how to flush a spilled chemical from the eye is described with the care of burns in Chapter 11.

Toothache

Toothache is usually caused by such tooth problems as tooth decay, an abscess or misalignment of the teeth. Tooth pain may also result from direct trauma to the mouth. In some cases tooth pain may result from a condition elsewhere in the mouth or head, such as a nerve problem.

The pain may be continuous or may come and go. It may be steady or throbbing, and hot or cold food or liquid may make it worse.

Follow these guidelines to care for toothache:

1. See a dentist or doctor immediately if the person has experienced a mouth injury or a tooth has been knocked out. (See Chapter 12 for the care of a displaced tooth.)

2. Encourage the person to see a dentist or doctor soon for the care of any toothache.

3. Avoid hot or cold food and liquid.

4. Victims may take their own pain-killing medication.

Neck Ache

Neck pain may result from a variety of factors or conditions. Neck pain which occurs after a traumatic injury should be evaluated by a doctor because of the possibility of serious spinal injury or a pinched nerve related to an injury. When a nerve is pinched as a result of arthritis or an injury, pain may extend down the arm or be associated with tingling or numbness.

Another potentially serious cause of neck pain associated with a stiff neck, headache, fever and sometimes nausea and vomiting is meningitis, an infection which can be life threatening. A person experiencing these symptoms should seek medical attention as soon as possible.

Neck pain may also result from strain of the neck muscles, caused by activity, tension or sitting or sleeping in the same position for too long. Cold or flu may also cause generalised neck pain.

Follow these guidelines to care for neck pain:

1. Seek immediate medical aid if the victim has any of the following symptoms or signs:
   * pain following trauma
   * very stiff neck
   * nausea or vomiting
   * altered conscious state
   * swelling in the area

2. Encourage the person to seek prompt medical attention for neck ache with any of the following symptoms or signs:
   * persistent neck pain.
   * fever
   * headache
   * pain extending down the arm
   * tingling or numbness

3. Treat minor neck pain with a hot water bottle wrapped in cloth or a heating pad held against the painful area.

4. Victims may take their own pain-killing tablets.

Backache

Back pain may result from injury, muscle strain or a chronic condition such as a disc problem or poor posture. Many people develop chronic pain from work or leisure activities which put a strain on the back.

Follow these guidelines to care for back pain:

1. Seek immediate medical aid if the victim has any of the following symptoms or signs:
   * back pain related to injury such as a fall or blow to the back
   * bleeding
   * blood in the urine
   * inability to move
   * loss of sensation in the legs
   * fever

2. Encourage the person to seek prompt medical attention with any of the following symptoms:

   • pain extending down the leg

   • persistent pain

   The doctor may establish a long-term management plan to allow the back to heal and to prevent re-injury.

3. Treat minor back pain related to muscular strain as for any other muscular strain (see Chapter 14).

4. Victims may take their own pain-killing tablets.

5. Encourage the person to rest as much as possible, to avoid activity which puts additional strain on the back and to sleep on a firm bed without using a pillow.

Abdominal Pain

Abdominal pain can result from many minor conditions not requiring medical assistance, or may be an indication of a serious underlying condition. Less serious causes include indigestion, constipation and menstrual cramping. More serious causes include injury to the abdomen, **appendicitis**, an **ulcer** and conditions affecting other organs.

Abdominal pain that lasts less than 30 minutes and is not associated with other symptoms or injury is likely to be minor and not require medical assistance. Care depends on the nature of the pain and the presence of any other symptoms.

Follow these guidelines to care for abdominal pain:

1. Seek immediate medical aid if the victim has any of the following symptoms or signs:

   • injury to the abdomen

   • vomiting of black or bloody material

   • stools that look black and tarry

   • very severe pain

   • the person is or could be pregnant

2. Encourage the person to seek prompt medical attention with any of the following symptoms or signs:

   • persistent pain

   • fever

   • diarrhoea

3. For pain related to menstrual cramps, the person may experience relief from walking about. Such persons may take their own pain-killing tablets.

4. Position the person half-sitting with shoulders and head supported and knees bent, or in the position of greatest comfort, often curled up.

5. Put a hot water bottle wrapped in cloth or a heating pad over the painful area.

6. Position a person who vomits, or seems likely to, on the side.

Summary

- Pain is a symptom of an illness, condition or injury.
- The general principles of pain management are to:
  - —assess the person's pain in the secondary survey after first caring for any serious problems.
  - —look for the cause of pain.
  - —help manage the victim's pain after caring for serious conditions, while waiting for the ambulance.
  - —recognise that the victim's pain response may not indicate how serious the injury or illness is.
  - —remember that the expression of pain is influenced by many cultural and individual factors.
  - —reassess pain frequently because changing levels of pain may indicate a change in the victim's condition.
- General techniques of pain management include:
  - —Reassuring the victim that help is on the way.
  - —Positioning the victim or part of the body to minimise pain.
  - —Controlling the environment to minimise factors that increase the victim's perception of pain.
  - —Helping the victim maintain privacy and dignity to minimise discomfort.
  - —Using distraction and relaxation techniques to diminish the victim's awareness of pain.
  - —Minimising shock.
  - —Assisting a victim with their own analgesics when appropriate.
- In addition to general techniques for managing pain, assess pain in specific body areas and consider any accompanying symptoms and signs to determine whether the victim should receive medical assistance.
- With minor pains not accompanied by significant other symptoms and signs, care may include use of a heating pad, the person's own pain-killing tablets and other specific steps for the particular body area.

Study Questions

1. *An important principle of pain management is to always help the victim relieve pain before going on to check for other problems such as bleeding. True or false? Briefly explain your answer.*

2. *The severity of the victim's response to pain does not always reflect the severity of the condition. True or false? Briefly explain your answer.*

3. *When you reassure a victim after calling an ambulance, you should always say:*
   a. "Don't worry—you'll be okay."
   b. "Help is on the way, and I'm going to stay with you."
   c. "I've had first aid training, and your condition is not too bad."
   d. All of the above.

4. *Immobilising an injured body part involves:*
   a. preventing movement of the area, which can aggravate the injury and increase pain
   b. helping the victim support the injured area in the most comfortable position
   c. using a bandage or sling or improvised material for immobilisation.
   d. All of the above.

Answers are in Appendix A (page 363).

Procedures at Major Incidents

MAJOR INCIDENTS are situations in which there are multiple victims requiring first aid or situations involving hazardous environmental conditions. These range from traffic collisions to natural disasters, to scenes of potential violence. Knowing what to do in such situations is important. Being prepared for natural disasters such as bushfires or floods involves advance planning for prevention and action if the disaster occurs.

This chapter will help you to be prepared for a wide variety of major incidents in which your safety or that of others may be threatened.

For Review

A basic understanding of the emergency action principles that first aiders should follow in all emergencies (Chapter 3) will help your understanding of the chapter.

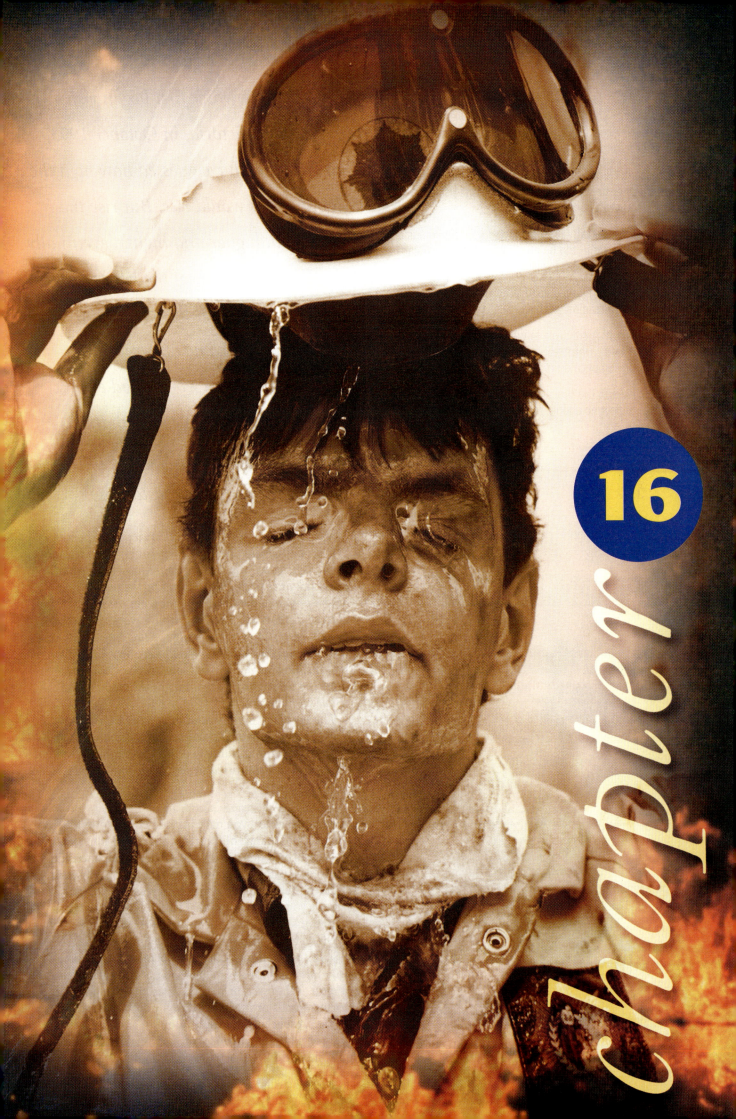

chapter

16

Key Terms

Cyclone: A severe tropical storm system characterised by high to extreme winds and often heavy rain.

Flash flood: Flood which results from surface water run-off after heavy rains; usually with fast-rising water levels and swift currents.

Hazardous material: Any substance, including liquids and gases, used in the home or workplace which can cause injury or illness if spilled or improperly handled.

Hostage: A person held involuntarily, usually by someone committing a criminal act.

Major incident: A situation in which several victims need care or in which abnormal environmental conditions complicate first aid management.

Triage *(tree-arj)*: The process of assessing multiple victims to determine who should receive care first.

When the water first began rising in Benalla, Victoria, in October 1993, no one could have guessed how high the flood waters would rise. But rise the water did, higher and higher, eventually flooding two-thirds of the houses and most of the land in this community. Gradually it became apparent that this was Victoria's worst flood ever. Only later would it be seen that, historically, this was Victoria's most devastating natural disaster.

Although there was massive destruction of homes, property, roads and bridges, surprisingly few injuries resulted from all this devastation. Many people had made advance preparations, and as the waters rose others prepared for the flood following the instructions of local authorities. The community worked together to help keep people safe during the flooding—and kept working together with the Flood Recovery Centre for months afterward, assuring safe drinking water, restoring utilities and attending to the needs of the whole community.

The people of Benalla and other communities in Victoria demonstrated that even in a natural disaster causing damage totalling over $500 million, injury and illness can be minimised when people pull together.

In earlier chapters you have learned how to provide first aid for a wide range of injuries and sudden illnesses. In most cases only one person needs care, which often allows you to give your full attention to that victim. However, in other situations, there may be several victims needing care, or you may have to deal with environmental conditions which complicate first aid management or which become emergencies in themselves.

Such situations are called major incidents. These situations may involve vehicles, hazardous materials or electrical power, or natural disasters such as severe storms, floods or bushfires. Also under this heading are fires, especially in large buildings, and, finally, situations of potential violence, such as suicide or when a person is held hostage.

As explained in Chapter 3, the first emergency action principle is to ensure your safety and that of others before entering the scene. In many kinds of incidents or natural disasters, the scene may be dangerous because of fumes, fire, spilled chemicals, moving water or other factors. This chapter describes principles for managing these specific situations.

SAFETY

Safety is a concern in all major incidents—safety for yourself, for bystanders and for the victim.

You cannot help a victim if you become injured yourself by entering a dangerous scene. Approach cautiously and evaluate the situation. If you are in a vehicle, park a safe distance away to avoid obstructing traffic or posing a risk to yourself or others. As you walk toward the scene, look for anything which may indicate a risk: other vehicles or machinery in motion, fumes, spilled petrol or any chemicals, fallen power lines, deep or fast-moving water, an unstable structure or even a violent or potentially violent person on the scene. If you see, hear or smell any such danger, do not enter the scene. Call for, or send someone else to call for, emergency help. Retreat to a safe location if necessary.

Most importantly, never attempt a rescue for which you have not been trained. Well-meaning first aiders have been injured or killed when taking chances to try to rescue someone or by entering an unsafe scene. Your call for emergency help will bring professional rescuers with the equipment and training necessary to rescue a victim in an unsafe situation.

Look out for the safety of others. Keep friends, family and bystanders away from an unsafe scene. Bystanders who want to help can be sent to call for assistance or be asked to keep others back.

Finally, in your desire to help, don't forget the victim's safety as well. Remember that a victim of serious injury or illness should not be moved unless necessary. If the scene is dangerous, first try to remove the danger from the victim. If the danger cannot be removed, then remove the victim from the danger if you can do so quickly and safely. (Chapter 17 describes emergency lifting and moving.) If the scene is dangerous and you cannot remove the victim, then you must move to safety yourself.

Examples of dangerous scenes include:

- Fire or the danger of fire.
- The presence of explosives or hazardous materials.
- An unstable situation such as a structure about to collapse.

> ## Remember:
> *Your aim at all times must be to avoid making the situation worse.*

MULTIPLE VICTIMS

Major incidents often involve more than one victim with injuries. If several first aiders are present on the scene, you may be able to focus your attention on just one victim at a time. In some cases, however, you may face the dilemma of two or more victims needing your care. You then have to decide who to care for first.

As a general principle, care first for a victim with serious injury and let victims with lesser injuries wait for help to arrive, *unless* the care you give one victim is unlikely to help that person but may allow other victims to die who might have been saved. For example, a car crash might result in three victims: one with massive head, chest and abdomenal injuries whose heart is not beating, and two others who are bleeding profusely but still breathing. Giving CPR to the first victim may not save that person's life, whereas you can possibly control bleeding in both the others and save both their lives.

This is not an easy decision to make, but it can be a necessary one. Professional rescuers and ambulance personnel must also make decisions like this, in a process called **triage.** The same principle is true for professional rescuers as for first aiders: do that which gives the greatest chances of survival to the greatest number of victims.

INCIDENTS

Incidents requiring special attention include traffic collisions, hazardous materials incidents and incidents involving electricity. In all cases, remember the principles of safety and the general rule to remove the danger from the victim if possible and, if not, remove the victim from the danger.

Traffic Collisions

A victim of a road traffic collision may be found inside or outside the vehicle. Be sure the scene is safe before approaching. Check the scene carefully for any dangers before approaching the crash site (Figure 16-1). With a victim either in or out of the vehicle, remember to avoid moving the victim unless it is essential to save life. Ask bystanders to help stop or divert traffic to reduce the risk of further collisions. Use warning triangles, if available, on the road at least 200 metres from the scene.

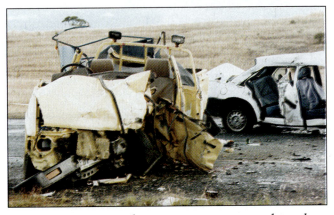

FIGURE 16-1 *A car crash scene may present many hazards.*

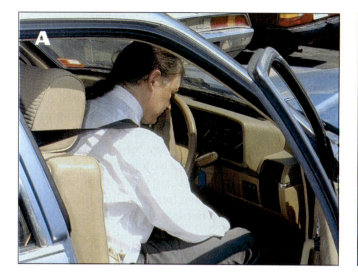

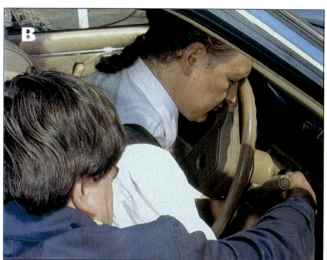

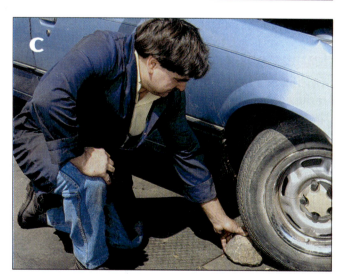

FIGURE 16-2 *Be sure the car is safe and cannot move before giving first aid (see description).*

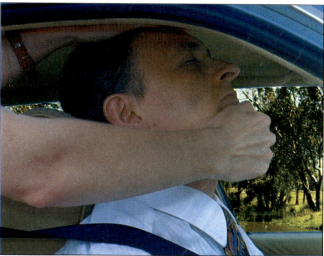

FIGURE 16-3 *For a victim trapped in a car, use head tilt and jaw support to keep the airway open, and monitor the person until the ambulance arrives.*

Move the victim from the vehicle only if necessary to get away from a danger at the scene, such as fire, or if the victim requires expired air resuscitation (EAR) or cardiopulmonary resuscitation (CPR). Otherwise, leave the victim in the vehicle and follow these guidelines:

1. Check for any hazardous materials at the scene (Figure 16-2A).

2. Send someone to call an ambulance immediately.

3. Open the vehicle's door or reach in through the window to switch off the engine and activate the hazard lights (Figure 16-2B). Also, disconnect the battery if you know how, as fires can be caused by damaged wiring even after the engine is switched off.

4. Take other steps to prevent fire. Do not let anyone smoke nearby. Ask bystanders to obtain a fire extinguisher, if possible, and have it ready. Remember, if there is a fire under the bonnet, release the bonnet catch but do not open the bonnet fully. Aim the fire extinguisher through the gap towards the flames. With a diesel truck or bus, shut off the emergency fuel switch outside.

5. Be sure the car cannot move. Secure the handbrake, put the transmission in gear if it is not already, and block the wheels (Figure 16-2C).

6. Check in and around the vehicle for other victims, such as children who may not be visible in or around the car. Ask any conscious victim how many people were in the car.

7. Quickly assess the response, airway, breathing and circulation of a victim inside the car. Unless it is necessary to provide EAR or CPR, leave the victim in the vehicle and care for injuries there.

8. If the person is trapped in the car, for example, by being pressed up against the steering wheel, provide care as best you can. It may be possible to relieve pressure on the chest by moving the car seat back carefully. Use head tilt and jaw support to keep the airway open, and monitor the person continually while waiting for the ambulance (Figure 16-3).

9. If a victim inside or outside a vehicle must be moved to escape danger or for you to give care, do so carefully and gently because of the risk of spinal injury or increased bleeding. Use the techniques described in Chapter 17.

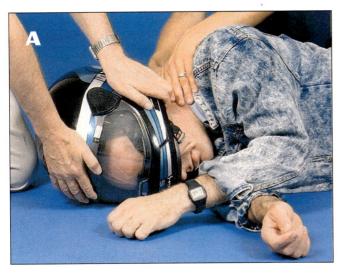
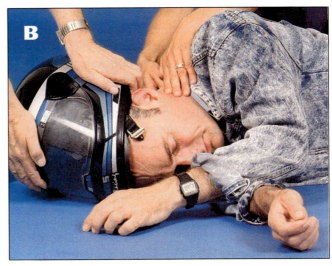

FIGURE 16-4 A *Lift the helmet so that it clears the chin,* **B** *then ease it over the base of the skull.*

Removal of Protective Helmets

A traffic collision or other incident may involve a victim who is wearing a motorcycle helmet or other type of protective headgear. The victim may remove the helmet if it does not cause pain to do so. The first aider should not remove a protective helmet unless the victim:

- is unconscious; or

- is vomiting.

If you need to remove a helmet to provide care, follow these guidelines:

1. Place the person on the side in the lateral position, supporting the head.

2. Maintain the victim's head in line with the body. If possible, avoid forward flexion or rotation of the head.

3. Unfasten a fabric chin strap; cut it if necessary.

3. Take pressure off the head by pulling the sides of the helmet apart with your hands. If possible a second person should support the victim's neck while the helmet is being removed. With a full-face helmet, this process should be performed by two people.

4. With the helmet sides pulled apart, lift the helmet back from the head. First tilt the helmet back and lift it so that it clears the chin (Figure 16-4A), then ease it forward to clear the base of the skull (Figure 16-4B), and then lift it off.

Hazardous Materials Incidents

Hazardous materials are common in vehicles, storage facilities, industrial sites and even the home. In any scene involving a vehicle crash, check for the presence of hazardous materials as part of checking the scene before approaching. Watch for clouds of vapour, any spilled liquids or solids, bottles or gas cylinders knocked over at the scene, and any unusual odours. Be careful to avoid any sparks, flames or cigarettes in the vicinity which may trigger a fire or explosion.

Vehicles and storage containers holding hazardous materials must display notices or signs indicating the contents along with appropriate warnings (Figure 16-5). Give the code number on such a sign when you call for emergency help. Avoid coming into contact with any spilled substance or breathing toxic fumes. Remember that fumes can be odourless and invisible. If you suspect toxic fumes are present, try to stay upwind from the spill.

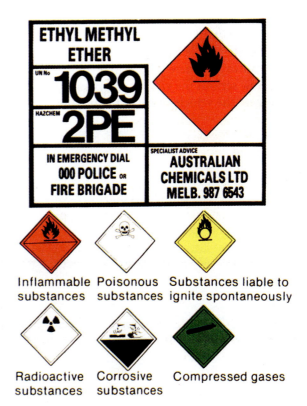

FIGURE 16-5 *Hazardous materials warning signs provide information on how to handle an emergency.*

Even in the home, be aware of the possibility of hazardous materials. For example, you may come upon an unconscious victim who you think possibly had a heart attack, when actually carbon monoxide from a faulty heater has poisoned the person. Look for anything unusual in the scene which may indicate danger. In one case, for example, a professional rescuer was about to give EAR to a non-breathing victim on the scene—when suddenly he saw the victim's dog also lying unconscious in a corner. He immediately removed both the victim and himself from the house to the fresh air outside.

Incidents Involving Electricity

Electricity poses a serious threat in any scene where high-voltage power lines have fallen or, in a setting indoors, where wires or a damaged electrical appliance can expose a person to a low-voltage electric current.

High-voltage power lines may be knocked down by a collision of a vehicle with the power line pole, by high winds in a storm, by lightning or by other causes (Figure 16-6). Follow these guidelines if you see fallen power lines:

1. Stay back, and move bystanders back, from the cables to a distance of at least 6 metres, because high-voltage electricity can arc up to 6 metres (see Chapter 7).

2. Do not attempt to move the cable, even with a non-conductive implement, again because of the risk of the electricity arcing. Some cables are so well insulated with rubber that they can spring back to the victim if pushed away by an untrained person.

3. Send a bystander to call both the fire service and the electricity supply authority.

4. If the fallen cable is touching a car, tell anyone inside the car to stay there until help arrives. Regardless of how serious the victim's injuries may be, do not go near the vehicle or try to remove the person.

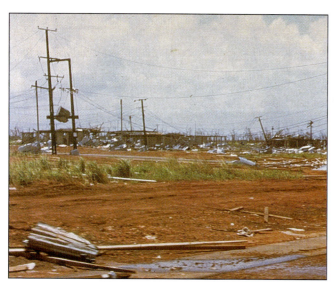

FIGURE 16-6 *Stay at least 6 metres back from fallen high-voltage power lines.*

5. Stay clear of a metal fence or structure, or body of water, which may be in contact with the fallen cable.

A loose wire, frayed or broken power cord or faulty electrical appliance can also pose a low-voltage electric shock risk in the home or workplace. Stay clear of the wire or appliance when approaching the victim. If the person is still in contact with the electrical source, shut off the power at the fuse box or main circuit breaker before touching the victim.

NATURAL DISASTERS

Natural disasters result from the impact of hazards which include severe storms, cyclones, floods, heat waves, bushfires and other natural phenomena, including earthquakes, landslides and volcanic eruptions. Natural disasters can result in injury to people directly because of the forces involved. This situation can be very serious in widespread natural disasters because ambulances and other emergency personnel cannot respond at once to every call for help. The first aider may need to care for a victim of a natural disaster for a longer period of time before emergency help arrives than would normally be the case.

Although conscious of the destructive forces of natural disasters, more injuries and deaths actually occur from the after-effects of the disasters, such as electrical currents, hazardous materials, rising waters and other dangers. Preventing injury and death may therefore depend on following safety guidelines, such as those below, for survival after a disaster impact:

1. Know how to turn off the electricity, gas, and water in your home or place of work.

2. Keep your first aid kit, a torch and a portable radio in a secure place where anyone in the house can find them.

3. Stay in your house unless it is dangerous to remain there. If you must leave, work out a safe route to a safe destination and wear protective shoes and clothing.

4. Follow the official instructions broadcast from the local radio station.

5. If it is safe to go out check on nearby neighbours, who may need help. However, avoid unnecessary trips out and sightseeing because extra traffic will slow emergency vehicles.

6. Use the telephone only for an emergency.

Severe Storms

Severe storms cause more damage in Australia than floods, bushfires or earthquakes. Tropical cyclones and tornadoes, which sometimes result from severe thunderstorms, are the most destructive (Figure 16-7). Injuries result from falling tree limbs, collapsing structures, blown debris, lightning strikes and capsizing boats. Your actions before the storm season, as a storm approaches, during the storm and after the storm can help prevent or minimise injury. Following are severe storm action guidelines from the Disaster Awareness Program of Emergency Management Australia (EMA):

Before the storm season:

- Trim tree branches well clear of your house.
- Have a portable radio and torch with fresh batteries.
- Keep a first aid kit (and acquire basic first aid knowledge).
- List emergency contact numbers.
- Clear your yard of loose objects.
- Clean and check the roof, guttering and downpipes.
- Familiarise your family with the steps to take before and during a storm.
- Keep masking tape (for glass), plastic sheeting and large garbage bags (for emergency rain protection).

As the storm approaches:

- Listen to local radio for information.
- Shelter and secure pets and animals.
- Shelter vehicles or cover them with tarpaulins or blankets.
- Disconnect all electrical appliances.
- Tape (in an X cross fashion) or cover large windows.

When the storm strikes:

- Stay inside and shelter well clear of windows, in the strongest part of the house (the bathroom or a cellar).
- If necessary, cover yourself with a mattress, blanket, quilt or tarpaulin, under a table, etc.
- Listen to a portable radio for storm updates.
- If outdoors, find emergency shelter (but not under a tree).

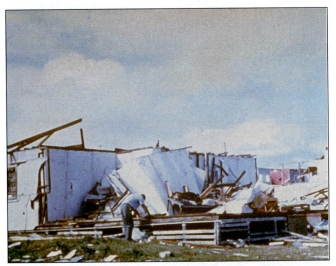

FIGURE 16-7 *The wind and rain from a cyclone can cause major damage.*

- If driving, stop clear of trees, power lines or streams
- Avoid using the telephone during the storm.

The "eye" of the cyclone may pass over, causing a lull in winds lasting from a few minutes to an hour or more, after which the storm forces will resume. Stay in shelter during and after the passing of the eye.

After the storm passes:

- Check your house for damage.
- Listen to local radio for official warnings and advice.
- If you do not need help yourself after the storm, check your neighbours.
- Beware of fallen power lines, damaged buildings and trees and flooded watercourses.
- Don't go sightseeing; stay home and help others.

In addition, if you are caught outside during a thunderstorm, take steps to avoid being hit by lightning. (See pages 117–118 for first aid for electrical injuries.)

If you are travelling in a caravan when high winds are expected, follow the manufacturer's instructions for securing the caravan. EMA recommends positioning the caravan with the narrow end facing the wind, chocking the wheels, using chassis and roof tie-downs and making outside equipment safe.

Floods

Flooding is a potential problem throughout Australia. Although low-lying coastal and inland river areas are more at risk for periodic flooding caused by storms and heavy rains, flash flooding can occur in almost all parts of Australia. Flash floods occur from intense bursts of rainfall and pose a great risk because they may occur in populated and urban areas and may occur with little or no warning. Flooding can also occur at a point well downstream from the actual rainfall.

If you live or work in an area subject to flooding, take precautions and know what to do if flooding occurs. EMA recommends the following:

Ask your local State or Territory emergency service:

- What do the terms major, moderate and minor flooding mean in your area and at what official river height will your home become isolated or inundated.
- Details of the local flood plan, whether you may need to evacuate and how to get to the nearest safe location.

Keep an emergency kit. During and after a flood you will need:

- A portable radio and torch with fresh batteries.
- Candles and waterproof matches.
- Stocks of fresh water and tinned food.
- A first aid kit and first aid knowledge.
- Good supplies of essential medication.

- Strong shoes and rubber gloves.

- A waterproof bag or bags for clothing and valuables.

- A list of emergency contact numbers.

Act on flood warnings:

- Listen to your local radio or TV for further information.

- Check that your neighbours know of the warning.

- Stack furniture and possessions above the likely flood level, on beds and in the roof (electrical items on top).

- Move garbage, chemicals and poisons to a high place.

- Protect or relocate valuable stock and equipment.

- Move livestock to higher ground.

- Check your car and fill it with fuel.

- Check your emergency kit and fresh water stocks.

If you need to evacuate:

- Empty freezers and refrigerators, leaving doors open to prevent floating and subsequent damage.

- Collect and secure personal valuables, papers, money, photo albums and family mementoes.

- Turn off electricity, gas and water.

- Don't forget to take your emergency kit.

During and after the flood:

- Keep your emergency kit safe and dry.

- Do not eat food which has been in contact with flood water, and boil all tap water until supplies have been declared safe.

- Don't use gas or electrical appliances which have been flood affected until they have been safety checked.

- Beware of snakes or spiders which may move into drier areas in your house.

- Avoid wading, even in shallow water, because it may be contaminated. If you must enter shallow flood water, wear solid shoes and check the depth with a stick.

- Check with police for safe routes before driving anywhere, and don't enter water without checking the depth and the current.

- Keep listening to your local radio and TV station and heed all warnings and advice.

Even those who do not live in a flood area need to know what to do in case of a flash flood. Flash floods cause more injuries and deaths than other types of floods. The depth and current of flood water is difficult to estimate, and often people attempt to drive, swim or walk through the water and are swept away. Flood waters also often carry debris and objects which may strike a person in the water, increasing the risk of drowning. *Never drive or walk into flood waters* (Figure 16-8). If your car becomes stuck in water flowing over the road,

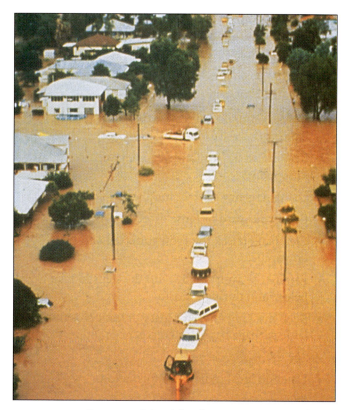

FIGURE 16-8 *Because of the risks of strong currents and debris swept by the water, you should never walk or drive into flood waters.*

leave it immediately if the water is still very shallow, because the water may be rising fast. If the water is deep or moving very fast, it is usually better to stay with the vehicle and wait for rescue or for the water to recede.

Bushfires

Bushfires can be terribly destructive in many areas of Australia (Figure 16-9). If you live in an area at risk, it is very important to know what precautions to take and what to do if a bushfire occurs.

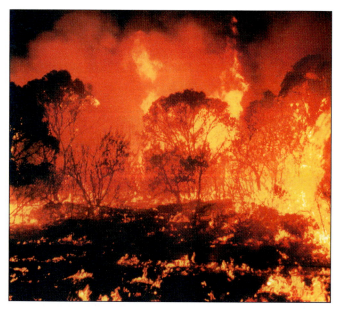

FIGURE 16-9 *Bushfires can be terribly destructive.*

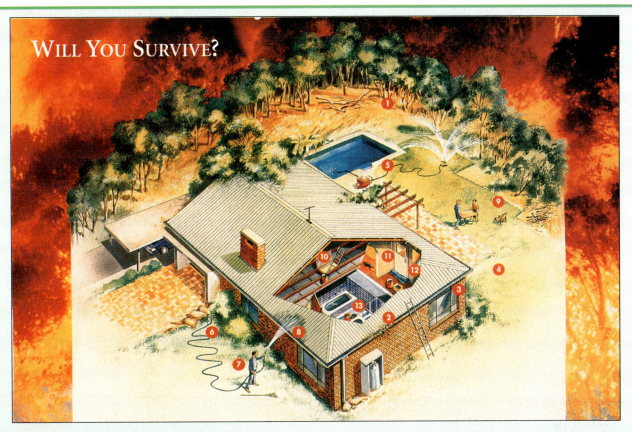

WILL YOU SURVIVE?

BEFORE THE BUSHFIRE SEASON

1. Clear a fuel break between your property and any nearby bush, incorporating natural breaks like roads, creeks, dams and gravel driveways. In most cases, a 20–30 metre circle of safety is recommended… Once established, it's important to keep fuel breaks cleared down to the ground.

2. Clean out gutters and clear dry vegetation, over-hanging branches, rubbish and any flammable liquids from around the house. Clear undergrowth from fences and keep woodheaps and other combustibles uphill and well away from buildings.

3. Seal open eaves and spaces under the house. Fit wire screens to windows, doors, vents and chimneys to protect glass and stop sparks entering the house.

4. Keep lawns short and grass healthy.

5. Ensure that you have clear access to water. Consider installing a sprinkler system with an independent water supply (swimming pool, tank or dam) and a petrol- or diesel-powered pump.

6. Check that garden hoses and firefighting equipment inside and outside the house are in good working order and that pump engines are fuelled. Ensure that hoses reach all parts of the house.

IF FIRE APPROACHES

7. Cover as much exposed skin as possible with cotton or woollen clothing—no synthetics. Wear gloves, long trousers, a long-sleeved shirt and sturdy footwear. It is likely to be very smoky, so wrap a wet cloth over your nose and mouth if needed.

8. Plug downpipes with plastic bags filled with sand, soil or a large wet sponge and tape them securely in place. Fill gutters with water to help prevent spot fires igniting. If you have enough time and water, hose dry underfloor areas and any crevices in the house where sparks and burning embers may enter., Dampening the ground around the house where there might be flammable fuels like bark or dry garden mulch will also help protect the home.

9. Disconnect garden hoses and any plastic tap fittings and take them inside the house, along with mats and any other flammable items. Start auxiliary pump if you have one, connect it to your independent water supply and turn on sprinklers. Switch gas and power off at the mains. Make sure gas-cylinder safety valves point away from the house.

10. Once inside, put a ladder through the ceiling trapdoor so you can regularly check the roof space for fire or sparks, and have a bucket of water on hand.

11. Ensure that all people and pets are in the house and close all windows, shutters, vents and doors…

12. Block gaps under doors and around windows with wet, rolled towels. Remove blinds, close curtains and push furniture away from windows.

13. Fill buckets, basins, baths and sinks with water in case you need to extinguish spot fires. Wet towels and woollen blankets for personal protection.

Source: Courtesy of *Australian Geographic*, supplement to January–March 1995 issue.

Start by contacting the local fire authorities to learn about regulations, risks, the warning system and emergency plans for the area. The local fire service should have information bulletins which will help you to plan your actions in the event of a fire. Follow these general guidelines:

1. In the fire danger months of summer do not light fires in the open. Be very careful with cigarettes, barbecues and any other flames. Observe total fire ban warnings.

2. Keep the area around your house clear of flammable materials. Remove dry vegetation, and clean out the guttering. Tan bark, heavy mulch and woodpiles should be removed from areas close to the house. Maintain fuel reduction throughout the summer. Keep lawns mowed and green.

3. Keep available a water hose which can reach all around the house and any outbuildings. You cannot always rely on supplied water during a bush or grass fire; if you have a suitable pump, use water from a nearby tank, dam or swimming pool.

4. During high-risk periods, regularly tune into a radio or TV station to learn of any alerts.

5. Plan for your own personal safety. If you plan to stay with your house, put together a kit of protective clothing for everyone. Include sturdy leather shoes or work boots, a broad-brimmed hat and goggles. A wet towel around your neck can be used over the face to assist breathing in heavy smoke.

Most importantly, decide in advance whether or not to evacuate your house if a bushfire approaches. Many lives are lost when people stay behind to defend their home against the fire but then make a last-minute panic-stricken decision to flee and are caught in the fire. It is recommended that you decide for yourself, based on questions such as the following:

• Are you physically able to defend your home?

• Are you mentally and emotionally prepared to face fire?

• Should any household members (the very young, ill, elderly or disabled) be evacuated?

• Are you prepared to stay with the house to continue watching for smouldering flames even hours after the bushfire has passed?

• Is your property a high fire risk? Have you done preventive work?

• Are you equipped to fight fire, and do you have a plan of action?

If you decide evacuation is your best course of action, follow these guidelines:

1. Plan in advance:
   —Where to go.
   —When to leave (but never at the last moment when flames are close).
   —How to travel (plan what vehicle to use and have a planned and alternate route).
   —What to take with you.
   —What to do if family members are separated.

2. Listen to issued warnings and leave as early and quickly as you can once you decide it is appropriate to evacuate. Be sure to take survival equipment with you (wool blankets, drinking water, medicines).

3. Wear appropriate heavy clothing and shoes, even though you do not plan to be close to the fire.

4. Close doors and windows behind you as you leave.

If you decide to stay and defend your home, follow these guidelines if the bushfire comes near:

1. Put on your planned heavy clothing and shoes, even in hot weather, as protection against the radiant heat of the fire.

2. Shut windows and doors.

3. Turn off electricity and gas at the main supply.

4. Make sure water hoses are connected to taps and ready to use.

5. Plug downpipes and fill guttering with water.

6. Keep ready full water buckets and wet bags outside the house in key areas. Fill baths and sinks with water. Soak towels and woollen blankets with water.

7. Watch for burning leaves or twigs blown ahead of the fire. Put out any flames immediately. Keep the side of the house facing the fire as wet as possible.

8. Drink water frequently to prevent dehydration.

9. Stay outside to monitor conditions until flames approach or the radiant heat increases, and then go inside. *Resist the urge to flee at this time.* Stay in shelter inside the house, going outside only to check for flames on the house if the radiant heat is bearable.

10. If flames inside the house force you to flee, wrap yourself in a woollen blanket and seek protection outside behind a solid object such as a brick garden wall.

You may be in an open area when a bushfire approaches. If in a car, close the windows, cover your body to shield against radiant heat and lie down low until the fire passes; then leave the car in case the wind blows the fire back. If you are in the open, cover your body as best you can with fire-resistant clothing or material (not synthetics), and cover your face with a wet cloth.

Earthquakes

The 1989 Newcastle earthquake, which resulted in 13 fatalities and 150 injuries, is a reminder that Australia is not immune to significant earthquakes. Most fatalities and injuries occur because a building collapses or debris falls onto the victim. Although earthquakes occur with little or no warning, there are things you can do now to prevent injury if an earthquake does occur, and you should know what to do during and after an earthquake to minimise risks. The following guidelines are from Emergency Management Australia (Disaster Awareness Program).

Be prepared:

- Keep ready a torch with fresh batteries, a battery-operated radio, your first aid kit and book and a list of emergency numbers.
- Plan how family members will reunite if separated.
- Know the safe areas to move to if shaking starts: against inside walls or under sturdy furniture.
- Know dangerous areas to avoid: near windows or mirrors, beneath hanging objects, next to fireplaces.
- Know how to turn off your electricity, water and gas.
- If you live in an earthquake-prone area:
  —Check the chimney, walls, roof and foundations for stability.
  —Secure the water heater and appliances which could topple or rupture utility lines.
  —Secure tall, heavy furniture which may topple.
  —Secure any heavy hanging objects.
  —Keep flammable and hazardous liquids on bottom shelves or cupboard floors.

If an earthquake begins:

- If indoors, stay there. Take cover under an interior door frame or sturdy furniture. Keep away from windows, chimneys and hanging objects.
- Do not use a lift.
- In a crowded public place, do not rush for the doors. Move away from overhead objects or shelves containing heavy objects.
- If outdoors, stay back from buildings, walls, power lines, trees, etc. In a city street of tall buildings, seek refuge under a strong archway or doorway.
- If in a vehicle, pull off the road into a clear area, avoiding bridges and overpasses. Watch out for power lines overhead.

After an earthquake:

- Check for injuries and give first aid.
- Do not use the telephone unless there is a serious injury or fire.
- Turn off stoves and heaters.
- Do not light matches until you check for gas and fuel leaks.
- Check for water leaks, broken electrical cables and gas leaks. Turn off any leaking utility at the supply.

- Check the building for cracks and damage, including roof, chimneys and foundation. If serious damage has occurred, evacuate the building and do not return until it has been checked by an authority. Aftershocks can cause the collapse of a damaged structure.
- Check food and water supplies. Conserve water because the supply may be interrupted.
- Listen to the radio for instructions and co-operate with emergency personnel.
- In order to keep the streets clear for emergency personnel, do not drive unless it is necessary to seek medical attention.
- Be prepared for aftershocks.

BUILDING FIRES

Fires in a large building can burn and spread very quickly. If there is a fire in a multi-storey building, unless you are certain you can immediately put it out with an available fire extinguisher, you should call emergency services immediately and act to get everyone out of the building as quickly as possible. Ensure any fire alarms have been activated to warn others to leave. Close doors and windows to help contain the fire and slow its progress. *Never attempt to fight a fire unless you are trained and are not in danger.*

The smoke and fumes from the fire are often more dangerous than the flames themselves. You can easily be overcome by smoke, and many synthetic materials used in curtains, carpeting, furniture and other items give off toxic fumes when burning. Get out as quickly as you can, and do not go back into the building. If there is smoke, crawl low to escape because smoke rises and any breathable air is close to the floor (Figure 16-10). If you are trapped inside, go to a room with a window. Shut the door and block off door cracks and vents with towels,

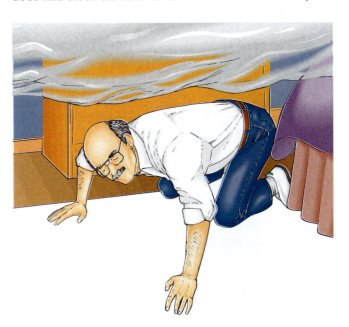

FIGURE 16-10 *Whenever there is smoke in a room, stay close to the floor.*

rags or clothing. Call for help from a window. If a phone is available, call the fire department—even if rescuers are already outside—and tell the dispatcher your location.

As a general rule, never enter a burning structure unless you know the location of someone inside who needs assistance getting out. *Follow these guidelines if you can enter without endangering yourself:*

1. Use a cord tied around your waist for a lifeline and have a signal system so that you can be pulled back out to safety if needed.

2. Before opening any door, feel it with the back of your hand and check for hot air coming out beneath the door. Do not open the door if it is hot.

3. If it is safe to enter, take deep breaths of air before opening the door. Keep your face averted as you open the door.

4. If there is smoke inside, put a wet cloth over your mouth and nose and stay close to the floor. Move quickly because there may be little air present for breathing.

5. Drag the victim out with arms extended alongside the head. When safe outside, check the victim's response, airway, breathing and circulation, and provide needed care following the Basic Life Support flow chart (see page 35).

If in any situation your clothing catches on fire, remember to **Stop, drop and roll.** Stop whatever you are doing, drop to the floor or ground, and roll over and over until the flames are extinguished. If someone else's clothing catches on fire, do not allow the person to run. Get the person on the ground and smother the fire with a blanket or other available non-flammable material.

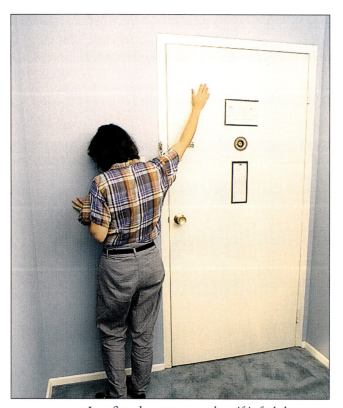

FIGURE 16-11 *In a fire, do not open a door if it feels hot.*

A fire in a large building such as a hotel can be especially dangerous. Knowing how to get out could save your life. Locate the fire exits and extinguishers on your floor. If you hear an alarm while in your room, feel the door first and do not open it if it is hot (Figure 16-11). Do not use the lift. If the hall is relatively smoke free, use the stairs to exit. If the hall is filled with smoke, crawl to the exit. If you cannot get to the exit, return to your room. Turn off the ventilation system, stuff door cracks and vents with wet towels, and telephone the front desk or the fire service to report the fire and your location.

Chapter 20 describes steps you can take to prevent fires and to practise fire safety awareness in the home and work place.

POTENTIAL VIOLENCE

Major incidents in which first aid may be required also include scenes potentially involving violence. Always follow the emergency action principles and do not enter the scene if it may be unsafe. However, in some instances you may already be on the scene when the potential for violence arises or becomes apparent, and in this case you should act in a way which ensures safety for yourself, any victims and bystanders.

Crime scenes are a special situation. Do not approach the scene until you are sure it is safe. In a crime scene the victim may have injuries from a shooting, stabbing or other violence. If the scene is safe, provide care for the injury, but be careful not to touch anything unnecessarily. Law enforcement authorities will need to gather evidence at the scene.

Hostile Situations

A hostile situation involves someone acting in a hostile or threatening manner. This includes the victim, family members or bystanders.

A victim's hostile behaviour may result from the effects of an injury or illness or from fear, use of alcohol or other drugs, or even a lack of oxygen. If the victim is hostile to you, stay calm and explain that you only want to help. Hostility usually disappears once the person realises you are not a threat. However, if the victim remains hostile, do not argue or try to force care on the person. A friend or family member may be able to calm and convince the person to accept your care. Remember, you cannot give care without the victim's consent. If the hostility persists, withdraw from the scene.

Emotional family members or friends may also become hostile if they feel the victim's well-being is threatened or they are frightened. Be understanding and explain how you want to help. If you stay calm, often they will also calm down.

If a bystander or a crowd at the scene becomes hostile, withdraw and wait for law enforcement and ambulance personnel to arrive. Never approach a hostile crowd.

Suicide

If a victim has committed or attempted suicide, be careful about entering the scene. If you see that the person is obviously dead, do not disturb the scene unnecessarily but wait for police and ambulance personnel. If the victim may still be alive, give emergency care if it is safe to enter the scene.

Do not approach a suicidal person who has a weapon. Withdraw from the scene and wait for the arrival of police. If the person has attempted or is threatening suicide by a method which does not threaten your personal safety, such as by swallowing pills, call an ambulance immediately and remain at the scene as long as it is safe to do so. Stay with the person and be calm and reassuring. Listen to what the person is saying and be understanding. Do not argue with, contradict or trivialise anything the person says. Do not leave the person alone. You cannot restrain or give first aid to a person who refuses your offer to help, but if the person becomes unconscious, you can and should provide emergency care.

Hostage Situations

If you encounter a hostage situation, your priority is to avoid becoming a hostage yourself. Do not approach the scene, but call police immediately. If you are taken hostage, give first aid to other hostages if the hostage-taker allows, but do not attempt heroics or put yourself at risk.

CRITICAL INCIDENT STRESS

In addition to providing care to injured victims during a major incident, first aiders should be aware of their own needs and responses.

Stress is a physical, mental or emotional state which causes tension, distress or disruption to a person's mental or emotional balance. Critical incident stress is a term used for the reaction that can occur after an emergency. It is likely to occur to a first aider after a situation in which a victim dies or is seriously injured, or in any event which threatens the first aider. When this stress becomes too great, it often has negative effects. It can cause sleeplessness, anxiety, depression, exhaustion, restlessness, nausea, nightmares and other problems. Some effects might not occur right away but appear days, weeks or even months after the event.

Critical incident stress is a normal reaction to a very stressful situation. First aiders experiencing this response need to recognise it in order to cope with it. If you do not identify and accept it, serious long-term effects can occur. Do not ignore it, or feel you are weak or abnormal for experiencing it. Because critical incident stress is so common, there are professionals trained to help you understand and cope with it. Do not hesitate to ask your health care provider for help.

Summary

- Any emergency scene can be dangerous, but the scene at a major incident is more likely to involve hazards or risks. Your personal safety is always your first concern. Whenever you are unsure whether the scene is safe or whether special equipment or training may be necessary to handle the situation, withdraw from the scene and wait for properly trained personnel or the ambulance.

- Specific major incidents involve particular hazards. The general guidelines for dealing with these hazards are summarised in Table 16-1.

Table 16-1

RESPONDING TO MAJOR INCIDENTS

Type of incident	Appropriate behaviour
Multiple victims	Care for victims with the most life-threatening conditions first, or provide care to help save the greatest number of victims.
Traffic collisions	Keep the scene safe from other moving vehicles. Turn off the engine, prevent fire and stabilise the vehicle before giving care. If possible provide care without moving the victim.
Hazardous materials	Stay a safe distance away, upwind and uphill. Prevent sparks or flames. Notify fire and emergency personnel immediately.
Electricity	Assume any fallen cables are dangerous. Do not try to move fallen cables. Do not touch any metal fence or structure or body of water contacting fallen wires. Notify fire officials and the electricity supply authority. In the home, shut off power before touching faulty appliance cords or wires.
Storms	Take preventative action when storm warnings are issued. Shut off power, gas and water mains. Stay indoors and follow official broadcast instructions.
Floods	Take preventative action and have an emergency kit and supplies ready. Monitor official broadcasts and be prepared to evacuate if ordered. Never drive or walk into moving water.
Bushfires	During the danger season, keep your house and yard prepared to lower the risk of fire spreading. Have water and equipment ready if a bushfire threatens. Be prepared for evacuation.
Earthquakes	Check the earthquake history of your area with local authorities by obtaining a risk map. Ask your local council how you can make your home safer during an earthquake. Have a standard emergency kit on hand. Know your safe areas during an earthquake and form a plan with your family.
Fire	Never enter a burning structure. If caught inside, stay low, do not open hot doors or use lifts, and exit immediately or call for help. Do not attempt to rescue a victim unless it is safe for you to enter the area.
Crime scene	Do not enter the scene until you are sure it is safe. Do not touch anything unless it is essential to give care.
Hostile situations	Try to calm and reassure the victim. Retreat to safety if threatened. Do not try to restrain, argue with or force care upon a victim.
Suicide	Withdraw from the scene if a weapon is brandished. Do not touch anything at the scene unless this is essential to give care. If you are not at personal risk, stay with a suicidal person and offer them understanding.
Hostage situation	Stay out of the scene if possible, and call for police.

Study Questions

1. **How close can you safely come to fallen high-voltage power lines?**
   a. Stay back at least 1 metre.
   b. Stay back at least 6 metres.
   c. Move them if you are wearing leather gloves.
   d. Touch them only with your shoe.

2. **When the "eye" of a cyclone arrives and the high winds diminish, you should:**
   a. go outside to assess the damage
   b. drive your car away to a more secure location
   c. judge by the cloud formations how to act
   d. stay in a safe location to wait out the rest of the storm

3. **If smoke and flames reveal a fire under the bonnet of a car, you should:**
   a. release the bonnet latch and shoot the fire extinguisher beneath the bonnet without raising it
   b. use a stick to raise the bonnet in order to use the fire extinguisher directly on the flames
   c. do nothing but wait for fire personnel to arrive
   d. try to push the car to a location where flames will not spread to nearby objects

4. **After an earthquake:**
   a. it is safe to enter buildings that seem to be structurally sound, in order to gather your possessions
   b. it is not safe to enter any buildings because aftershocks may continue to put the building and those in it at risk
   c. it is safe to enter if you carry the end of a rope so that you can be pulled out to safety if necessary
   d. it is safe to enter as long as you cannot smell leaking gas fumes

5. **You should only remove the helmet of an injured motorcyclist if:**
   a. the victim is unconscious or vomiting
   b. the victim is wearing a full-face helmet
   c. the victim is unable to remove the helmet because of pain
   d. a bystander instructs you to do so

Answer are in Appendix A (page 363).

Handling and Moving Victims

THROUGHOUT THIS BOOK you have been learning how to give first aid to victims with serious injuries or sudden illness, in situations where help is on the way. In some circumstances, however, you will need to move the victim—whether in an emergency such as a fire or risk of explosion, or in a less urgent situation such as the removal of an athlete with a sprained ankle.

This chapter describes those circumstances in which a victim can or should be moved, and how to do so in a manner safe for both the victim and the first aider.

For Review

A review of the emergency action principles first aiders should follow in all emergencies (Chapter 3) will help your understanding of the chapter.

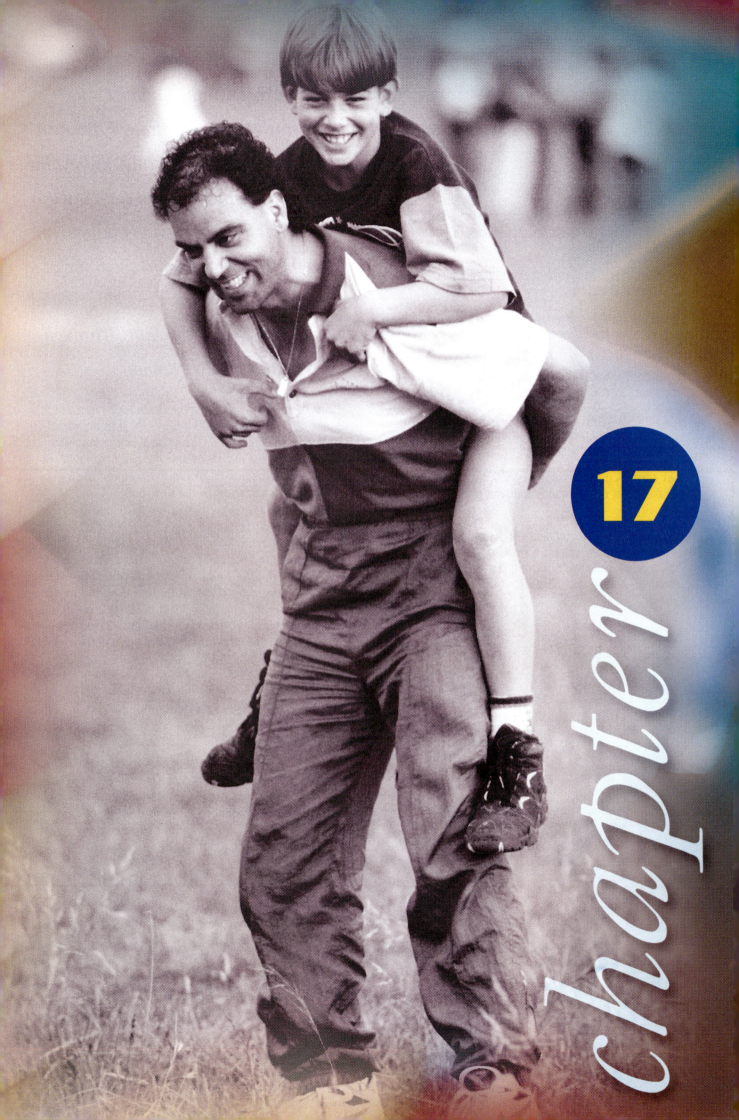

17

chapter

Key Terms

Ankle drag: An emergency move in which you pull the victim away from danger by the legs.

Assisted walk: A planned move in which you support and assist the victim to walk.

Body mechanics: The principles for moving and lifting in ways that prevent straining your body or putting yourself at risk for injury.

Chair lift: A planned move in which two first aiders carry the victim in a chair.

Clothes drag: An emergency move in which you pull the victim away from danger by clothing gathered behind the neck.

Emergency moves: Methods for quickly moving a victim to safety.

Fore and aft carry: An emergency move in which two first aiders carry a victim away from danger by lifting the victim under the arms and by the legs.

Seat carry: A planned move by which two first aiders make a seat of their hands and arms for carrying the victim.

Stretcher: Any of several different devices for lifting and carrying a victim, typically with a frame on which the person lies while two or more first aiders hold on to the frame or poles along the sides.

You wake up in the middle of the night smelling smoke through the open bedroom window. Something is burning outside the house, but you cannot tell where. You quickly get dressed and run from the bedroom toward the front door. There is a sudden crackling sound outside, followed by screams. Through the windows you see flames.

You rush outside and see the neighbour's house ablaze. A man carrying a young child staggers through the door and collapses to the ground in the doorway. Smoke is blowing over him and the child. You can see flames inside the house. You hear the sound of sirens, but they are still far off in the distance.

You make a split second decision to help and run to the collapsed victims. Both the man and the child are semi-conscious and coughing. You recognise the immediate danger and the need to get them to a safer place. You pick up the child and run toward your house. Other neighbours begin to gather. You hand the child to one of them and run back to help the man. With a neighbour's help, you carry him away from the fire and into fresh air.

The house is nearly fully ablaze when the fire fighters arrive. Through the smoke and flames, you see that the place where the man and child once lay is now covered with burning debris from a collapsed wall. You made a fast decision to rescue two people. You did it quickly and probably saved two lives.

In earlier chapters, you learned how to care for victims of injury and illness at the scene when it is safe to do so. However, sometimes the victim is in a dangerous situation and must be rescued before you can give care. In this chapter, you will learn how to safely move victims without endangering or injuring yourself.

PRINCIPLES OF MOVING VICTIMS

Usually when you give first aid, you will not face hazards that require moving the victim immediately. In most cases, you can follow the Emergency Action Principles described in Chapter 3 and give care where you find the victim. Moving a victim needlessly can lead to further injury. For example, if the victim has a closed fracture of the leg, movement could result in the end of the bone tearing the skin. Soft tissue damage, damage to nerves, blood loss and infection are all possible results of unnecessary movement.

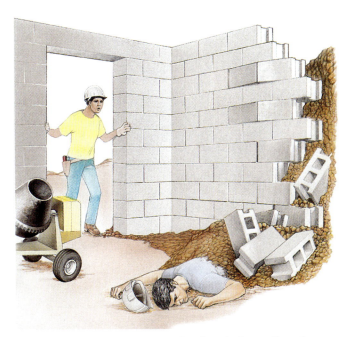

FIGURE 17-1 *Move a victim only when in immediate danger, such as from a collapsing structure.*

When to Move a Victim

You should move a victim *only if there is immediate danger* such as fire, lack of oxygen or the presence of poisonous fumes, risk of drowning, risk of explosion, a collapsing structure or uncontrollable traffic hazards (Figure 17-1).

Before you act, consider the following factors in order to ensure that you move a victim quickly and safely:

- Dangerous conditions at the scene.
- The size of the victim.
- Your own health and physical ability.
- Whether others can help you.
- The victim's condition.

Considering these factors will help you decide how to proceed. For example, if the victim is large and heavy and you have limited strength, or if you are injured or have a significant medical condition, you may be unable to move the person and will only risk making the situation worse. If you become part of the problem, ambulance personnel will now have one more person to rescue.

If any bystanders can help, never try to move a victim by yourself because of the risk of injury to both you and the victim. When working with others to move a victim, be sure everyone knows what to do before starting.

Protecting the Victim During a Move

To protect the victim during any move, follow these guidelines:

- Only attempt to move the victim if you are sure you can comfortably handle the person's weight. A victim who falls or slips could be further injured.
- Walk carefully using short steps to keep the victim as steady as possible.

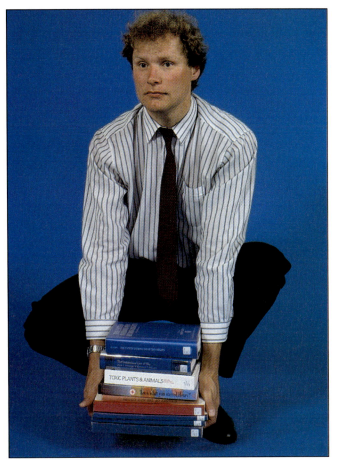

FIGURE 17-2 *Use good body mechanics when lifting: keep the back straight, knees bent, feet spread apart and one foot forward.*

- When possible, move forward rather than backward to avoid bumping into anything.
- Always look where you are going in order to keep an even footing and prevent jarring the victim.
- Support the victim's head and spine, maintaining alignment.
- Avoid bending or twisting a victim with a possible head or spine injury.

Protecting Yourself When Moving a Victim

It is important to protect yourself when moving the victim. Use good body mechanics to prevent straining your body or putting yourself at risk of injury. The back is especially vulnerable to injury caused by bending, twisting, lifting and carrying heavy weights.

Follow these guidelines:

- Only attempt to move the victim if you are sure you can comfortably handle the person's weight. Musculoskeletal injuries can result from attempting to lift or move too great a weight.
- When lifting, bend at the knees and hips and lift with your legs, not your back. Keep your back straight and head erect. Keep your centre of gravity low and your feet spread about shoulder width apart, with one foot slightly forward (Figure 17-2).

- Hold the weight close to your body for greater stability.

- When carrying or lifting use your whole hand, as this will strengthen your grasp.

- Walk carefully using short steps. This helps you keep your balance and prevents sudden strains.

- When possible, move forward rather than backward.

- Face the direction of any body movement to prevent twisting your back.

- Be especially careful when lifting a victim in an awkward situation, such as raising a child onto your shoulders or a victim over a wall or through a window. Avoid twisting or any sudden lurching movements.

Choosing What Move to Use

When you have decided to move a victim, your choice of method depends firstly on whether you need to move quickly in an emergency, or can take the time to plan the move and secondly on whether you can use the assistance of others or equipment such as a chair or blanket. Never rush a move if the situation does not require it.

EMERGENCY MOVES

There are several ways to quickly move a person to safety in an emergency. But there is *no one best way.* As long as you can move the person to safety without injuring yourself or causing further injury to the victim, the move is successful.

Different emergency moves are used depending on the circumstances and whether another person is available to help you move the victim.

One-Person Moves

If the person is conscious and does not have a serious injury, you may be able to assist the victim in walking away from the danger (see Assisted Walk on page 314). However, if the victim is unconscious or has a serious injury and you are alone, you need to drag the person from danger using one of the following methods.

Ankle Drag

For victims too large to carry or move in any other way, you can pull the victim by the legs, holding the ankles, as shown in Figure 17-3. The victim should be lying on the back. This technique is best used when dragging a victim over smooth ground, although it offers little protection to the victim's head and neck. However, for a victim without a head or neck injury, this drag is preferred when a first aider is working alone because it has less risk of back injury for the first aider and maintains traction on the body to keep bone ends apart if the victim has a fracture.

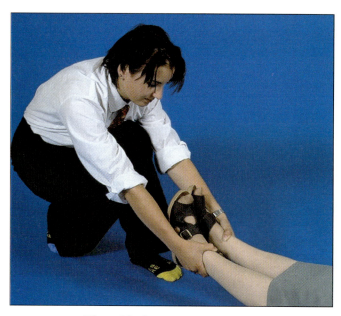

FIGURE 17-3 *The ankle drag.*

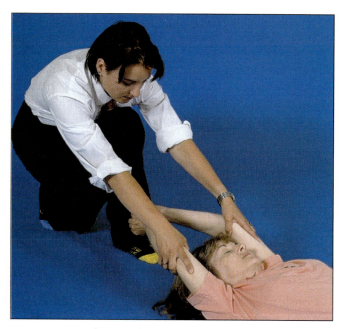

FIGURE 17-4 *The arm drag.*

Arm Drag

As an alternative to the ankle drag, you can drag the victim head first by pulling by the arms. The victim should be lying on the back. Raise the victim's arms above the head and hold them at the elbow, as shown in Figure 17-4. In this way you may be able to hold the arms against both sides of the head to provide some stability for the head and spine, and to prevent the head from bumping over rough areas. Do not lift the arms or head off the ground because this can aggravate a neck injury. If you are alone with a victim with suspected head or neck injury who *must* be moved from danger, use this method. This type of emergency move is exhausting and may result in back strain for the rescuer.

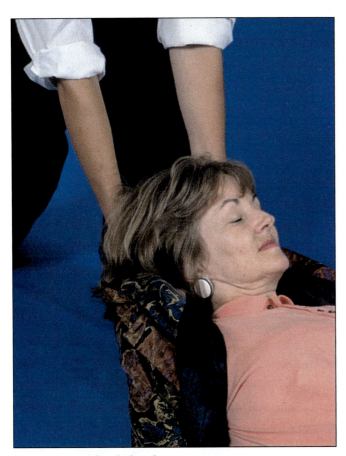

FIGURE 17-5 *The clothes drag.*

Clothes Drag

The clothes drag can also be used for moving a person not suspected of having a head, spine or other major injury. For a clothes drag, open the top buttons of the victim's shirt and jacket to avoid pressure on the throat when the clothes pull up, and gather the loose fabric in tight behind the victim's neck. Using the clothing, pull the victim to safety. During the move, the victim's head is cradled by both the clothing and the rescuer's hands (Figure 17-5). This type of emergency move is also exhausting and may result in back strain for the rescuer.

Two-Person Move

Two first aiders can move a victim much more safely than one. If the victim is conscious and can stand, both can assist the victim in walking away from danger (see two-person Assisted Walk on page 314). However, if the victim is unconscious or has serious injuries in any emergency situation which requires an immediate move, use the following fore and aft carry method.

1. From both sides, support the victim in a sitting position. Cross the victim's arms across the chest.

2. The larger or stronger first aider moves behind the victim and places one hand under each of the victim's armpits to reach forward and hold the victim's wrists. The victim must keep both arms folded across the chest.

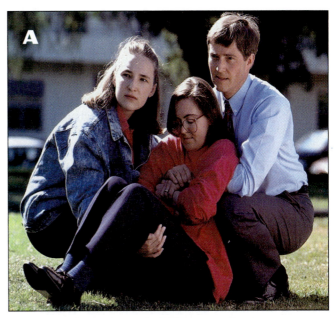

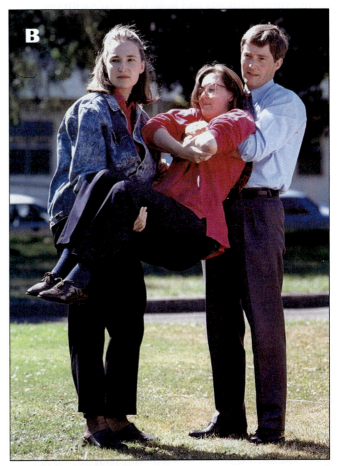

FIGURE 17-6 *The fore and aft carry (see description in points 3 and 4 below).*

3. At the victim's side, the other first aider puts one hand and forearm under the victim's thighs and knees and holds the thighs firmly. The other arm is placed around the victim's back (Figure 17-6A).

4. On the signal from one first aider, both stand, lifting the victim (Figure 17-6B).

Use this method to carry the victim quickly from danger or to transfer a victim to a chair or wheelchair in a non-urgent, planned move.

PLANNED MOVES

When there is no immediate danger or threat to life but you must still move the person to seek medical attention, take the time to plan the move that is safest not only for the victim but for you and other first aiders as well. This could happen in a remote area where help cannot be brought in.

Planned moves include the one- or two-person assisted walk, the seat carry, the chair lift and the use of a stretcher.

Assisted Walk (Human Crutch)

The most basic move is the assisted walk which can be used with a conscious victim who can stand in either an emergency or a planned move. Do not use this method for a victim with an upper arm, shoulder or rib injury. Stand at the victim's injured side. Place the victim's arm across your shoulders and hold it in place with one hand (Figure 17.7A). Support the victim with your other hand around the victim's waist (Figure 17.7B). In this way your body acts as a "crutch", supporting the victim's weight while you both walk.

Two-Person Assisted Walk

The two-person assisted walk is like the one-person human crutch, but the second person supports the victim in the same way from the other side (Figure 17-8). This method is commonly used to help injured athletes from the playing field.

Four-Handed Seat Carry

The four-handed seat carry by two first aiders is used for conscious victims who cannot put weight on either leg to use the assisted walk, or whose injury or illness does not allow the person to stand upright The victim must be able to use one or both arms to hold on to one or both first aiders. If the victim is unconscious or disorientated, unable to hold on or injured in the upper body, use the two-handed seat carry instead.

Follow these steps for the four-handed seat carry:

1. Both first aiders face each other behind the victim's back. Make the four-handed seat by both grasping your own left wrist with your right hand, and the other's right wrist with your left hand, as shown in Figure 17-9A).

2. Stoop or crouch down, keeping the back as straight as possible, and slide the four-handed seat under the victim.

3. Ask the victim to put both arms (if able) around your necks and settle into the seat (Figure 17-9B).

4. Both first aiders should stand at the same time. Be sure you have a secure, firm grip and good body position before starting to move. Take the first step with the outside leg, and then walk with ordinary steps.

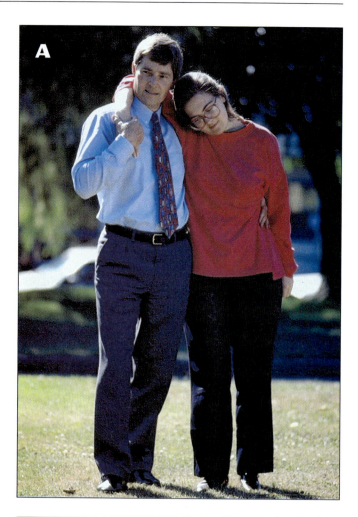

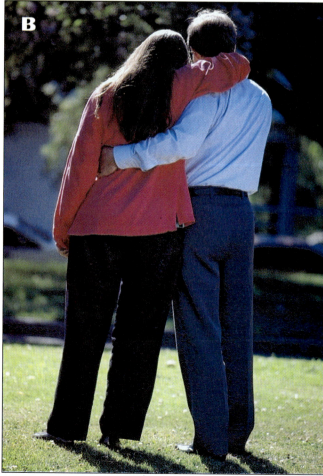

FIGURE 17-7 *The one-person "human crutch" assisted walk.*

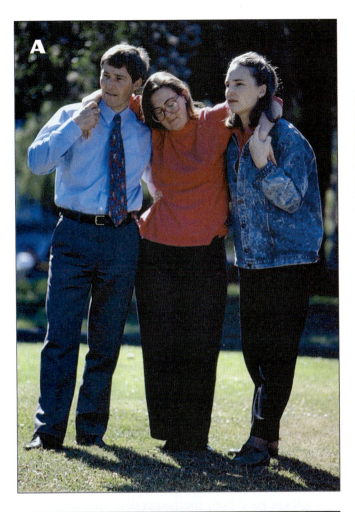

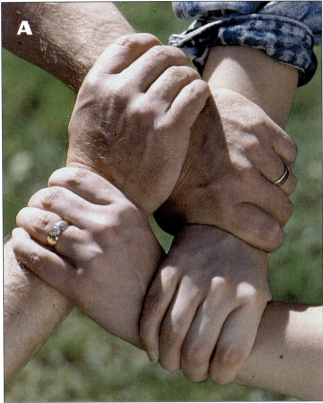

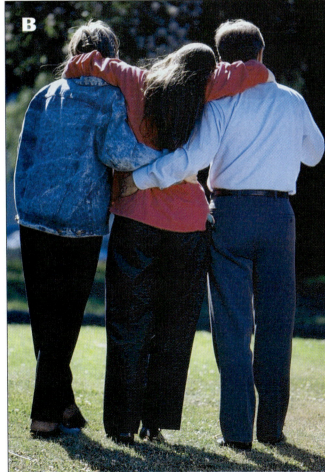

FIGURE 17-8 *The two-person assisted walk.*

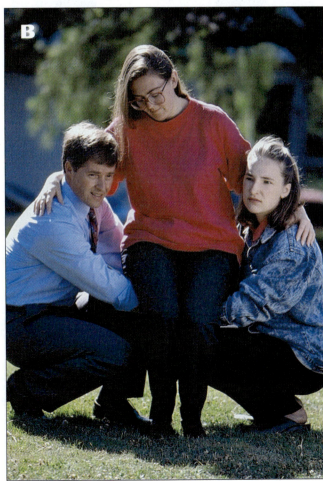

FIGURE 17-9 *Four-handed seat carry.*

Two-Handed Seat Carry

The two-person seat carry is used for a victim who is unconscious or disoriented, injured in the upper body or arms, or unable to help hold on for any other reason. Follow these steps:

1. Both of the first aiders face each other behind the victim. Put one arm under the victim's thighs and the other across the victim's back.

2. Grasp each other's wrists under the victim's legs. (Figure 17-10A shows how the arms are positioned; Figure 17-10B shows positioning of the arms around the victim.)

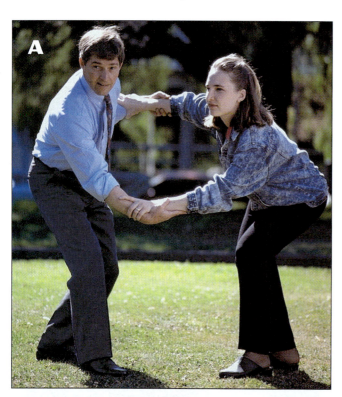

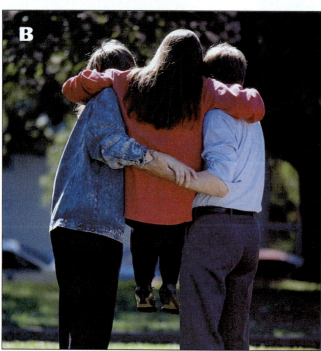

FIGURE 17-10 *The two-handed seat carry.*

3. Both of the first aiders should stand at the same time. Be sure you have a secure, firm grip and good body position before starting to move. Take the first step with the outside leg, and then walk with ordinary steps.

Chair Lift

The chair lift method is used to move a victim without serious injuries along a passageway or up or down stairs. Almost any ordinary chair can be used as long as it is sturdy and safe. Follow these steps:

1. Check that the chair is strong enough to hold the victim and that the parts by which it will be lifted are secure. Move any obstructions from the stairway or passageway.

2. Position the victim in the chair, and if necessary secure the person with a broad bandage around the waist or other non-injured area and around the chair.

3. Support the chair from the back as the other first aider, holding at the top of the chair's front legs, tilts the chair backward to prevent the victim from sliding forward (Figure 17-11). (If the stairway or hallway is wide enough, both of the first aiders can stand at the sides of the chair, each holding the back and front of the chair, and walk sideways.)

4. Both first aiders lift together, following the principles of good body mechanics described earlier.

5. Move slowly in the direction the victim is facing.

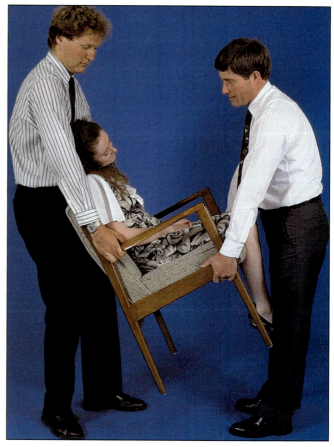

FIGURE 17-11 *The chair lift.*

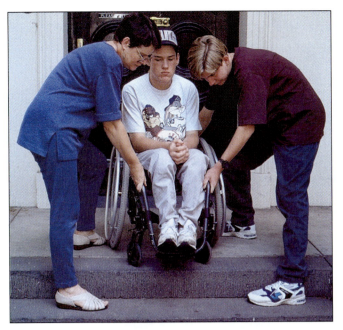

FIGURE 17-12 *When lifting a person in a wheelchair, lift the wheelchair carefully, holding non-moveable parts.*

Wheelchair Lift

When it is necessary to carry a wheelchair up or down stairs or in any other circumstances when it cannot be wheeled, you can adapt the chair lift method as follows:

1. Explain to the person and the other first aider what you are about to do.

2. Put on the wheelchair's brakes (ask the person to show you if you are unsure how to work the brakes).

3. Make sure the person is seated well back in the wheelchair.

4. Determine what part of the chair it is safe to lift. Do not lift it by removable arm rests or side supports because these may come loose during the move. Do not lift it by the wheels.

5. Lift and carry the chair using good body mechanics and moving slowly forward (Figure 17-12).

Stretcher Moves

If a seriously injured or ill victim must be moved, a stretcher is the safest way to reduce the risk of causing additional injury. Several kinds of stretchers are commonly used, including the standard stretcher, Donway lifting frame (formerly called Jordon frame) and scoop stretcher. In addition to these, you may see ambulance personnel use other specialised types of stretchers.

Before putting the victim on any type of stretcher, test it to ensure it has not been damaged and is still able to bear the weight of a victim. One person should lie on the stretcher while each end is lifted independently, and then both ends together, to test that the stretcher is sturdy and secure.

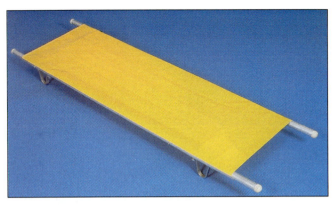

FIGURE 17-13 *The standard (Furley) stretcher.*

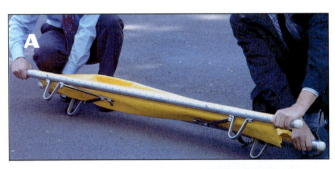

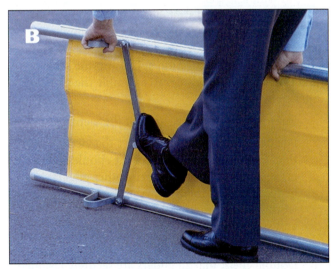

FIGURE 17-14 *Opening the standard stretcher.*

Standard (Furley) Stretcher

The standard or Furley stretcher has a canvas section stretched between two metal or wooden poles with handles at each end (Figure 17-13). Beneath the canvas near each end is a traverse which opens to lock the poles in place. Runners on the bottom of the poles hold the stretcher up off the ground.

Take care when opening the stretcher. Release any straps or fastenings, hold it on its side and pull the poles apart (Fig 17.14A). Use your shoe—not your hand—to push the traverses open all the way (Figure 17-14B). Then you can lay the stretcher down on its runners.

To close the stretcher, turn it on its side. With the heel of your shoe—not your hand—push the joints of the traverses inward to release the catch. Pull out the canvas as you bring the poles together, fold up the canvas and secure the straps or fastenings.

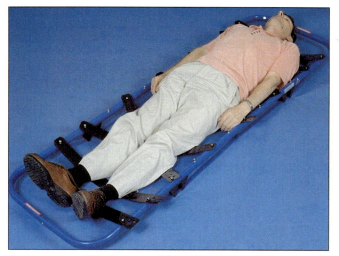

FIGURE 17-15 *The Donway lifting frame.*

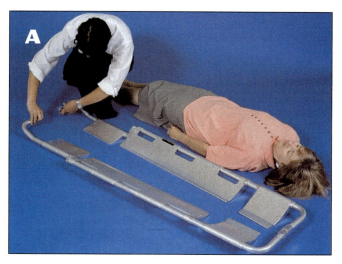

Donway Lifting Frame

The Donway lifting frame is a particular type of stretcher which can be assembled beneath a victim, eliminating the need to lift the victim onto it as with a standard stretcher. This stretcher should not be used for a victim with a suspected spinal injury because it is not as rigid as the standard stretcher.

The Donway lifting frame consists of a tubular frame and plastic gliders which are passed beneath the victim and hooked at both ends onto spigots on the sides of the frame. Follow these steps to assemble the stretcher under the victim:

1. Put together the frame around the victim.

2. Position the widest glider under the victim's head first. Cross two gliders under the shoulders for greater strength, then slide the other gliders beneath the natural hollows of the body and legs, working down toward the feet. Use all the gliders and space them out to support the body weight appropriately (Figure 17-15).

3. Double check that all gliders are securely fastened.

4. Raise the victim by holding the frame at either the sides or the ends, using good body mechanics.

5. If the victim is raised and lowered repeatedly on the stretcher, check the glider fastenings each time.

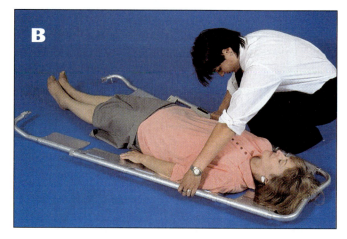

Scoop Stretcher

The scoop stretcher can be used to lift a victim onto an ambulance stretcher or to carry an injured person. It is assembled under the victim without having to lift the victim onto it and can therefore be used for lifting a person with suspected internal injuries. Its length is adjustable.

Follow these steps to use the scoop stretcher:

1. With the stretcher alongside the victim, adjust its length for the height of the victim (Figure 17-16A).

2. Detach the stretcher frame at both ends. Slip the stretcher halves under the victim from both sides, and attach the head of the frame (Figure 17-16B).

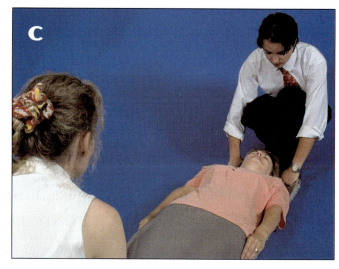

FIGURE 17-16 *Using a scoop stretcher (see description in text below).*

3. A second first aider reattaches the foot of the frame while the first keeps the victim's head stable.

4. Lift the stretcher using good body mechanics (Figure 17-16C).

Alternatively, the stretcher can be used in a "V" fashion by leaving the head of the stretcher attached when it is positioned and working the scoop inwards under the victim. Care should be taken to avoid pinching or pulling the victim's skin, hair or clothing.

Blanket Lift

The blanket lift is used to lift a victim onto an ambulance stretcher when a Donway lifting frame or scoop stretcher is not available. The blanket is first placed under the victim, then the victim is raised on it. At least 6 people are needed to perform this lift safely.

1. First make sure the blanket is strong enough. One person should lie on it while two others lift it.

2. Prepare the blanket for placement by rolling it in half lengthwise.

3. Lay the blanket with the rolled part beside the victim on the more severely injured side.

4. Three or four rescuers should co-ordinate to turn the victim on the side facing away from the blanket. Pull the rolled part of the blanket up against the victim's back (Figure 17-17A).

5. Carefully lay the victim back down onto the blanket past the rolled part, which should be eased out flat.

6. Tightly roll both sides of the blanket up to the victim's sides. (If available, poles can be rolled into the blanket on both sides for greater support.)

7. With the first aiders on each side facing each other across the victim, all squat down and hold the blanket with palms down and fingers inside the blanket's rolled edge. The first aiders position their hands to support the head and shoulders, the torso and hips and the legs (Figure 17-17B).

8. As directed by a first aider at the victim's head, all stand in a co-ordinated move, raising the victim. The blanket should be pulled tightly along each side and each end to ensure good support for the victim. Initially it may help for the first aiders to lean out slightly to keep the blanket under the victim (Figure 17-17C). If another first aider is available, a stretcher can be placed under the victim. If no other first aider is available, the six can carry the blanket carefully to the stretcher.

9. On instructions from the first aider at the head, the six carefully lower the victim onto the stretcher.

Remember:

The blanket lift, Donway lifting frame and scoop stretcher should never be used where serious internal injuries or a fractured spine are suspected. Wait for ambulance personnel to direct care unless it is a life-threatening situation.

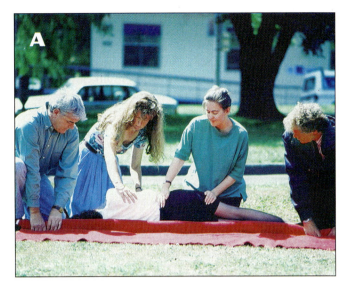

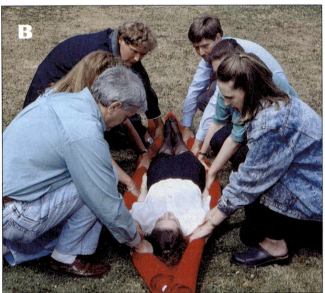

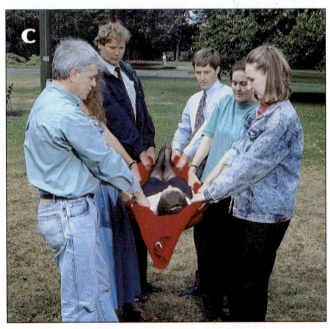

FIGURE 17-17 *The blanket lift (see description in text opposite).*

Carrying a Stretcher

Once the victim is secure on the stretcher, it can be carried to the ambulance or other site for continuing care. Four first aiders or bystanders should carry the stretcher when possible, although two trained people can do it when necessary.

It is important that those carrying the stretcher move in a co-ordinated manner. A trained person at the head of the stretcher should be in charge and give instructions to the others.

Follow these steps to lift and carry the stretcher:

1. All first aiders face forward, squat down, and hold the stretcher handles as shown in Figure 17-18A, using good body mechanics.

2. The first aider at the victim's head asks if everyone is ready and gives the instruction to lift. All stand together and hold the stretcher level or with the head slightly raised (see exceptions below).

3. The first aider in charge gives the instruction for everyone to walk forward. The group should intentionally walk out of step to avoid bouncing the stretcher (Figure 17-18B).

4. Follow the instructions of ambulance or other personnel to load the victim into the ambulance or other site.

As a general rule, the stretcher should be carried with the victim's head higher than the feet, unless the victim is in shock or has hypothermia; a victim of hypothermia must be kept horizontal at all times. The victim should be moved feet first except in certain circumstances.

Carry the victim head first only:

- when carrying a victim to a bed or into the ambulance

- when climbing up steps or a hill as long as the legs are not injured

- when going down steps or a hill when the lower limbs are injured

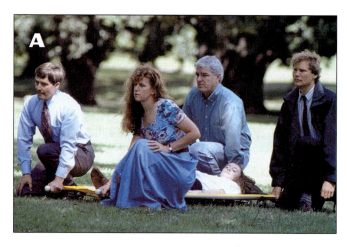

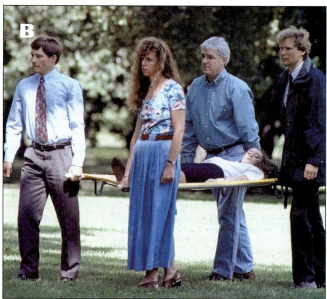

FIGURE 17-18 *Lifting and carrying a stretcher (see description in text opposite).*

Summary

- Be careful never to move an ill or injured person unnecessarily. Take the time to survey the scene for life-threatening or potentially life-threatening situations.

- If you must move a victim, choose the emergency move that is safest and easiest to rapidly move the person without injury to either you or the victim.

- Whenever lifting or carrying a weight, follow the principles of good body mechanics to prevent injury to yourself.

- Emergency moves include the ankle drag and arm drag, clothes drag and the two-person fore and aft carry.

- Planned moves include the one- and two-person assisted walk, the two- and four-handed seat carries, the chair lift, the use of stretchers and the blanket lift.

Study Questions

1. *List 4 situations in which it may be necessary to move a victim.*

2. *Name 4 common types of moves.*

3. *List the principles of good body mechanics which should be used when lifting.*

4. *Which of the following lifts should be used by two first aiders to transfer a helpless victim to a chair or wheelchair?*

   a. The two-person assisted walk.

   b. The four-handed seat carry.

   c. The fore-and-aft carry.

   d. The clothes drag.

Answers are in Appendix A (page 363).

Pregnancy and Childbirth

CHILDBIRTH usually occurs with a doctor or midwife in attendance, but sometimes the woman goes into labour unexpectedly. Childbirth is not an emergency just because a doctor or midwife is not present—childbirth is a natural process which in most cases can proceed safely without trained professionals. However, in some cases an emergency may occur which threatens the life of the mother or the newborn, and first aid care is needed until the ambulance arrives.

This chapter describes normal childbirth and what you can do to help the mother in an emergency.

For Review

A review of the emergency action principles for all emergencies (Chapter 3), infection control (Chapter 12) and cardiopulmonary resuscitation for infants (Chapter 4) will help your understanding of the chapter.

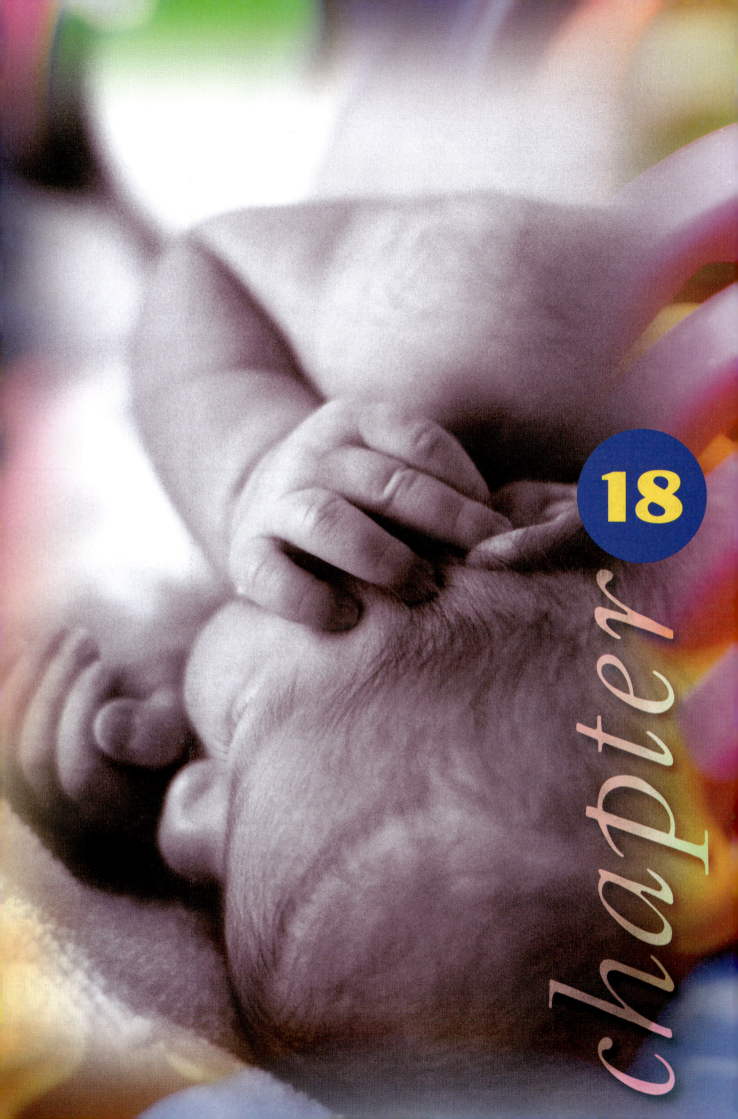

18

chapter

Key Terms

Amniotic *(am-nee-ot-ic)* **sac:** A fluid-filled sac that encloses and protects the developing foetus in the uterus; commonly called the bag of waters.

Birth canal: The passageway from the uterus to the vaginal opening through which a baby passes at birth.

Breech delivery: The delivery of a baby with feet or buttocks first.

Cervix: The upper part of the birth canal, between the vagina and the uterus.

Childbirth: The process of a baby being born, starting with labour.

Crowning: The time in labour when the baby's head shows at the opening of the vagina.

Delivery: The part of the childbirth process when the baby emerges from the birth canal.

Labour: The birth process beginning with the first contraction and lasting through delivery and stabilisation of the mother after delivery of the placenta.

Miscarriage: The spontaneous loss of a foetus before the 28th week of pregnancy, usually due to an abnormality of the foetus; also called a spontaneous abortion.

Placenta *(pla-sen-ta)*: The organ attached to the uterus and to the unborn child via the umbilical cord, for delivering nutrients to the baby in the uterus.

Prolapsed cord: A complication of childbirth in which a loop of umbilical cord protrudes through the vagina before the delivery of the baby.

Toxaemia *(tok-see-mee-a)* **of pregnancy:** A condition a woman may experience in late pregnancy which may lead to seizures; also called eclampsia.

Umbilical *(um-bil-iy-cal)* **cord:** The cord-like structure attaching the baby to the placenta while in the uterus and for a short time after delivery.

Uterus: The organ in the woman's pelvis where the baby develops; commonly called the womb.

Jane was looking forward to the birth of her second child in a week or so. On this day she had gone shopping with her mother, and she went to bed with an aching back and feeling very tired. She woke in the middle of the night with her backache worse and was unable to get comfortable. Then she felt a contraction and realised she was in labour. She wasn't worried about getting to the hospital in time because her previous labour had lasted for many hours.

Jane woke her husband Tom and asked him to call her sister to come over to look after their two-year-old Alice. While they waited for her to arrive from across town Jane's waters broke, and within minutes the contractions grew stronger and closer together. Tom went to get the car ready, but her sister still hadn't arrived. Jane timed her contractions and was surprised they were now only 3 minutes apart—they might not have time to get to the hospital! Tom decided to call an ambulance instead of trying to drive her there in a rush.

Jane lay in a comfortable position on the bed, and Tom helped her with the breathing exercises they had learned together in the antenatal classes. They couldn't believe the birth was happening so quickly. Tom started to gather clean towels and sheets and other supplies they might need.

The ambulance arrived within 15 minutes, just as Jane felt the urge to push. The ambulance officers prepared for the delivery just as the baby's head was first appearing. Tom helped Jane concentrate on her breathing, and she followed their instructions to push during contractions and rest between. Mark James was born a few minutes later, alert and crying loudly. Tom wrapped him in a clean towel and helped Jane hold him to her breast.

They hadn't planned it to happen this way, but Jane and Tom were happy. The childbirth had gone well and the baby was fine. They went to the hospital just to make sure there were no problems, the three of them staying together the whole time.

If you have never experienced or seen childbirth, your expectations of what it is like probably come from what others have told you and other accounts you have seen or heard. You probably think of childbirth as stressful, painful and perhaps frightening. It is understandable, therefore, to be apprehensive if you find yourself in an unplanned situation with childbirth approaching.

You should take comfort in the fact that things rarely go wrong. Childbirth is a natural process. Thousands of babies are born all over the world every day, without complications during the delivery and in areas where no medical assistance is available for childbirth.

By following a few simple steps, you can effectively assist in the birth process. This chapter describes the birth process, and how you can assist with the delivery of the baby and care for both mother and baby. For those rare instances where a problem does arise for the mother or baby, you will also learn what care to give until the ambulance arrives.

NORMAL PREGNANCY AND CHILDBIRTH

In the great majority of cases, childbirth proceeds as a normal, natural process—not as an emergency situation. Understanding the birth process and the stages of labour will help you know what to do and what not to do if your assistance is needed.

The foetus grows and develops in the mother's uterus, surrounded by the amniotic sac (also called the "bag of waters"). The foetus is linked to the mother through the umbilical cord, which attaches to the placenta, a special organ attached to the mother's uterus. Nutrients and oxygen reach the foetus through the umbilical cord. Figure 18-1 shows the mother and foetus at 40 weeks.

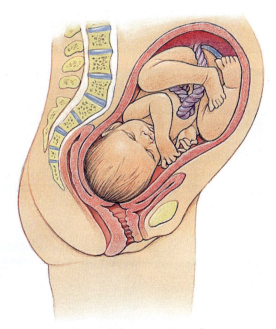

FIGURE 18-1 *Mother and foetus at 40 weeks.*

Usually at about 40 weeks (9 months) the childbirth process begins with the onset of contractions as the mother begins labour. Labour is the birth process, starting with the first contraction of the uterus and ending after birth when the placenta has been delivered and the mother has been stabilised. Although it is a continuous process, labour is typically considered in three stages: contractions preparing the birth canal, birth of the baby and delivery of the placenta (also called afterbirth). These stages are described in the following sections, outlining the care and assistance the first aider can provide both to the mother and baby throughout this normal process. Problems and emergencies which may arise through this process are described later in the chapter.

Stage One

The first stage of childbirth begins with contractions of the uterus, often called "labour pains". Muscles in the uterus contract with a wave-like action, each contraction building to a peak and then subsiding. Contractions may occur every 10 to 20 minutes at first, gradually becoming closer together and stronger. This stage may last as long as 16 hours or longer for a woman's first child, or 10 hours or less for later children, usually providing enough time for the woman to reach her planned place for delivery. When contractions are less than 3 minutes apart, childbirth is normally near.

When contractions first begin, the mother may feel a low backache. A "show of blood" occurs about this time or before labour begins, as the mucus plug in the cervix comes free. Usually near the end of the first stage the "waters" break, as the amniotic sac breaks. About half a litre of fluid may pour or trickle out through the vagina. It is usual for contractions to become more forceful once the "cushion" of fluid is no longer present. An ambulance, midwife or doctor should be called because it is important for the mother to receive trained supervision as she prepares to deliver her baby.

The first aider's role in the first stage is to help the mother be as comfortable as possible and to provide emotional support. If it is possible that childbirth may occur before the ambulance arrives, you should also be preparing to assist in the childbirth.

Stage Two

Stage Two is the act of birth itself, beginning when the cervix is completely dilated and ending when the newborn is outside the mother's body. This stage usually takes from 30 to 60 minutes.

As the contractions become stronger and the mother begins to strain with each one, help the mother into the position most comfortable for her and prepare for imminent childbirth. Often the mother is most comfortable lying on her back, propped up with knees bent, but some women find other positions, such as lying on the side or squatting, more comfortable.

Preparing for Birth

Preparing for birth means preparing yourself as well as the mother and the setting. Remember that the great majority of childbirths are normal and do not become emergencies. However, childbirth does normally involve blood loss and strong emotions. Try to relax and focus on helping the mother. Remember that she is the one who is having the pain and doing the work, and who needs reassurance.

Help the expectant mother by reassuring her and maintaining a calm atmosphere. She will be feeling increasing pain or discomfort with the contractions. Irregular breathing, fear and feeling alone or not knowing what to expect can all increase her pain. Help her relax by focusing on breathing regularly, slowly and deeply in through the nose and out through the mouth. Ask her to look at one object in the room while breathing evenly through the contractions. Be confident and encouraging.

Prepare the room for the childbirth. Request unnecessary people to leave the room, but ask a female relative or friend as well as the father to stay with the mother.

Cover the mattress or floor with plastic sheeting, towels, newspaper or other covering to protect it from the bleeding which occurs normally with childbirth. Outside the home, the mother can lie on any flat surface such as the ground or car seat. In a public area, ask others to move away in order to provide privacy.

Unless she prefers another position, assist the mother onto her back with head and upper back raised, not lying flat. The knees should be drawn up and apart. Remove any clothing that will be in the way during delivery, but keep the mother warm with blankets or sheets. Place folded sheets, blankets or towels under her buttocks. Have sanitary pads or other dressings available to absorb secretions and blood, and a large plastic bag or towel to hold the placenta after delivery.

Prepare for the newborn by finding a clean warm towel or blanket to wrap the baby in after birth. Prepare a cot by lining a basket, drawer or box with towels or other warm cloths.

Be prepared to cut the umbilical cord after birth if necessary (see later section). Sterilise a pair of scissors by boiling them for 10 minutes. Prepare three sterile ties or pieces of string 25 centimetres long to tie the cord; boil these also for 10 minutes or soak them for 10 minutes in methylated spirits. Also have available some sterile dressings for the cord after it is cut.

Preventing Infection

It is important to prevent infection for both the mother and child. Do not let anyone with a cold or other respiratory infection, a sore throat or dirty hands come near. Wash your hands and forearms thoroughly with soap under running water, scrubbing your nails as well. Wear latex gloves and a face mask if available.

Delivery

As contractions become more intense, encourage the mother to grasp her knees and push during each contraction. She should rest and relax between contractions.

Most babies are born head first. As the moment of birth approaches, the top of the baby's head appears at the dilated opening of the birth canal. This is called **crowning**. When this happens, ask the mother now to stop pushing and to "pant like a dog." Place one hand on the baby's head to steady it as it emerges. If the baby were to suddenly "shoot out", injury could result. Hold one hand steady on the baby's head but do not twist or pull on it; allow the head to emerge slowly and gently. With your other hand, hold a clean pad under and against the mother's anus to prevent a bowel movement from touching the baby or birth canal.

As the head emerges, the baby rotates to one side to let the shoulders and body emerge (Figure 18-2A). Look to see if the umbilical cord is looped around the baby's neck. If so, ease it over the baby's head to release the tension, but do not pull on it. If it cannot be slipped over the head, slide it over the baby's shoulders as they emerge, and let the baby slide through the loop.

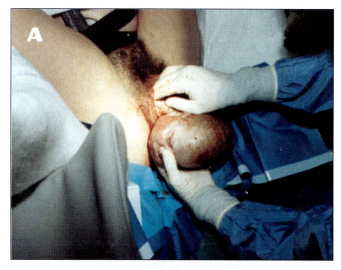

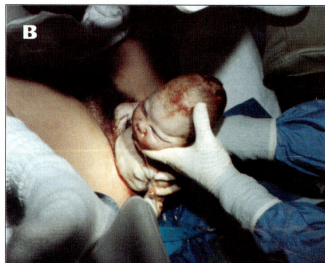

FIGURE 18-2 *Steps of childbirth (see description in text above and on the next page).*

If the amniotic sac did not break earlier in labour as it usually does, you may see a membrane covering the baby's face as it emerges. Tear this membrane with your fingers and pull it away from the baby's face immediately to let the baby breathe.

Support the baby's body as it emerges, and guide the shoulders out one at a time if necessary (Figure 18-2B). Catch the body on a clean towel, and turn the baby on its side. Place it on the mother's abdomen and chest, with head slightly lower than the trunk. Take care to avoid pulling on the cord.

Care of the Newborn

Immediately open the baby's mouth and wipe out any mucus or fluid that is present. Keep the face pointing down to let fluid drain from the mouth and nose. Usually the baby's breathing starts spontaneously, and the baby will be crying.

If the baby has not made any sounds, flick your finger on the soles of the feet to stimulate the crying response, but do not slap the baby. Crying helps the baby to clear the airway of fluids and mucus and promotes breathing. Check to ensure the airway is clear (Figure 18-3). If the baby is still not breathing after one minute, expired air resuscitation (EAR) or CPR may be needed. Give care following the Basic Life Support flow chart (see page 35).

Be sure to keep the baby warm by wrapping it in a blanket or towel. If the mother wishes, the baby may be positioned at her breast.

Care of the Mother

Care for the mother once you are sure the baby is breathing well and is warm. Allowing the mother to nurse the baby will stimulate the uterus to contract, helping to slow bleeding. The mother usually continues to bleed for a while after the placenta is delivered. Gently clean the birth canal area with clean towels or gauze pads.

Stage Three

Mild contractions will continue until the placenta is expelled, usually within 30 minutes. Have a clean towel or plastic bag ready to catch it. Keep the mother in the birth position, and encourage her to push it out. Do not pull on the cord.

Do not tie or cut the umbilical cord between the placenta and the baby unless it will be a long time before the ambulance arrives. Keep the placenta with the mother and baby for transport. The doctor will want to examine the placenta to ensure all of it has been delivered, because even a small piece left inside the uterus can cause later problems for the mother.

Some bleeding will continue. Place a sanitary pad or towel over the vagina, but do not insert anything inside the vagina or otherwise attempt to stop the bleeding by pressure.

The new mother typically experiences shock-like symptoms and signs such as dizziness, shivering and cool, pale, moist skin. Keep her positioned on her back until the ambulance arrives, and raise her legs as for shock.

Stabilisation of Mother and Infant

The final stage of the childbirth process involves the initial recovery and stabilisation of the mother and baby (Figure 18-4). During this period, normally lasting about an hour, the mother should not be moved except by health professionals. The uterus contracts to control bleeding, and the mother gradually recovers from the stresses of childbirth. The baby who is breathing well and is warm needs no additional care during this time. However, stay with the mother and child and continue to monitor both.

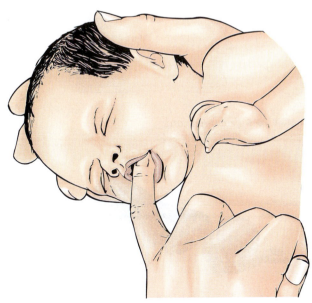

FIGURE 18-3 *Clear the newborn's airway.*

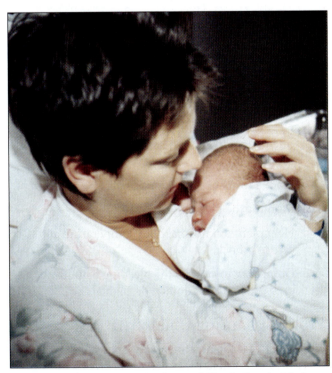

FIGURE 18-4 *Mother and infant stabilised after the birth.*

PROBLEMS REQUIRING FIRST AID

Although the great majority of women have no serious difficulties through pregnancy and childbirth, emergencies can occur in which the first aider may need to provide care for the mother or infant. The following sections describe first aid for the mother with problems occurring during pregnancy or childbirth and for the newborn.

Problems During Pregnancy

Emergencies directly related to pregnancy are rare. However, a pregnant woman who experiences any sudden illness or injury may require special care or handling. For example, CPR for a pregnant woman is slightly varied by tilting her pelvis to the left (see Chapter 4). As a general principle, first aid for a pregnant woman is always based on her symptoms and signs, following the Basic Life Support flow chart (page 35) as usual. Sometimes a pregnant woman develops a condition known as toxaemia of pregnancy, in which seizures may occur. If the woman has a seizure, an ambulance should be called and care given as for seizures (see page 150). Another potential emergency a pregnant woman may experience is miscarriage.

Miscarriage

A miscarriage is a spontaneous abortion. It occurs before the 20th week of pregnancy, usually due to an abnormality of the foetus. As many as 20 percent of pregnancies end with miscarriage. A miscarriage can cause abdominal pain and bleeding, which can persist or become profuse. The foetus or other tissue may be expelled.

Do not be concerned with trying to diagnose the pregnant woman's problem. Any pregnant woman experiencing abdominal pain and/or bleeding from the vagina needs immediate medical attention.

While waiting for the ambulance, give the following first aid to a pregnant woman experiencing vaginal bleeding:

1. Help the woman into a comfortable position, often lying down with head and shoulders slightly raised.

2. Place a towel or sanitary pad over the vagina.

3. Monitor the bleeding and the pulse.

4. Help maintain normal body temperature and care for shock.

5. Do not try to control the bleeding by putting pressure on the abdomen or vaginal area.

Problems During Childbirth

Remember that the great majority of all childbirths occur without problems. However, an emergency can occur which will be stressful and in some cases life-threatening for the mother or baby. The following sections describe first aid for three problems which may occur during childbirth: prolapsed cord, massive bleeding and breech delivery.

Prolapsed Cord

A prolapsed cord occurs if a loop of the umbilical cord protrudes from the vagina before the birth occurs (Figure 18-5). This is a life-threatening situation for the baby because the cord will be compressed during childbirth, stopping the flow of oxygenated blood to the baby. The baby may then die within minutes.

If you see a prolapsed cord, call for an ambulance immediately if one is not already on the way. Do not try to push the cord back into the birth canal. Position the expectant mother in a knee-chest position (Figure 18-6), which helps take the pressure off the cord.

If the baby's head begins to emerge, position the mother in the usual position and help deliver the baby as quickly as possible. Be prepared to resuscitate the baby.

Massive Bleeding

Persistent vaginal bleeding is the most common problem of childbirth. Call an ambulance immediately if one is not already on the way. Give care to minimise shock. Help the woman to assume the same knee-chest position as for a prolapsed cord. Do not put pressure on the abdomen or vaginal area in an attempt to stop the bleeding.

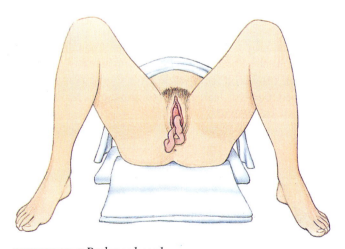

FIGURE 18-5 *Prolapsed cord.*

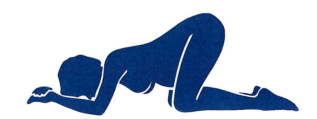

FIGURE 18-6 *The knee-chest position reduces pressure on a prolapsed cord.*

Breech Delivery

Most babies are born head first, although in rare situations the baby's feet or buttocks may emerge first. This is called a breech delivery (Figure 18-7).

A breech birth can become a life-threatening emergency for the baby if the head lodges in the birth canal, because the cord will be compressed between the head and the canal. Follow these steps to assist with a breech delivery:

1. Position the mother at the edge of the bed or other support, with buttocks at the edge and feet supported off the bed on boxes, chairs, etc. (Figure 18-8A). This is to allow the baby's legs and body to hang down as it emerges.

2. Be ready to support the baby's legs and body as it emerges. Keep the baby's body warm because a cool temperature might stimulate the baby to breathe before the head emerges.

3. Let the baby hang down from the birth canal as it emerges (Figure 18-8B). Do not handle the baby's body as it emerges, as this could stimulate it to breathe while the head is still in the birth canal.

4. If the head does not emerge within 3 minutes after the shoulders are out, you need to make sure air can reach the baby's mouth and nose. Raise the baby by the legs and feet, keeping the head in the

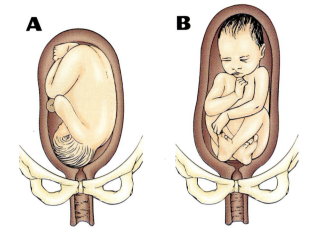

FIGURE 18-7 A *Normal position of a baby before birth.* **B** *Breech position.*

birth canal. The head will rotate inside the birth canal so that the mouth and nose are free of the opening (Figure 18-8C).

5. Wipe mucus and fluid from the baby's nose and mouth to open the airway.

6. Do not pull on the body to try to speed the delivery of the head, because this could cause damage. If the baby can breathe through the nose and mouth, delivery can proceed on its own.

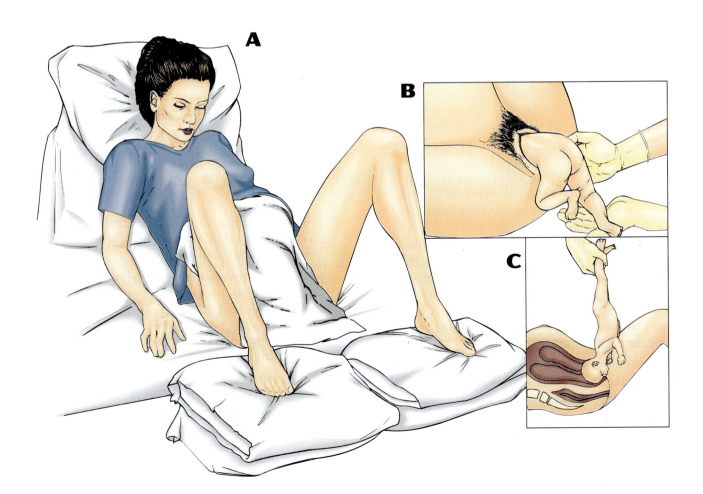

FIGURE 18-8 *Steps for a breech delivery (see description above).*

Problems After Childbirth

A problem or emergency may occur after childbirth as well. Problems affecting the mother include bleeding or an undelivered placenta. Problems involving the newborn include situations in which the cord needs to be cut and non-breathing or sick babies.

Problems with the Mother

Massive Bleeding

Bleeding normally stops soon after delivery of the baby or the placenta. A small amount of bleeding is not unusual.

If the bleeding is more severe, gently massage the mother's lower abdomen (just below the navel). This helps stimulate the uterus to contract, which will slow or stop the bleeding. Continue this gentle massaging until the ambulance arrives. Give care to minimise shock.

Undelivered Placenta

In rare cases the placenta may not be delivered soon after the delivery of the baby. If the placenta has not delivered 30 minutes after childbirth and the ambulance has not arrived, the cord should be cut. Do not pull on the cord in an effort to pull the placenta out. In an isolated area, follow telephone or radio instructions from the ambulance service or other medical personnel.

Problems with the Infant

Problems with newborns are rare, but you should know what to do in situations when the umbilical cord should be cut or the newborn does not start breathing.

Cutting the Cord

As described earlier, in most cases you do not need to be concerned about tying or cutting the umbilical cord. Leave it attached to the baby and protect it from possible damage. Even after the placenta has been delivered, you can leave the umbilical cord in place between the baby and the placenta for a short time until the ambulance arrives.

In an isolated area in which the ambulance may not arrive soon, you should be prepared to cut the cord about 20 to 30 minutes after the placenta is delivered. In addition, cut the cord if the placenta has not been delivered by 30 minutes after the childbirth. Check first to see that pulsation in the cord has stopped, then follow these guidelines:

1. Have prepared 3 sterile ties or boiled pieces of string and scissors which have been sterilised by boiling, and a sterile dressing.

2. First tie the cord tightly about 15 centimetres from the baby's abdomen. Tie the cord a second time about 20 centimetres from the baby's abdomen (Figure 18-9A).

3. Use sterile scissors to cut the cord between the two ties (Figure 18-9B).

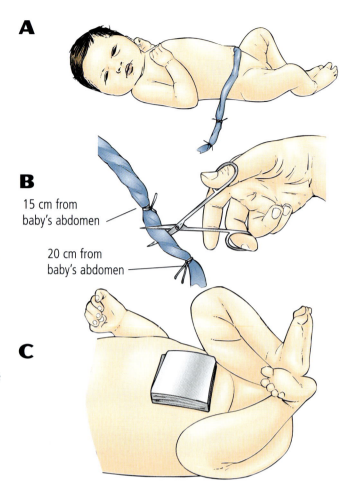

A

B

15 cm from
baby's abdomen

20 cm from
baby's abdomen

C

FIGURE 18-9 *Steps for tying and cutting the umbilical cord (see description in text below).*

4. Put a sterile dressing over the cut end at the baby's abdomen (Figure 18-9C). Do not apply an anti-septic or any other substance over the cut end of the cord. If the placenta has not yet been delivered, also cover the other end of the cord with a sterile dressing.

5. After 10 minutes, check the cord end for bleeding. Tie the cord a third time about 10 centimetres from the baby's abdomen.

6. When you are certain that there is no bleeding, put a sterile dressing over the cord end, and secure the dressing in place with a nappy or clean cloth wrapped around the baby.

Non-Breathing Newborn

Sometimes a newborn is not breathing at the immediate moment of childbirth. As described in the earlier section on normal childbirth, you need to remove any mucus and fluid from the mouth and nose to open the airway, and you may need to stimulate breathing by flicking the soles of the feet.

If the baby does not start breathing, you will need to give EAR or CPR (Chapter 4). Follow the Basic Life Support flow chart (see page 35).

Problem Babies

In most childbirths, if the baby is breathing well there are no other problems requiring immediate medical attention. However, some babies simply are not as strong or are sickly. Babies born prematurely or with a low birth weight, for example, are more likely to be sick and need medical care. Seek emergency care as soon as possible for a baby which looks very small or sickly, and monitor the baby continuously. Be sure the baby is kept warm. Be prepared to give EAR or CPR if needed, following the Basic Life Support flow chart (see page 35).

Summary

- Childbirth is a natural process which normally occurs without emergency problems.

- During Stage One, once labour begins, help prepare the expectant mother and provide emotional support.

- During Stage Two, the birth itself, help the mother with breathing, cleanliness and infection prevention, and the delivery process itself. Support the baby as it emerges, clear the airway and ensure breathing, and keep the baby warm.

- During Stage Three, the delivery of the placenta, assist the mother who has continued bleeding and is displaying shock-like symptoms.

- Problems during pregnancy are rare. Care for a miscarriage by positioning the woman and giving care to minimise shock until the ambulance arrives.

- Problems may occur during childbirth:
  - For a prolapsed cord, position the mother to take pressure off the cord.
  - For massive bleeding, position the mother to minimise bleeding and care for shock.
  - For a breech delivery, assist the baby to breathe by positioning its body as it emerges to allow air to reach the mouth and nose.

- Problems may occur after childbirth:
  - If profuse bleeding occurs, massage the abdomen to stimulate the uterus to contract.
  - For an undelivered placenta, cut the cord after 30 minutes and seek medical advice as soon as possible.
  - Cut the cord, using a sterile technique, if the ambulance will not arrive soon or the placenta has not been delivered.
  - Care for a non-breathing newborn by attempting to stimulate breathing and giving EAR or CPR as appropriate.
  - Give supportive care to sickly babies until the ambulance arrives.

Study Questions

1. **Usually childbirth involves:**

   a. medical emergencies
   b. bleeding by the mother
   c. bleeding by the newborn
   d. a need for drugs to be administered

2. **How long do contractions usually last before childbirth?**

   a. 10 to 30 minutes.
   b. 1 to 2 hours.
   c. 4 to 6 hours.
   d. 10 to 16 hours.

3. **When the expectant mother's "bag of waters" breaks, this may signal that:**

   a. there is an emergency for which you should immediately call an ambulance
   b. childbirth may occur soon
   c. there has been a miscarriage
   d. labour is just beginning

4. **If the newborn is not crying or breathing after being born, you should:**

   a. flick the soles of its feet with your finger
   b. slap it on its buttocks
   c. start CPR immediately.
   d. a and c.

5. **If a pregnant woman in her 4th month is bleeding heavily and has abdominal pain, the first aid you should give is to call for an ambulance and:**

   a. bandage her tightly over the vagina
   b. squeeze her legs together
   c. give care to minimise shock
   d. help her into the knee-chest position

6. **If the expectant mother has a prolapsed cord, you should:**

   a. position her in the knee-chest position
   b. massage her abdomen
   c. push hard on the cord to move it back up into the uterus
   d. pull hard on the cord to get the placenta out

7. *For a breech delivery, you should:*

    a. position the expectant mother in the knee-chest position

    b. hold the mother's legs together to delay childbirth until the ambulance arrives

    c. push hard on the baby to turn it around in the uterus

    d. raise the baby to position the head in the birth canal so that the baby can breathe

8. *Cut the baby's umbilical cord:*

    a. about 10 minutes after birth in all cases, if the ambulance has not arrived

    b. only in cases when the mother dies during childbirth

    c. in cases when the placenta has not delivered within 30 minutes of the childbirth

    d. if the umbilical cord looks blue

9. *Which of the following is a correct action to take when you cut the umbilical cord?*

    a. Tie the cord in two places and cut in between.

    b. Cut the cord and then tie the end of the cord itself in a knot.

    c. Cut the cord as close to the abdomen as possible to shape the belly button well.

    d. Cut the cord first, and tie it with a string only if it bleeds.

Answers are in Appendix A (page 363).

Substance Abuse

IN OUR SOCIETY people are increasingly using medications, alcohol and other drugs, and many other substances which can have powerful effects on the body. Although many of these substances have an appropriate use when taken in correct amounts, they have adverse or toxic effects when misused or abused. To help someone experiencing the adverse effects of a substance, you need to understand the common substances misused or abused and to recognise the symptoms and signs of a person needing assistance.

This chapter also discusses prevention of substance abuse and misuse.

For Review

A basic understanding of the functions of the central nervous system (Chapter 2) and the care for altered conscious states (Chapter 9) will help your understanding of the chapter.

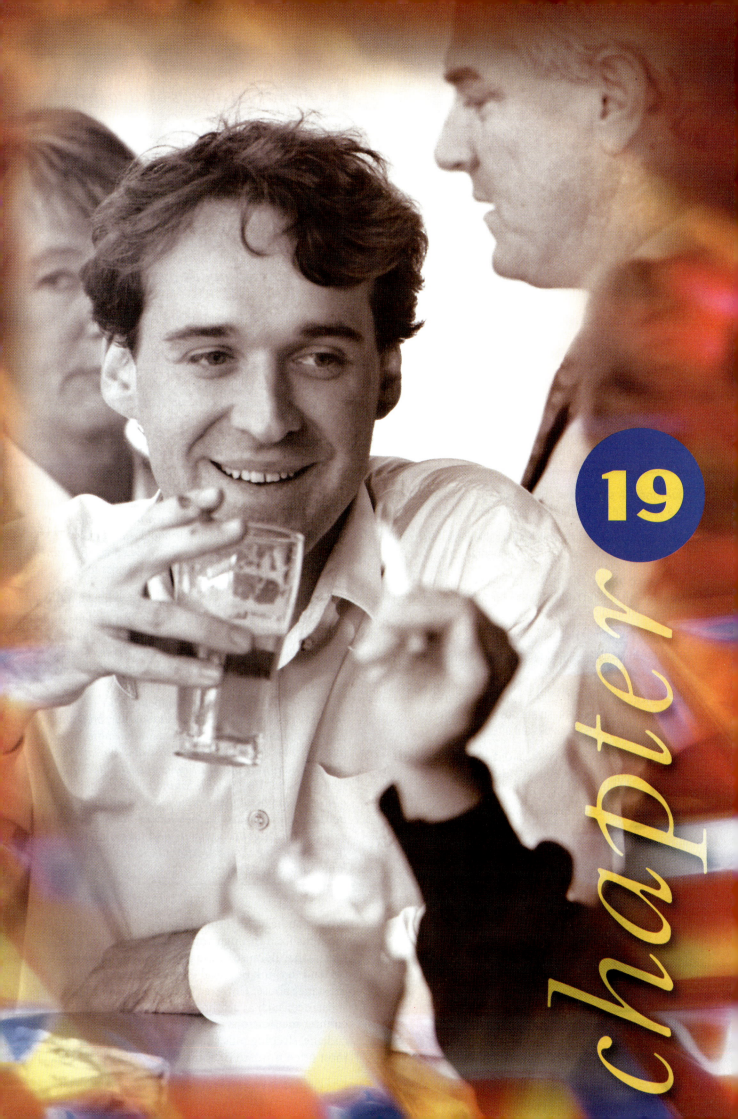

chapter

19

Key Terms

Addiction: The compulsive need to use a substance. An addicted user initially suffers mental, physical, social and emotional distress after stopping.

Dependency: The desire to continually use a substance.

Depressants: Substances which affect the central nervous system to slow down physical and mental activity and alleviate anxiety.

Drug: Any substance other than food which affects the functions of the body.

Hallucinogens *(hal-oo-sin-o-jenz)*: Substances which affect mood, sensation, thought, emotion and self-awareness; alter perceptions of time and space; and produce delusions.

Inhalants *(in-hay-lants)*: Substances (their gas or fumes) inhaled to produce an effect.

Medication: A drug given to prevent or correct the effects of a disease or condition or otherwise enhance mental or physical welfare.

Overdose: A situation in which a person takes enough of a substance that it has toxic (poisonous) or fatal effects.

Stimulants: Substances which affect the central nervous system to speed up physical and mental activity.

Substance abuse: The deliberate, excessive use of a substance without regard to health concerns or accepted medical practices.

Substance misuse: The use of a substance for unintended purposes or for intended purposes but in improper amounts or doses.

Tolerance: A condition which occurs when a user of a substance has to increase the dose and frequency of use to obtain the same desired effect.

Withdrawal: The condition produced when an addicted person stops using or abusing a substance.

Roberta had always liked to drink. In her university days she often went to parties and drank beer in great quantities, but she was careful never to drive when she was intoxicated and so she never worried about drinking too much.

After university, working long hours as a sales manager in a competitive industry, she now drank scotch and usually she had two or three drinks with lunch. She never thought about it—all her clients seemed pleased when she bought the drinks at business lunches and dinners, particularly the male executives. Her husband, a professor at the local university, never said a word about her missing dinner night after night as long as she called to tell him she would be late. After all, she brought home a good pay cheque. They had their weekends together, at least when she wasn't on a business trip.

Even when she started keeping a bottle in the filing cabinet in her office, she knew she didn't have a drinking problem. She never drove when really drunk, she never got sick—she just needed a boost to get through her stressful days.

One day, after losing a major contract and having an argument with her boss, she went to lunch alone and had two drinks before the food arrived. The food did not appeal to her, so she had another drink. There was no real point in rushing back to the office now, anyway…

She wasn't sure what had happened, but when she raised her head from her desk she saw her boss and secretary standing at the doorway to her office watching her. Her boss shook his head and walked away. She realised then that she must have passed out. She could imagine what they were thinking, what people in the office would gossip about now. Feeling rather ashamed, her first impulse was to reach for the bottle in her filing cabinet. It was gone. Someone had taken it. How dare they take it! she thought. After all, it wasn't as if she had a drinking problem!

When you hear the term substance abuse, what thoughts flash through your mind? Narcotics? Cocaine? Marijuana? Because of the publicity they receive, we tend to think of illegal **drugs** when we hear of substance abuse. However, in Australia today legal substances such as alcohol, tobacco and over-the-counter **medications** including aspirin, paracetamol, codeine, sleeping pills and certain stimulants are the most often misused or abused substances.

The term **substance abuse** refers to a broad range of improperly used medicinal and non-medicinal substances. Substance abuse costs Australian society huge sums each year in medical care, insurance and loss of productivity. Even more important, however, are the lives lost or permanently impaired each year from injuries or medical emergencies related to substance abuse or misuse.

This chapter will teach you about common forms of **substance misuse** and abuse, how to recognise these problems, and how to care for the victims. In an emergency caused by substance abuse or misuse, the care you give can save a life.

EFFECTS OF SUBSTANCE MISUSE AND ABUSE ON HEALTH

Substance abuse and misuse poses a very serious threat to the health of many Australians. In 1992 about 200 deaths occurred in Australia due to unintentional poisoning by drugs and medicinal products. Half of these cases involved opiates and related drugs, and pain-killers and prescribed drugs misused or abused accounted for many other deaths. Alcohol poisoning caused by excessive drinking resulted in many deaths, and many other alcohol-related deaths occurred in car collisions and other preventable injuries.

The number of emergency department patients saying they have used illegal substances has risen dramatically. The greatest increase in Australia is in the number who admit to using cocaine, amphetamines ("speed") and marijuana. In addition, Hepatitis B and the human immuno-deficiency virus (HIV) which causes AIDS, are now transmitted more commonly through intravenous drug use than ever before, because of shared, unclean needles.

FORMS OF SUBSTANCE MISUSE AND ABUSE

Many substances that are abused or misused are not illegal. Other substances are legal when prescribed by a doctor. Some are illegal only for people who are under age. Figure 19-1 shows some misused and abused substances.

A drug is any substance other than food taken to affect body functions. A drug used to prevent or treat a disease or otherwise enhance mental or physical welfare is a medication. Any drug can cause **dependency**. Dependent people feel that they need the drug to function normally. Those with a compulsive need for a substance and who would suffer mental, physical and emotional distress if they stopped taking it are said to have an **addiction** to that substance.

When a person continually uses a substance, its effects on the body decrease—a condition called **tolerance.** The user then has to increase the dose and frequency of substance use to obtain the desired effect.

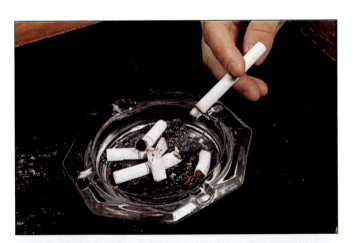
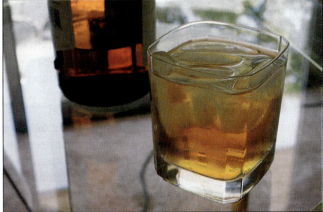
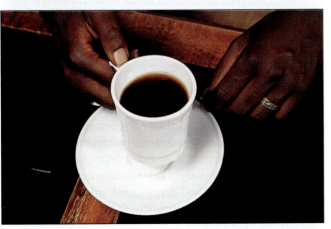
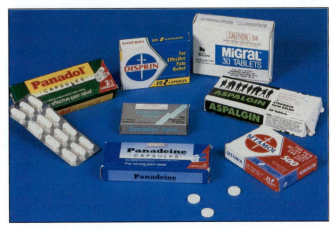

FIGURE 19-1 *Substance abuse and misuse involves a broad range of improperly used medical and non-medical substances.*

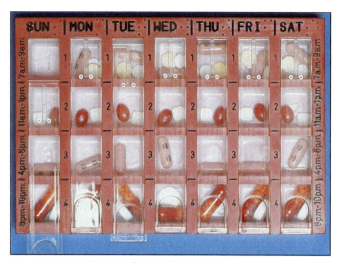

FIGURE 19-2 *Misuse of a medication can occur unintentionally for an elderly person or a person with failing eyesight. Use of a dosette can help prevent this problem.*

An **overdose** occurs if someone takes too much of a substance and experiences poisonous effects. An overdose may occur if the person intentionally or unintentionally takes more than is needed for medical purposes. An elderly person, for example, may not remember taking the medication and then take another dose, or a person with failing eyesight may mistake one medication for another. People may also misunderstand the instructions for taking a medication and may take it at the wrong times or in the wrong amount. Use of a dosette may help such a person keep track of the medications taken (Figure 19-2).

An overdose may also be intentional, such as a suicide attempt. Sometimes the suicide victim takes a sufficiently high dose of a substance to be certain to cause death. Other times, to gain attention or help, the victim takes enough to need medical attention but not enough to cause death.

The term **withdrawal** describes the condition produced when an addicted person stops using or abusing a drug. This may occur as a deliberate decision or because the person is unable to obtain the specific drug. Withdrawal from certain substances, such as alcohol, can cause severe mental and physical discomfort and become a serious medical condition.

COMMONLY MISUSED AND ABUSED SUBSTANCES

Substances are categorised according to their effects on the body. The basic categories are **stimulants, hallucinogens** and **depressants.** A drug's category depends mostly on its central nervous system effects. Some substances depress the nervous system, whereas others speed up its activity. Some are not easily categorised because of their multiple effects.

Drugs also affect different people in different ways. Individual effects may depend on the dosage taken, whether the person is also taking some other drug, different ratios of body fat to muscle, and so on.

Stimulants

Stimulants affect the central nervous system to speed up physical and mental activity; they have limited medical value. They produce temporary feelings of alertness, improve task performance and prevent sleepiness. They are sometimes used for weight reduction because they suppress appetite.

Many stimulants are ingested as pills, but some can be absorbed, injected or inhaled. Amphetamine, dextroamphetamine and methamphetamine are stimulants. Their street (slang) names include uppers, bennies, black beauties, speed, crystal, meth and crank. One of the most recent and dangerous new stimulants is called ice, which is a smokable or injected form of methamphetamine that is extremely addictive.

Cocaine is one of the most publicised and powerful stimulants. The most common method of using cocaine is sniffing the powder form, known as "snorting", wherein the drug is absorbed into the blood through capillaries in the nose. A more potent form of cocaine is crack, which is injected or smoked. The vapours which are inhaled into the lungs reach the brain within 10 seconds, causing immediate effects. Crack is highly addictive.

The most common stimulants in Australia are legal. Caffeine is present in coffee, tea, many kinds of soft drinks, chocolate, diet pills and pills used to combat fatigue. Nicotine, another stimulant, is found in tobacco products. Other stimulants used for medical purposes are inhaled to treat asthma.

Hallucinogens

Hallucinogens do not have a medical use. They cause changes in mood, sensation, thought, emotion and self-awareness. They alter the person's perception of time and space and produce delusions.

Among the most widely abused are lysergic acid diethylamide (LSD), commonly called acid; psylocibin, called mushrooms; Australian mushrooms, called gold tops or blue meanies; phencyclidine (PCP), also known as angel dust; and mescaline, otherwise referred to as peyote, buttons or mesc. These substances are usually ingested, but PCP is also often inhaled.

Hallucinogens sometimes cause what is called a "bad trip", producing intense fear, panic, paranoid delusions, vivid hallucinations, profound depression, tension and anxiety.

Depressants

Depressants affect the central nervous system to slow down physical and mental activity. Some depressants are prescribed for depression and alleviation of anxiety or as a muscle relaxant. Common depressants are barbiturates, benzodiazepines, narcotics, alcohol and various **inhalants.** Most depressants are ingested or injected; their street names include downers and reds. All depressants alter the conscious state to some degree. They relieve anxiety, promote sleep, depress respiration,

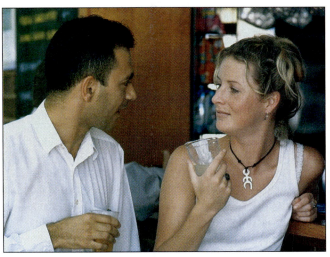

FIGURE 19-3 *Alcohol is one of the most widely used and abused substances in Australia. The tangible and intangible costs are staggering.*

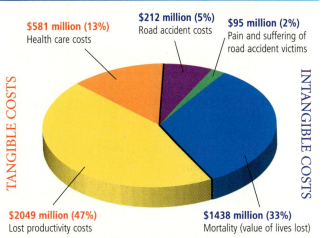

Costs of Alcohol Abuse

TANGIBLE COSTS

INTANGIBLE COSTS

$581 million (13%)
Health care costs

$212 million (5%)
Road accident costs

$95 million (2%)
Pain and suffering of road accident victims

$2049 million (47%)
Lost productivity costs

$1438 million (33%)
Mortality (value of lives lost)

Source: "Estimating the Cost of Drug Abuse in Australia," Monograph Series No. 15, Australian Government Publishing Service, Canberra, 1988.

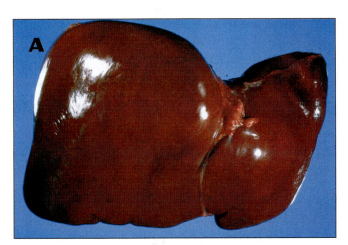

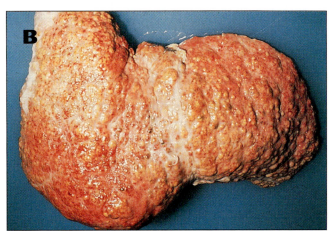

FIGURE 19-4A *Healthy liver.* B *Chronic drinking can result in cirrhosis, a disease of the liver.*

relieve pain, relax muscles and impair co-ordination and judgment.

Narcotics have effects similar to those of other depressants. They are powerful and are used to relieve anxiety and pain. All narcotics are illegal without a prescription, and some are not prescribed at all. The most common narcotics are morphine, codeine and heroin. All are highly addictive.

Alcohol is the most widely used and abused drug in Australia (Figure 19-3). In high doses, its effects can be toxic. Alcohol is like other depressants in its effects and the risks for overdose. Alcohol is often used to loosen inhibitions and is thus often mistakenly considered a stimulant. Frequent drinkers may become dependent on the effects of alcohol and increasingly tolerant of them.

Alcohol taken in large or frequent amounts has many unhealthy consequences. Alcohol can cause the oesophagus to rupture or can injure the stomach lining, causing the victim to vomit blood. Chronic drinking can affect the brain and cause a lack of co-ordination, memory loss and apathy. Other problems include irritated bowel, heart disease and liver disease such as cirrhosis (Figure 19-4).

In addition, many psychological, family, social and work problems are related to chronic drinking. Chronic drinking is frequently a contributing cause in problems within the home such as spouse or child abuse or family stress. Personal productivity declines as a result of habitual drinking, leading to lower performance in school or in the workplace. Although the indirect effects are not easily measured, chronic drinking is frequently cited as one of the most serious and pervasive problems in our society.

Solvents and Aerosols

Substances inhaled to produce an intoxicating effect are called inhalants. These may also have a depressing effect on the central nervous system and may damage the heart, lungs, brain and liver. Solvents such as acetone, toluene and butane, found in glues, petrol, kerosene, lighter fluid, paints, nail polish and remover and aerosol sprays, have all been inhaled. The user at first appears to be drunk. Some young people tend to inhale in groups when sharing these drugs.

How Much Drinking Is Safe?

Is any amount of drinking safe? There is no easy answer to this question. Medical research clearly shows that at a certain level, drinking is definitely harmful. However, that does not mean that drinking below that level is always safe. After all, even one or two drinks can affect one's judgment in a way that, in certain circumstances, could result in actions leading to death. In general, you should never think of drinking as completely safe, although social drinking at certain levels in certain situations can be done responsibly.

For reasons of overall health, drinking an average of more than four drinks a day for men, or two drinks a day for women, is clearly associated with major health risks. Similarly, drinking more than five days a week can lead to chronic health problems. A drink is defined as 300 ml (10 oz) of beer, 120 ml (4 oz) of wine or 30 ml (1 oz) of spirits.

These guidelines are averages and must be adjusted for the individual person and circumstances. Following are guidelines for specific situations.

Pregnancy: Even drinking as little as one or two drinks a week can have adverse effects on the foetus. Total abstinence is recommended by most medical experts.

Driving: Although the legal limit for alcohol in the blood means it is legal to drive after drinking a limited amount of alcohol, that does not mean it is safe to do so. Judgment, reaction time and complex skills are affected by even very small amounts of alcohol in the blood, making driving a more dangerous activity. Experts recommend not driving after any drinking. This also holds true for boating, as alcohol is involved in many boating injuries and fatalities.

Social Drinking: Follow the above guidelines for maximum safe amounts to drink, but also drink responsibly for the situation:

- Avoid heavy/binge drinking sessions.

- Decrease your drinking if other factors put you at combined risk for adverse effects, including: use of other drugs, family history of alcohol problems, past hepatitis B infection, smoking, stomach disease or surgery, diabetes or psychiatric illness.

- Do not drink while operating machinery.

- Arrange in advance for a designated non-drinking driver.

- Avoid or decrease your drinking in hazardous environments such as before swimming or water sports, in cold environments, or in any potentially dangerous situation.

- Drink slowly: your body can handle only one drink an hour. There are many things you can do to slow the pace of drinking, such as:
  —Don't eat salty foods, which make you more thirsty.
  —Dilute your drinks to lower the alcohol content.
  —Eat while you drink.
  —Order small sizes of drinks.
  —Offer to serve yourself later if you have not finished your drink.

Sources included: Is There a Safe Level of Daily Consumption of Alcohol For Men and Women?, the National Health and Medical Research Council, (1992), the Australian Government Publishing Service; and Should You Stop Drinking Alcohol, CEIDA, the NSW Centre for Education on Drugs and Alcohol (1986).

Other Substances

Other substances with mixed effects include designer drugs, marijuana, steroids and also over-the-counter substances which can be purchased without a prescription.

Designer Drugs

Designer drugs are variations of medically prescribed substances such as narcotics and amphetamines. Street chemists modify them into extremely potent and dangerous street drugs; hence the name "designer drug". One designer drug, a form of the commonly used surgical anaesthetic "Fentanyl", can be made 2000 to 6000 times stronger than its original form.

When the chemical make-up of a drug is altered, the user can experience a variety of unpredictable and dangerous effects.

One of the more commonly used designer drugs is "Ecstasy" (MDMA). Although Ecstasy is structurally related to stimulants and hallucinogens, its effects are somewhat different from either. Ecstasy can evoke a euphoric high which makes it popular among young adults, although it can be followed by deep depression and paranoia. Ecstasy produces stimulant-like effects including high blood pressure, rapid heartbeat, profuse sweating and agitation, as well as the hallucinogen-like effects of paranoia, visual distortion and erratic mood swings.

Marijuana

Marijuana is derived from the plant Cannabis sativa. It is typically smoked in cigarette form or in a pipe. The effects include feelings of elation, distorted perceptions of time and space and impaired judgment. Marijuana irritates the throat, reddens the eyes and causes a rapid pulse, dizziness and often an increased appetite, sometimes called "the munchies".

Many young people smoke marijuana from a "bong", a type of water pipe often made from a bottle. This form of smoking can cause hyperventilation and lung collapse. Emergency departments in hospitals commonly see collapsed lungs in people in extreme respiratory distress who have been "bonging".

Anabolic Steroids

Anabolic steroids are an appropriate medical drug for specified diseases and conditions. Their medical uses include bringing about weight gain for persons unable to gain weight naturally. They are different from corticosteroids, which are used to counteract the toxic effects of poisons such as poison ivy. Anabolic steroids are sometimes used by athletes trying to enhance performance and increase muscle mass (Figure 19-5). They are also used by non-athletes to increase body size, that is, to get "the look", to improve body image. Chronic use of anabolic steroids can lead to sterility, liver cancer and personality changes such as aggressive behaviour. Steroid use by younger people may also disrupt normal growth.

Over-the-Counter Substances

Aspirin, paracetamol, laxatives, cough medicines and antihistamine sprays are commonly misused or abused over-the-counter substances. Aspirin is an effective anti-inflammatory drug and minor pain reliever found in a variety of medicines. People use aspirin for many reasons and conditions. As useful as aspirin is, misuse can have a poisonous effect on the body. Typically, aspirin can cause inflammation and bleeding of the stomach and small intestine, which results in bleeding ulcers. Aspirin can also impair normal blood clotting.

Laxatives, another over-the-counter substance, are used to relieve constipation. They come in mild and strong forms. If used improperly, laxatives can cause uncontrolled diarrhoea which can result in dehydration. The very young and the elderly are particularly susceptible to dehydration.

Antihistamines, such as nasal sprays, can help relieve the congestion of colds or hay fever. If misused, they can cause physical dependency. Using the spray over a long period can cause nosebleeds and changes to the mucous membrane lining of the nose, making it difficult to breathe without the spray. Some antihistamines claim to be "non-drowsy" and presumably safer when driving, but this is not always the case.

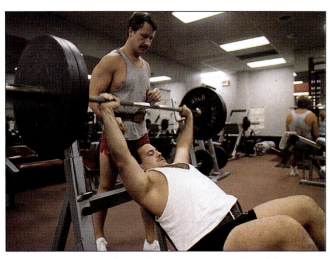

FIGURE 19-5 *Steroids are drugs sometimes abused by athletes to enhance performance and increase muscle mass.*

SYMPTOMS AND SIGNS OF SUBSTANCE MISUSE OR ABUSE

Many of the symptoms and signs of substance misuse and abuse are similar to those of other medical emergencies. You should not necessarily assume, for example, that someone who is stumbling is disoriented or has a fruity, alcohol-like odour on the breath is intoxicated by alcohol, because the person may be a victim of a medical emergency or disease. Always ask the person if any substance has been used.

The misuse or abuse of stimulants can have many unhealthy effects on the body. Following are some symptoms and signs which may occur:

- moist or flushed skin
- sweating
- chills
- nausea, vomiting
- fever
- headache
- dizziness
- rapid pulse
- rapid breathing
- high blood pressure
- chest pain
- cyanosis
- dry mouth
- lack of appetite

In some instances, stimulants can cause respiratory distress, disrupt normal heart rhythms or even cause death. The victim may appear very excited, restless, talkative or irritable or suddenly lose consciousness. Stimulant use can lead to dependency and can cause heart attack or stroke.

STEROIDS: BODY MELTDOWN

You've seen Arnold Schwarzenegger and you want to look just like him. If you think steroids are the answer, think again. These drugs may build up bodies on the outside, but they can cause a body meltdown on the inside.

Anabolic steroids are synthetic chemicals which mimic the hormone testosterone, which gives the male his masculine characteristics —his deeper voice, his beard and moustache and other sex characteristics. Steroids also help create proteins and other substances used to build muscle tissue, which is why they are popular with athletes.

The problem is that some young athletes and bodybuilders are listening to their gym friends rather than their doctors. Steroids are being used in greater doses than ever before and at earlier ages. Doctors do not know what these dosages will do to the body.

Most doctors do not prescribe anabolic steroids except for certain medical problems. Before you listen to some gym guru's opinion of steroids, consider these effects:

> **If you think steroids are the answer, think again. These drugs may build up bodies on the outside, but they can cause a body meltdown on the inside.**

- **Stunted growth:** In children, steroids cause the growth plates in the bones to close prematurely. As a teenager you may have been destined to be tall, but steroid use can cause permanently stunted growth.

- **Heart disease and stroke:** Steroids cause dangerous changes in cholesterol levels. Dramatic drops in the amount of good cholesterol, which helps remove the fatty deposits on the artery walls, are possible with steroid use. There may also be dramatic increases in bad cholesterol, which clogs the arteries and causes heart problems. Your steroid-doped body may look fine on the outside, but inside your body may look like that of a man in his 50s whose arteries are so clogged that he needs heart surgery.

- **Aggressive personality and psychological disorders:** Some men who take anabolic steroids become unnaturally aggressive. A few have developed documentable mental disorders. In a *Sports Illustrated* article,[1] a South Carolina football player on steroids described his nightmare with steroids. He described how he pulled a gun on a pizza delivery boy in his dorm and how his family intervened when he began threatening suicide. Many doctors feel the psychiatric effects of steroids may be the most threatening side effect.

- **Lowered white blood cell count:** Taking steroids also affects the number of white blood cells in the body. With fewer white blood cells your body has fewer antibodies to fight against infections, including cancers and other diseases.

- **Sexual dysfunction and disorders:** Synthetic steroids cause the body to cut off its own natural production of steroids, which can result in shrinking testicles and shrinking sexual interest. Women may grow facial hair and experience a decrease in breast size and a permanent deepening of the voice; men may also develop enlarged breasts.

- **Disabled liver:** Steroids seriously affect the liver's ability to function. They act as an irritant to the liver, causing tissue damage and an inability to clear bile. Doctors have also found blood-filled benign tumours in the liver after steroid use.

There are also dangers beyond the physiological side effects. Because steroids are often sold on the black market, they are increasingly sold by drug traffickers who obtain their wares from unsanitary laboratories. Health problems related to this include substitution of veterinary steroids and use of impure substances.

Doctors are also concerned that sharing needles to inject steroids increases the danger of transmission of diseases such as hepatitis B and HIV which causes AIDS. Doctors and other public health officials are particularly concerned about the long-term effects of high doses.

Arnold Schwarzenegger maintains the size of his massive biceps and quadriceps naturally. He used steroids in his early bodybuilding days, but that was before doctors knew the risks. "It was an experimental thing in the 60s and 70s", Schwarzenegger says. "Then we didn't have the knowledge which we have now. Now we know that it is harmful."

"With steroids, it's not bodybuilding", he adds, "it's body destroying."

1. T. Chaikin and R. Telander, "The Nightmare of Steroids," *Sports Illustrated*, 69(1988):18. ■

The symptoms and signs of hallucinogen abuse may include:

- sudden mood changes
- flushed face
- seeing or hearing something not present
- anxiety, fear, distress

The symptoms and signs of alcohol and other depressant abuse may include:

- drowsiness
- confusion
- blurred speech
- slow heart and breathing rates
- poor co-ordination
- an alcohol abuser may smell of alcohol

The symptoms and signs of alcohol withdrawal, a potentially dangerous condition, include:

- confusion
- restlessness
- trembling
- hallucinations

Always call for an ambulance if you suspect a person is suffering from alcohol withdrawal or from any form of substance abuse.

Remember that, as in other medical emergencies, you do not have to diagnose substance misuse or abuse to provide care. However, you may be able to find clues that suggest the nature of the problem. Often these clues will come from the victim, bystanders or the scene itself. Always ask the person if some substance was taken. Look for containers, drug paraphernalia and symptoms and signs of other medical problems. Try to get information from the victim or from any bystanders or family members. Because many of these physical symptoms and signs of substance abuse mimic other conditions, you may not be able to determine that a person has overdosed on a substance. To provide care for the victim, you need only recognise abnormalities that may indicate a condition requiring professional help. These include:

- breathing that is too fast or too slow
- pulse that is increased or decreased
- altered skin colour (especially cyanosis), temperature or moisture
- behaviour changes
- other symptoms and signs of poisoning (see Chapter 10)

When you are not sure whether a person is suffering from substance abuse, how should you provide care?

FIRST AID FOR SUBSTANCE MISUSE OR ABUSE

Because substance abuse or misuse is a form of poisoning, care follows the same general principles. Your initial care for substance misuse or abuse does not require that you know the specific substance taken. Follow these general principles as you would for any poisoning:

- Survey the scene to be sure it is safe to help the person.
- Carry out a primary survey and care for any life-threatening conditions.
- Call the Poisons Information Centre or your local emergency telephone number, and follow their directions.
- Question the victim or bystanders during your secondary survey to try to find out what substance was taken, how much was taken and when it was taken.
- Calm and reassure the victim.
- Help maintain normal body temperature.
- Withdraw from the area if the victim becomes violent or threatening.
- If you suspect that someone has used a designer drug, tell ambulance personnel. This is important because a person who has overdosed on a designer drug may not respond to normal medical treatment.

PREVENTING SUBSTANCE ABUSE

Preventing substance abuse is a complex process, one not yet well understood or successfully carried out. Just educating people about substances and their effects on health or attempting to instil a fear of penalties for illegal use has not proved successful. Prevention efforts must involve an understanding of the person as an individual and the person's own environment. In Australia, younger teenagers (aged 12 to 14) are increasingly becoming substance abusers.

Understanding the many factors which can lead a person to substance misuse and abuse is an important step toward prevention. These factors may include:

- lack of parental supervision
- the breakdown of traditional family structures
- a wish to escape unpleasant surroundings and stressful situations
- widespread availability of substances
- thrill-seeking, experimentation
- rebellion
- peer pressure
- low self-esteem
- media glamourising, especially of alcohol and tobacco

Perhaps one of the most compelling factors is the belief that using substances can cause a person to feel good and have fun.

Each point below has a bearing on an individual's behaviour regarding substance use:

- Substance abuse is frequently linked to past and present home and community environments.

- Self-destructive behaviour such as substance abuse is linked to how people feel about themselves. People with positive feelings of self-worth are less likely to become substance abusers.

- Young people may model the behaviour of peers and older adults. Before adults "light up" or have a drink, or misuse or abuse a substance, they should be aware that their actions may influence others, especially impressionable young people.

- The more that is known about substances, their effects and the penalties for their use, the more chance there is to make educated choices about behaviour regarding them.

A person's best defence against substance misuse or abuse is one's own values and beliefs. Values and beliefs result from upbringing, and from life experiences and choices. Preventing substance misuse and abuse in life begins by examining knowledge, values, attitudes and beliefs. Furthermore, discussing values with others can help to strengthen convictions and lower the chances of becoming a victim of substance misuse or abuse. Completing the Substance Misuse and Abuse table (opposite) may help clarify feelings about substance misuse and abuse.

Many resources offer help to victims of substance abuse. Community-based programs offered through schools and churches often provide help and access to hotlines and local groups which give help and support for substance abuse problems. For help in locating such a program, ask your health care provider.

PREVENTING SUBSTANCE MISUSE

Not all substance misuse is intentional. By being careful, it is possible to prevent unintentional misuse or overdose.

- Use common sense with all medications.

- Read the product information and use only as directed.

- Ask your doctor or pharmacist about the effects, side effects and possible contra-indications or interactions if you are taking other medications.

- Never use another person's prescribed medications; what is right for one person may not be right for another.

- Always keep medications in their appropriate, marked containers.

- Because time can alter the chemical composition of medications, causing them to be less effective and possibly even toxic, destroy all out-of-date medications. For example, aspirin hydrolises over time and forms the toxic substance salicylic acid.

SUBSTANCE MISUSE AND ABUSE

- I view substance abuse as…

  _____

- The thought of using an illegal substance…

  _____

- Substance abuse begins…

  _____

- The thought that alcohol, tobacco and caffeine are drugs…

  _____

- Substance abusers should…

  _____

- If I found out that a close friend was abusing an illegal substance, I would…

  _____

- Substance abuse treatment programs are…

  _____

- Those abusing substances while pregnant should…

  _____

- If I were faced with a situation of providing emergency care to a known intravenous drug user, I would feel…

  _____

- If I could change something about myself, I would…

  _____

- How do I feel about myself? I feel…

  _____

- The greatest fear I would have about seeking help for a substance abuse problem is…

  _____

2 *Describe three situations which represent substance misuse.*

Summary

- Substance abuse and misuse may produce a variety of symptoms and signs, some of which are common to other medical emergencies.

- Look for clues that may indicate the nature of the problem. Try to get information from the victim, bystanders or family members.

- If the victim's condition may have been caused by substance misuse or abuse, provide care for a poisoning emergency. Call your local emergency number and follow their directions. Call an ambulance if necessary.

- If a person under the influence of a substance becomes violent or threatening, retreat to safety and wait for the ambulance to arrive.

Answers to Application Questions

1. To provide care you must first recognise that a condition requiring professional help exists. Follow the Emergency Action Principles and provide care as for any poisoning emergency.

2. Examples of substance misuse include:
   - Taking somebody else's medication prescribed for similar symptoms.
   - Taking medication prescribed for you on a previous occasion.
   - Unintentionally mistaking one medication for another.
   - Putting more than one medication in the same container.
   - Ignoring directions concerning when and how to take medication.
   - Ignoring directions concerning alcohol use when taking a medication (including antibiotics).
   - Inappropriate use of laxatives, for example, to avoid weight gain.
   - Ignoring directions concerning driving or operating machinery when taking medication.

Study Questions

1. *Match each term with its definition.*

    a. Addiction.
    b. Dependency.
    c. Medication.
    d. Drug.
    e. Overdose.
    f. Substance abuse.
    g. Tolerance.
    h. Withdrawal.

_____ Deliberate, excessive use of a substance.

_____ A drug given to prevent or correct a disease or otherwise enhance mental or physical welfare.

_____ Any substance other than food which affects the functions of the body.

_____ Taking enough of a substance to produce a toxic or fatal effect in the body.

_____ The compulsive need to use a substance.

_____ The condition produced when an addicted person stops using or abusing a substance.

_____ A desire to continually use a substance, feeling that it is needed to function normally.

_____ A condition which occurs when a substance user has to increase the dose and frequency of use of a substance to obtain the desired effect.

2. *List four symptoms and signs which might indicate substance abuse or misuse.*

3. *List four commonly misused or abused legal substances.*

4. *List four things you can do to prevent unintentional substance misuse.*

5. *Describe the care for a victim of suspected substance misuse or abuse.*

6. *Match each type of substance with the effects it has on the body.*

   a. Depressants.

   b. Hallucinogens.

   c. Inhalants.

   d. Stimulants.

   ____ Produce psychological changes in mood, sensation, thought, emotion and self-awareness, alter perception of time and space and produce delusions.

   ____ Produce intoxicating effects similar to those of alcohol.

   ____ Alter the conscious state to some degree, causing relaxation, anxiety and pain relief and impaired judgment and co-ordination.

   ____ Speed up the physical and mental activity of the brain, producing temporary feelings of alertness and improved task performance.

In questions 7 and 8, circle the letter of the correct answer.

7. *Which of the following is true of substance abuse?*

   a. It occurs only among the elderly who are forgetful and may have poor eyesight.

   b. It is the use of a substance for intended purposes but in improper amounts or doses.

   c. It is the use of a substance without regard to health concerns or accepted medical practices.

   d. Its effects are minor and rarely result in medical complications.

8. *The effects of designer drugs are:*

   a. well known

   b. unpredictable

   c. sometimes dangerous

   d. easily controlled.

   e. b and c.

9. *List two clues at the scene of an emergency which might indicate substance abuse or misuse.*

Answers are in Appendix A (page 363).

Guide to a Healthier Life

CHAPTERS throughout this book have focused on first aid for different kinds of injuries and sudden illnesses. Along the way, prevention of many kinds of injuries has been discussed. Prevention is a key principle for living a healthy life: keeping an illness or injury from happening is much better than letting it occur and then hoping for full restoration to good health.

There are many things we can all do to live healthier lives and lower our risk of injuries and illness. Good nutrition, appropriate body weight, exercise and stress control all help us stay healthy. We may also need to break habits which put us at risk of illness, such as smoking or excessive drinking. We can take steps to prevent injuries by practising fire safety and following safety guidelines at work and in our recreation.

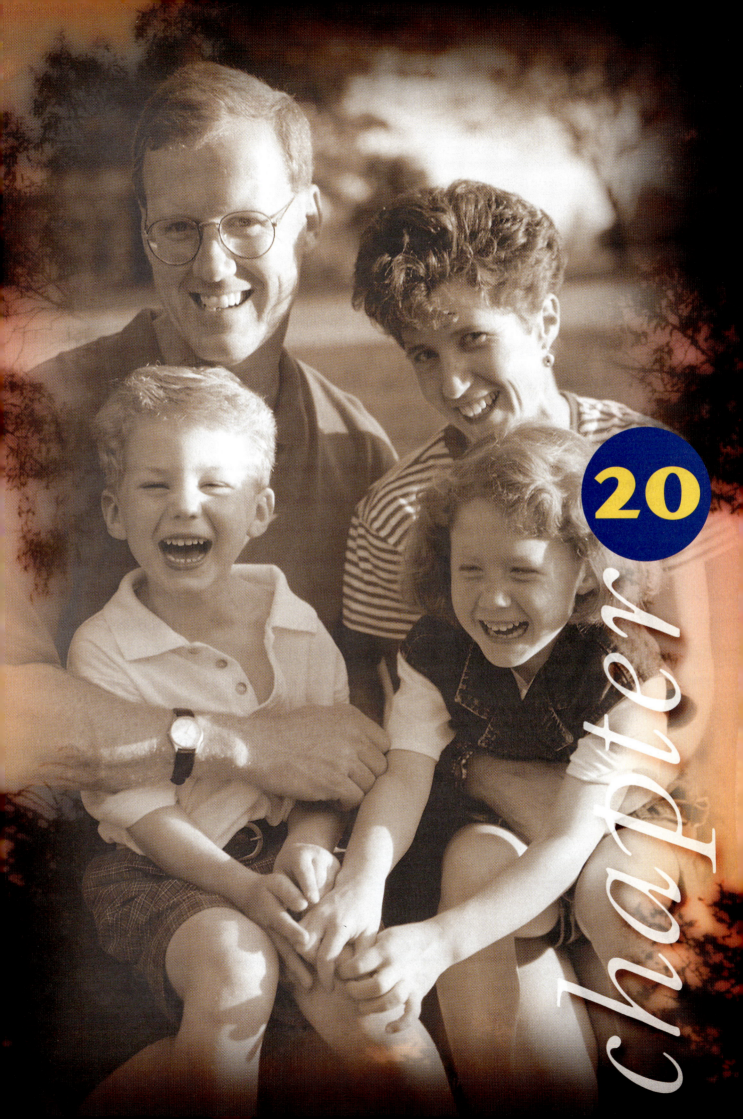

20

chapter

Key Terms

Cardiovascular *(car-dee-o-vask-yoo-lar)* **fitness:** A healthy condition of the heart and blood vessels, attained through diet, exercise and other good habits, in which cardiovascular disease is less likely.

Cholesterol: A dietary substance that in high levels in the blood can accumulate in blood vessels, contributing to cardiovascular disease.

Fibre: A dietary substance found in some foods, notably fruit and vegetables, that contributes to good health.

Obesity: Weighing 20 per cent more than desirable body weight, which increases the risk for certain illnesses.

Residual current devices (RCDs): Devices installed in appropriate places in the home to prevent accidental electrocution; sometimes called safety switches.

Saturated fat: A dietary substance found in some foods, such as meat and milk products, which in excessive quantities contributes to cardiovascular disease.

Stress: A general response of the body to demands upon it; uncontrolled stress over time can have unhealthy effects on the body.

Target heart rate: The heart rate maintained by continuous and vigorous exercise which gives the heart a healthy workout.

What is a healthy lifestyle? A healthy lifestyle combines beliefs and practices to form good habits in many areas of life, including nutrition, exercise and safety.

This book has so far described first aid basics, such as following the Emergency Action Principles. First aiders know the symptoms and signs of an emergency and what to do to help, how to give expired air resuscitation (EAR) and cardiopulmonary resuscitation (CPR), first aid for choking, and care for many emergency situations, including bleeding, fractures and burns. You have also read about how the body systems work together and about preventing injury and illness such as cardiovascular disease.

A healthy lifestyle builds on this knowledge. Everyone can adopt habits that lead to better health, more energy and a stronger feeling of well-being generally. Some of us may also decide to modify some existing behaviours to become healthier. This may be difficult to accomplish, because behaviour change often requires a change in attitudes and beliefs. Remembering that present and future health and well-being depend on preventing illness and injury can make it easier to change habits.

CARING FOR OUR BODIES

Caring for our bodies now can lead to great dividends in the future. How we treat our bodies in ordinary daily activities—eating, exercising, relaxing, working and sleeping—can be either beneficial or unhealthy.

Nutrition

One of the most important things we can all do to care for our bodies is to eat a healthy diet. A healthy diet is made up of balanced meals which provide nutrients essential to body maintenance, growth, development and repair. We also feel better and are happier when we eat well and are healthy.

However, many of us eat foods which tend to be too high in salt, fats and refined sugar, and too low in fibre and fluids. Changing eating habits need not be difficult. Paying attention to labels on foods before buying them is a good start. The goal is to eat foods which are low in salt, saturated fat and cholesterol. Package information is given per serving size, so the number of servings per package is important. Watch out for trade-offs such as diet products, including some diet soft drinks, which trade a few kilojoules for a lot of salt. Many products which are low in fat, cholesterol and kilojoules are high in salt.

Eating less of foods which are high in salt, fat and cholesterol can actually help prevent some diseases.

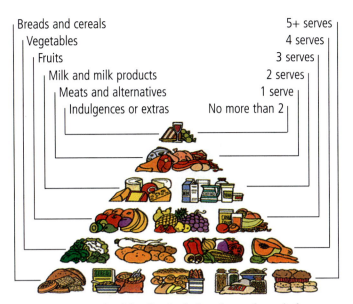

Breads and cereals	5+ serves
Vegetables	4 serves
Fruits	3 serves
Milk and milk products	2 serves
Meats and alternatives	1 serve
Indulgences or extras	No more than 2

FIGURE 20-1 *A healthy diet includes planned meals from the 12345+ food and nutrition plan.*

Try reducing salt intake by taking the salt shaker off the table. Limiting fat intake begins with eating or drinking only low-fat dairy foods and using unsaturated oils and fats for cooking and eating. Although it can be difficult, we also need to try to eat wisely at restaurants and fast-food places.

As we reduce our intake of less healthy foods, we should eat more of the healthier foods: fruits, vegetables and grains. A healthy, balanced diet requires every day the following from the five basic food groups: carbohydrates (breads and cereals), dairy products, protein (meat and fish), fruit and vegetables.

One way to understand and choose foods for a balanced diet is to follow the "12345+ Food and Nutrition Plan" developed by the CSIRO, Division of Human Nutrition (Figure 20-1). This plan shows the type and amount of each food needed for an adequate intake of important nutrients without eating too much of less healthy foods. The plan works as a guide by suggesting the number of serves you should eat on average from each of the food groups.

Following is a general guide for daily intake:

- 1 serve of lean red meat (60 to 100 grams a serve; or 120 grams fish/chicken).
- 2 serves of dairy foods (300 millilitres milk or 40 grams cheese or 200 grams yoghurt—preferably low-fat).
- 3 serves of fruit.
- 4 serves of vegetables (one green leafy; one red/yellow; one starchy).
- 5 to 12 serves of cereal foods (one serve = 1 slice of bread; or 1 bowl of cereal; or 1/2 cup cooked rice; or 1 cup cooked pasta, etc.).

Also included are "indulgences" or extra foods. You should aim to eat no more than 2 serves of these per day. Drinking fluids is also important for health. Everyone should try to drink at least 8 glasses of water each day, instead of coffee, tea or soft drinks.

Weight

Maintaining a good body weight also improves health and general well-being. We have more energy, feel better about ourselves and generally seem to enjoy life more when our body weight is in the healthy range. However, many adults are over- or underweight. Obesity—weighing 20 per cent or more than desirable body weight, contributes to diseases such as heart disease, high blood pressure, diabetes and gallbladder disease. However, the percentage of body fat cannot be determined simply from body weight—a health care provider knows the best methods for measuring body fat.

On the other hand, being too thin is also unhealthy and may be a sign that the body is not getting all the nutrients it needs.

Body weight generally depends on diet and exercise, so sometimes we can change our weight by changing our eating and activity habits. Most important is a healthy attitude about weight loss or gain goals. Becoming obsessed with trying to lose weight fast, for example, can also have unhealthy effects if the body does not get the nutrition it needs. Avoid fad diets and over-the-counter products which promise instant results. The best way to reach a weight goal is to adjust present habits to eat well and exercise regularly. This way, once new habits have been formed, it will be easier to reach a set goal and maintain the desired weight.

Weight loss and gain depend on the balance of caloric intake and energy output. Someone who takes in more kilojoules than they use will gain weight. Someone who uses more kilojoules than they take in will lose weight. There are several guides to weight control. Table 20-1 provides guidelines for achieving and maintaining the right weight. Remember that

Table 20-1

STRATEGIES TO ACHIEVE AND MAINTAIN AN APPROPRIATE WEIGHT RANGE

- Keep a log of the times, settings, reasons and feelings associated with eating.
- Set realistic, long-term goals (such as losing or gaining half a kilogram per week, instead of 2 or 3 kilograms per week).
- Have an occasional reward of a small amount of a special food.
- Eat slowly and take the time to enjoy the taste of the food.
- Stay physically active in daily routines. Take the stairs instead of the lift, and park farther away in the carpark.
- Have a reward upon reaching weight goals.
- Seek support from family and friends for losing or gaining weight.
- Keep a record of the food eaten each day.
- Have a weigh-in once a week at the same time, and record this weight. (Daily weighing can be frustrating.)
- Be prepared to deal with occasional plateaus when losing or gaining weight.

everyone is unique in metabolic rates and other factors which influence weight loss and gain. The best thing we can do is monitor our own habits and weight and learn to do what works best for us individually, realistically working to reach our goals.

Day-to-day fluctuations in weight reflect changes in the level of fluids in the body. One day and the same time each week should be used as a weigh-in time. Weight loss or gain should be tracked based on this weekly amount, not on day-to-day differences.

Weight loss or gain should always be combined with regular exercise—another part of a healthy lifestyle. Any activity—walking to the bus, climbing the stairs, cleaning the house—uses kilojoules. The more active we are, the more kilojoules we use. Activity allows eating a little more while still maintaining body weight.

As we grow older, we may also need to change our eating habits. A person who eats the same number of kilojoules between the ages of 20 to 40 and maintains the same level of activity during this time will be considerably heavier at 40 than at 20. As we grow older it is more important to eat foods which provide the body with essential nutrients but are not high in kilojoules.

Exercise

Research has shown that physical fitness dramatically lowers the risk of cardiovascular disease and many forms of cancer. Put simply, we live longer and have less illness when we are physically fit and have regular exercise combined with a good diet. Exercise is good for the heart, lungs and blood vessels and increases muscular endurance, strength and flexibility. Exercise also helps us feel more alive, more energetic and better about ourselves.

Different forms of exercise can affect the body in three different ways. Exercise helps muscles become stronger, joints become more flexible and the entire cardiovascular system become more fit. The first step in designing an exercise program is to set goals. Not everyone needs to increase muscular strength; however, in growing older, both strength and flexibility are generally lost, and some exercise to improve these areas may be beneficial. Anyone planning a change in exercise level should consult with a health care provider to avoid putting too much strain on the body too quickly, which increases the risk of injury.

Everyone benefits from exercise which leads to cardiovascular fitness, regardless of age or present activity level. Cardiovascular fitness can help us:

- cope with stress
- deal with daily activities with more enjoyment
- control weight
- ward off infections
- improve self-esteem
- sleep better
- accomplish personal fitness goals

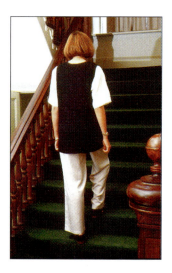
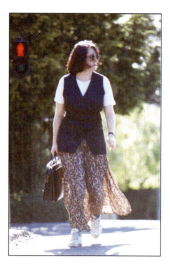
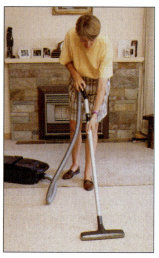
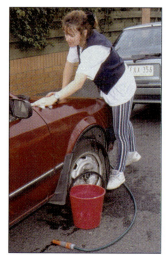

FIGURE 20-2 *Build exercise into your daily activities.*

Cardiovascular fitness depends on exercising the heart. To do this, we need to exercise at least three times a week for 20 to 30 minutes at a level which gives the heart a workout. This is sometimes called the "target heart rate". Exercise must be continuous and vigorous to maintain this rate. Health care providers can provide more information about this and demonstrate how to calculate one's target heart rate.

A simple way to ensure that exercise is vigorous enough to benefit the heart is based on the perceived level of exertion. Think of a scale of exertion from light activity to very hard exertion such as sprinting at top speed. About halfway between is activity which is somewhat hard. The best aerobic activity is to complete the full exercise period at a rate which is hard but less than the extreme of very hard. Breathing should be faster than normal, and the heart rate well increased. However, breathing should not be so hard that talking is difficult without gasping. Stop exercising immediately if any of the following occur: any pain or pressure in the chest, arm or throat; breathlessness or wheezing; dizziness, light-headedness or confusion.

As we build our cardiovascular fitness, we can eventually exercise for longer periods of time.

The "no pain, no gain" theory is not a good approach to exercise. In fact, someone who experiences pain usually is not exercising properly. Warm up before vigorous exercise and cool down afterwards. Also, we can all turn daily activities into exercise (Figure 20-2). Walk briskly instead of driving, whenever possible. Take the stairs instead of the lift or the escalator. Pedal an exercise bike while watching TV, listening to music or reading.

Someone who has been sedentary or who has health problems should see a doctor before starting an exercise program.

Stress Control

Everyone experiences some stress. Stress is a general response of the body to demands upon it. It can be pleasant or unpleasant, and it cannot be avoided. The stress of a deadline may help us work harder and make some people happier, but the unresolved stress of working in an unpleasant job, for example, can over time cause illness. The most important thing is to control stress rather than letting it take control.

Stress which is not controlled can have many unhealthy effects on the body. It can cause psychological problems and increase the risk of cardiovascular disease, cancer and ulcers.

Dealing constructively with stress helps us achieve a healthy lifestyle. Reaching a goal does not get rid of stress for very long; more stressful situations soon come along. After leaving school, for example, many of us look for a job; we may have to move and reorganise our lives; we may get married and make many life changes. All of these events can be stressful. Because stress never goes away forever, it is important to learn to manage it. People who do not learn to manage stress often develop negative habits such as smoking and overeating. Eventually, dependence on habits such as these can lead to poor health.

One of the best ways to handle stress is to develop habits and activities which divert attention to other things. For some people, this involves physical exercise. Another way is to avoid foods containing stimulants such as caffeine, found in coffee, tea, some soft drinks, chocolate and some pain relievers. Caffeine may increase stress or make it more difficult to control. When decreasing the amount of caffeine taken in every day, do so gradually to avoid the headaches which can occur with withdrawal.

Reducing stress through a change in lifestyle requires setting attainable goals. Goals which are not realistic may never be achieved, causing even more stress. To reduce stress, give yourself a reward of something special upon reaching goals or developing new habits.

Relaxation exercises are a form of focused meditation which help reduce stress by helping the body relax. These can be done by sitting or lying quietly in a comfortable position with the eyes closed. Begin breathing in deeply through the nose and exhaling through the mouth. Focus on breathing. Do this for about 10 minutes.

Breaking Unhealthy Habits

Smoking

During the past few decades, more people have become aware of the dangers of smoking. Smoking has been banned or restricted in many work sites, as well as on many airlines and in other public places (Figure 20-3). Cigarette smoking is the single most preventable cause of heart and lung disease. There is no doubt that cigarette smoking causes most cases of lung cancer. The risk of lung cancer starts to go down as soon as a smoker stops.

Increased cancer rates are not the only dangers of smoking. Smoking is also a major cause of heart disease, and smokers have a higher risk of heart attack and sudden cardiac arrest. A pregnant woman who smokes harms both herself and her unborn baby.

Users of smokeless tobacco also face serious risks. Chewing tobacco and snuff can cause cancer of the mouth and tongue, so these products should be avoided.

To stop smoking and stop using tobacco is difficult, but most ex-smokers and former users say they feel better physically and emotionally. Many programs have been designed to help the smoker break the habit. Following are things others can do to help a smoker quit, as recommended by the Quit campaigns run in all states and territories by the anti-cancer organisations.

- Offer real help, rather than preaching, smugness or criticism.

- Don't argue about the effects of smoking. Most smokers already know smoking is unhealthy, and arguments are likely to produce a defensive reaction.

- Don't nag the person about quitting, as this seldom achieves anything but only leads to both parties becoming angry.

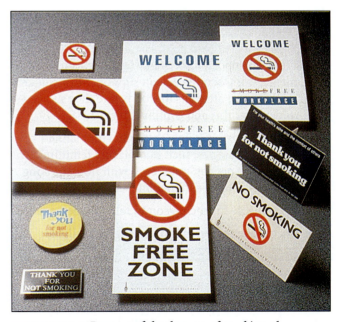

FIGURE 20-3 *Because of the dangers of smoking, the government and many private groups have taken steps to discourage or ban smoking.*

HABITS CAN BE HAZARDOUS

Sure, we should all stop smoking, or stop drinking, or stop eating overmuch, but how? Bad habits die hard. But we learned them at some point in our lives and we can unlearn them. It is never too late to try. Try these tips.

1. Break the chain. Be aware of linking a negative habit to other behaviours. If eating is associated with sitting and watching television, separate those two behaviours. Do not eat when watching television.

2. Control the stimulus. It's easier to stop drinking if there isn't a six-pack of beer in the fridge.

3. Restructure thinking. Stop thinking of a morning break as a cigarette break. Try something else to reduce stress, like taking a walk or drinking fruit juice. Have a plan of attack for tempting situations. For example, take chewing gum or lollies to work if that is a usual place for smoking.

4. Self-monitor. Keep close track of habits. By watching eating, drinking, and smoking habits, we can fight temptation. Recognising when and where it is most difficult to break a habit helps us find ways to circumvent the problem. For example, ordering a glass of water before lunch helps the stomach feel less empty, and we eat less.

5. Join a self-help group. Others facing the same issues can provide support. Sharing with a friend can help us through the rough times. Self-help groups, such as Overeaters Anonymous and Weight Watchers, have proven successful for countless people. ■

• Provide support, understanding and encouragement, even when the person slips up. Most smokers make several attempts to stop before they succeed— understand this and continue to encourage.

• Help the person follow through with planned quitting strategies, such as replacing tempting situations (parties, pubs, etc.) with non-smoking activities (exercise, film going, etc.).

• Be available for the person to talk to when needed.

• Encourage the person to investigate available group programs for quitting.

Alcohol

Alcohol is the most popular drug in Australia. Thousands of people drink beer, wine or distilled spirits.

In addition to the hazardous relationship between drinking alcohol and driving, consuming alcohol in large amounts has other unhealthy effects on the body, as described in Chapter 19.

Most important, regardless of the situation, drinking should be done responsibly. Always have a designated, non-drinking driver to return from a party or other event where drinking is anticipated. Pay attention to the rate of drinking, and if necessary slow down in order to stay in control.

Medical and Dental Care

Everyone should have regular medical, dental and eye check-ups, as preventing disease is far more effective than treating disease after it develops. With the rising costs of health care, prevention and early detection have increasingly become an important aspect of medical care. People need different types of medical examinations, depending on age, personal and family medical history and other factors. Your doctor, dentist and eye doctor can explain what tests to have and how often to have them.

PREVENTING INJURIES

Injuries are a major cause of death and disability in Australia, and can be prevented by using good safety practices. The following sections describe principles of safety for the home and motor vehicle, and at work and recreation.

Fire Safety

Fires can result from smoking, faulty heating equipment, appliances, electrical wiring, cooking and many other causes. Regardless of the cause, everyone needs to be aware of the danger of fire.

Plan and practise a fire escape route with family members.

The local fire department can provide additional safety guidelines. A smoke detector should be installed on every floor of a home. Many homes have smoke detectors which do not work because of old or missing batteries, according to a recent survey. A handy way to remember the batteries is to change them twice a year when resetting clocks for daylight saving time.

See Chapter 16 for additional information on what to do if a fire should occur.

Safety at Home

Thousands of injuries occur in homes each year. Removing hazards and practising good safety habits help make the home safer (Figure 20-4). Safety at home is relatively simple and relies largely on common sense. The following steps help to make the home a safer place:

• Keep emergency numbers as well as other important numbers near the phone.

• Make sure that stairs and hallways are well lit.

PREVENTING ACCIDENTS AT HOME

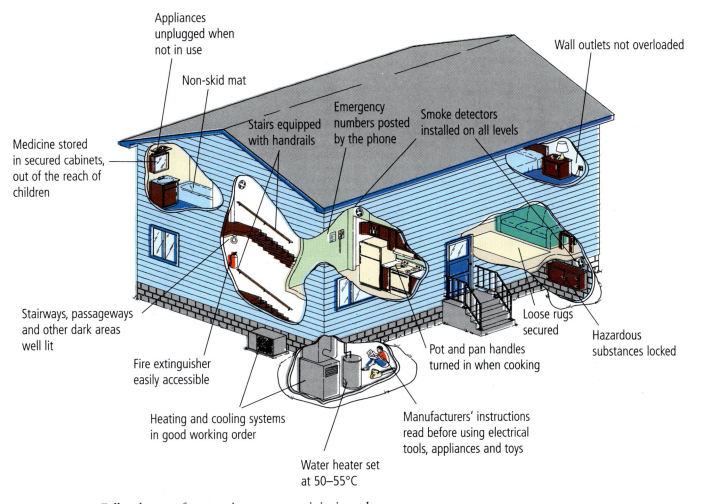

FIGURE 20-4 *Follow home safety practices to prevent injuries at home.*

- Equip stairs with hand rails. If elderly people live in the home, hand rails may be needed by the toilet and in the bath or shower area. For small children, put gates at the head and foot of the stairs.
- Install a residual current device (RCD) in appropriate places in the home to prevent accidental electrocution (Figure 20-5).
- Keep medicines and poisonous substances separate from each other and from food. They should be out of reach of children and in secured cabinets, if possible.
- Keep the heating and cooling systems and all appliances in good working order. Check heating and cooling systems annually before use.
- Read and follow manufacturers' instructions for electrical tools, appliances and toys.
- Turn off the oven and other appliances when not using them. Unplug certain appliances, such as an iron, curling wand or portable heater, after use.
- Make sure a working fire extinguisher is easily accessible. Place a fire blanket in the kitchen area to smother cooking fires.

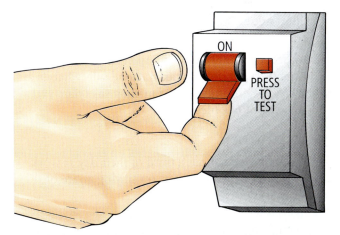

FIGURE 20-5 *Install a residual current device (RCD) in appropriate places in the home to prevent accidental electrocution.*

- Keep any firearms in a locked place, out of the reach of children, and in a separate place away from ammunition.
- Have an emergency fire escape plan and practise it.
- Have a torch with spare batteries.

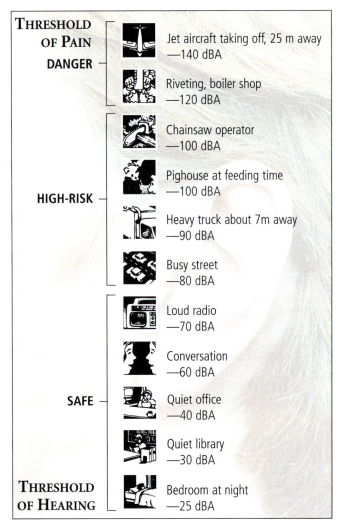

THRESHOLD OF PAIN

DANGER
- Jet aircraft taking off, 25 m away —140 dBA
- Riveting, boiler shop —120 dBA

HIGH-RISK
- Chainsaw operator —100 dBA
- Pighouse at feeding time —100 dBA
- Heavy truck about 7m away —90 dBA
- Busy street —80 dBA

SAFE
- Loud radio —70 dBA
- Conversation —60 dBA
- Quiet office —40 dBA
- Quiet library —30 dBA

THRESHOLD OF HEARING
- Bedroom at night —25 dBA

FIGURE 20-6 *Noise at too high a level or for a prolonged period can damage the hearing.*

- To prevent hearing damage, avoid exposure to loud noises (Figure 20-6).

This list does not include all safety measures for the home. For young children and elderly individuals, additional steps should be taken. Good safety habits at home lays the groundwork for making safety an integral part of our lifestyle.

Safety at Work

Most people spend about a third of their day at work. Safety at work depends in part on staying aware of the following:

- fire evacuation procedures
- the location of the nearest fire extinguisher and first aid kit

In a hazardous work environment, wear recommended safety equipment and follow safety procedures (Figure 20-7). Remember: safety is everyone's responsibility. Know the requirements for safety in the workplace. In all settings:

- don't take shortcuts
- don't take risks—the job isn't that important
- follow local requirements for safety precautions

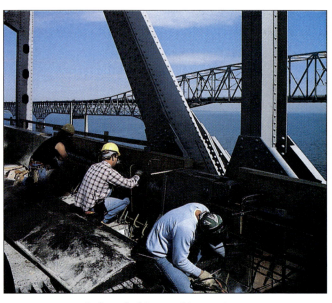

FIGURE 20-7 *Safety clothing and/or equipment are required for some jobs.*

Motor Vehicle Safety

Buckle up—always. Wearing a seat belt is the easiest and best way to prevent injury in a motor vehicle collision. Infants and children should always ride in approved safety seats. All states have regulations for the use of child safety seats. Safe driving habits are just as important. Don't take the car for granted—it's a lethal weapon!

Safety at Play

Make sports and other recreational activities safe by always following accepted guidelines for the activity (Figures 20-8, 20-9, 20-10).

When bicycling, always wear an approved helmet. Children should do likewise, even if they are still going along the footpath on training wheels. Most bike mishaps happen within a kilometre of home. The head or neck is the most commonly injured part of the body in most cycling fatalities. Wear an approved helmet. Keep off roads which are busy or have no shoulder. Wear reflective clothing and use reflectors on bike wheels for cycling at night.

With any activity in which the eyes could be injured, such as squash, wear protective goggles. Appropriate footwear is also important for preventing injuries. For activities involving physical contact, wear properly fitted protective equipment to avoid serious injury. Above all, know and follow the rules of the sport.

Those who do not know how to swim should learn how or always wear an appropriate flotation device in or around the water. Undercurrents can be dangerous even in shallow water. Be careful when walking beside rivers, lakes and other bodies of water. Two-thirds of all drownings happen to people who never intended to be in the water at all.

When exercising, remember to do appropriate warmup and cooldown exercises to help the body adjust and prevent injury.

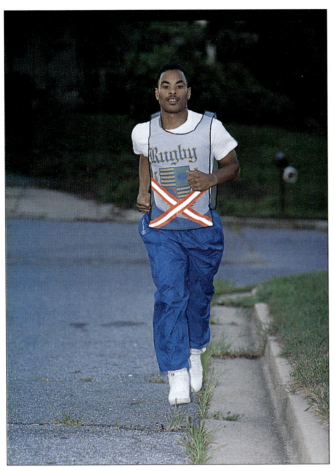

FIGURE 20-8 *Wear proper safety equipment during recreational activities.*

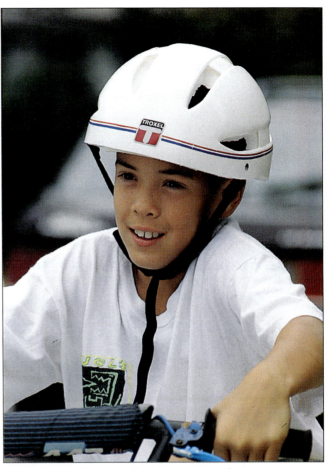

FIGURE 20-9 *When cycling, everyone needs to wear approved head protection gear, including children.*

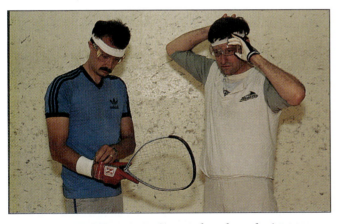

FIGURE 20-10 *Wear protective goggles when playing a sport such as squash, in which the eyes could be injured.*

Carefully plan a route for running, jogging or walking safely. Exercise only in well-lit, well-populated areas. Keep off busy roads. Wear reflective clothing and move facing the traffic if you must run or walk on the side of the road.

Whenever starting an activity which is unfamiliar, such as boating, skiing, motorcycle riding or any sport, take lessons to learn how to do the sport safely. Many mishaps result from inexperience. Make sure that equipment is in good working order. Ski bindings, for instance, should be professionally inspected, adjusted and lubricated before each season. Costly, yes—but so is a serious injury!

Summary

- Changing habits or acquiring new, healthier habits now help us live a better, longer life.

- Breaking unhealthy habits does not happen overnight, but becoming aware of them is an important first step.

- Good nutrition, weight maintenance and regular exercise all promote good health.

- Stopping smoking and avoiding excessive alcohol use lowers the risk of illness.

- Safety habits at home, in the car and at work will help prevent injuries.

Study Questions

1.   Describe two things people can do to improve their diet.

2.   List three healthy ways to handle stress.

3.   List two health dangers caused by the use of tobacco.

4.   List three ways a person can keep alcohol consumption under control.

5.   List three elements of a fire escape plan.

6.   List two things to pay attention to for safety at work.

7.   List four ways to prevent injuries during sports and recreational activities.

8.   List four ways to turn daily activities into exercise.

9.   Identify the most important action for avoiding injury in a motor vehicle crash.

10. List activities which improve cardiovascular fitness.

11. *Cardiovascular fitness increases muscular endurance, strength, and flexibility. It may also help us to:*

    a. sleep better

    b. ward off infections

    c. cope with stress.

    d. a and c.

    e. a, b and c.

12. *Which of the following helps a person sober up after having too much to drink?*

    a. Hot coffee.

    b. A cold shower.

    c. Time.

    d. a and b.

    e. a, b and c.

13. *List four ways to improve safety in the home.*

14. *Write a healthy meal plan for one day. Include breakfast, lunch, and dinner. Use actual foods, for example, "one slice of wholemeal toast," and use foods you like to eat.*

Answers are in Appendix A (page 363).

STUDY QUESTION ANSWERS

CHAPTER 1

1. b, c, e, d, a.

2. To preserve life; to protect the unconscious victim; to prevent the condition worsening and to relieve pain; to promote recovery.

3. Unusual noises—breaking glass; screeching tyres; moaning; calling for help; screaming; abrupt or loud unidentifiable noises; unusual odours—strong smell of petrol, chlorine, smoke, unidentifiable fumes; unusual appearance or behaviour—collapsed person; confused behaviour; breathing difficulty; slurred, hesitant, confused speech; uncharacteristic skin colour; sweating for no apparent reason; unusual sights—stalled vehicle; overturned pot; spilled medicine container; fallen electrical wires.

4. Presence of bystanders; uncertainty about the victim; nature of the injury or illness; fear of disease transmission; fear of doing something wrong.

5. Call for an ambulance; watch for and meet ambulance; keep area free of unnecessary traffic; get blankets or other supplies; provide information about incident or victim; help comfort victim and others.

6. Keep important information about yourself and your family in a handy place. Find out local emergency numbers; keep in a handy place. Keep medical and insurance records up to date. Keep a first aid kit stocked and easily accessible in your home, work, and recreation areas. Learn and stay practiced in first aid skills. Make sure your house or apartment number is easy to read. Develop a plan of action for emergencies that may occur, such as a fire, flood and cyclone. Wear a medical alert tag if you have a potentially serious medical condition.

7. g, a, b, c, e, f, d.

8. Screech of tyres, crash of metal; car smashed into pole; pole at odd angle; wires hanging from pole; vehicle stalled in middle of the street.

9. The emergency dispatcher may not have received the call until later because no one decided to act by calling 000 or the local emergency number, or because no one could get out of the traffic to call. The emergency dispatcher may have had a number of calls all coming in at the same time and been unable to dispatch the appropriate help. The dispatcher may not have been given the correct location of the emergency. The ambulance may have become stuck in traffic on the way to the crash because onlookers abandoned their vehicles. Once on the scene, ambulance officers may have evaluated a need for advanced medical help. Victims may have been trapped in vehicles, requiring extensive work to pry apart the wreckage.

CHAPTER 2

1. (a) respiratory (b) airway, lungs (c) circulatory (d) transports oxygen and other nutrients to cells and removes wastes (e) skin, hair, nails (f) helps keep fluid in, prevents infection, sweat glands and pores in skin help regulate temperature, helps make vitamin D, stores minerals (g) bones, ligaments, muscles, tendons (h) supports body, allows movement, protects internal organs and structures, produces blood cells, stores minerals, produces heat (i) nervous (j) brain, spinal cord, nerves.

2. o, d, l, m, g, c, k, i, a, e, h , f, j, b, n.

3. d.

4. c.

5. b.

6. d.

7. Any damage to the spinal cord or a nerve could interrupt or completely cut off the conduction of impulses to an area of the body. No nerve impulses would reach the area—it would be paralysed.

CHAPTER 3

1. b, a, d, b, d, d, c, a, b, a, b, a.

2. Survey the scene. Do a primary survey and care for life-threatening conditions. Call emergency personnel for help. Do a secondary survey, when appropriate, and care for other injuries or conditions that may need care.

3. Unconsciousness, altered conscious state; breathing problems; persistent chest or abdominal pain or pressure; no pulse; severe bleeding; vomiting blood or passing blood; poisoning; seizures; severe headache or slurred speech; injuries to head, neck, and back; possible broken bones.

4. (1) Is the scene safe? (2) What happened? (3) How many victims are there? (4) Are there bystanders who can help?.

5. Your exact location; telephone number from which the call is being made; caller's name; what happened; number of people involved; condition of victim(s); help that is being given.

6. Check conscious state; check for clear and open airway; check that the person is breathing; check that the person has a pulse; check for severe bleeding.

7. Do a secondary survey only when no life-threatening conditions exist. In a secondary survey, you look for other injuries or conditions that may need care.

8. (a) 6, (b) 4, (c) 1, (d) 5, (e) 2, (f) 3.

9. c.

10. b.

11. Because a motor vehicle is involved, ask if anyone has called emergency personnel. If not, ask someone to do so. Then follow the emergency action principles. Survey the scene. Traffic may be dangerous to you or others. Ask questions. Find out details such as what happened and how many people were involved. If you determine that it is safe to approach, do so. Once at the victim's side, begin a primary survey. Find out if the victim is conscious, has a clear airway, is breathing, has a pulse, or is bleeding severely. While you begin appropriate care, instruct other bystanders to redirect traffic, watch for the ambulance, keep onlookers from crowding in, get any materials you need, and help you provide care, if necessary.

CHAPTER 4

1. b, e, a, f, d, c.

2. e.

3. c.

4. b.

5. a, d, b, c, e.

6. Victim is unconscious, not breathing and has no pulse.

7. Another trained rescuer arrives and takes over. Ambulance personnel arrive and take over. You are physically unable to continue. The scene suddenly becomes unsafe.

8. e.

9. c.

10. b.

11. 2, 3, 1, 4, 5.

12. d.

CHAPTER 5

1. c, g, a, f, e, d, b, h.

2. Transports oxygen, nutrients, and wastes; protects against disease by producing antibodies and defending against germs; maintains constant body temperature by circulating throughout the body.

3. Blood spurting from a wound; blood that fails to clot after all measures have been taken to control bleeding.

4. Apply direct pressure using your hand. If a sterile gauze pad or other clean material is available, place it between the wound and your hand. Elevate the injured area if possible. Maintain pressure by applying a pressure bandage.

5. b, e, c, a, d.

6. History of injury or medical condition that could lead to internal bleeding; discolouration of the skin in the injured area; soft tissues, such as those in the abdomen, that are tender, swollen, or hard; anxiety or restlessness; rapid, weak pulse; rapid breathing; cool, moist skin or pale or bluish skin; nausea and vomiting; excessive thirst; declining level of consciousness.

7. 3, 4, 1, 2.

8. 4, 1, 2, 3.

9. A person who is close by could call emergency personnel, find materials for bandaging, reassure your father, watch for the ambulance, and get other materials, such as a blanket, that you might need to help maintain your father's body temperature.

10. a.

11. Place an effective barrier between yourself and the victim's blood. Wash your hands thoroughly with soap and water after providing care. Avoid eating, drinking, and touching your mouth, nose, or eyes while providing care or before washing your hands.

CHAPTER 6

1. b, c, a.

2. Restlessness; fast breathing; drowsiness; pale, cold, moist skin; rapid, weak pulse; unconsciousness; irregular breathing.

3. Medical emergencies: sudden illnesses and severe injuries; significant pain; fear.

4. Monitor the ABC. Care for any life-threatening problems. Help the victim rest comfortably. Help the victim maintain normal body temperature. Reassure the victim. Provide care for specific conditions.

5. e.

6. b.

7. a.

8. e.

9. b.

10. Shock is life-threatening because the circulatory system fails to circulate oxygen-rich blood to all parts of the body, causing vital organs to fail to function properly.

11. Elevating the legs helps to maintain blood flow to the vital organs.

CHAPTER 7

1. f, d, a, g, h, b, e, c.

2. Gasping for air; shortness of breath; breathing faster or slower than normal; making unusual noises such as wheezing, crowing, or gurgling; unusually deep or shallow breathing; unusually moist skin; flushed, pale, or bluish skin; dizziness or lightheadedness; pain in the chest; tingling in the hands or feet; apprehensiveness or fear.

3. Trying to swallow large pieces of poorly chewed food; drinking alcohol in excessive amounts before or during meals; wearing dentures; eating while talking excitedly or laughing, or eating too fast; walking, playing, or running with food or objects in the mouth.

4. Shortness of breath; wheezing when exhaling; dry or moist cough; thirst; increased pulse rate; drawing in of the spaces between ribs and above collarbone; cyanosis; collapse.

5. a.

6. b.

7. (a) T, (b) F, (c) F, (d)T, (e) F, (f) T, (g) T, (h) F, (i) F, (j) F.

8. a.

9. c.

10. b.

11. d.

CHAPTER 8

1. d, b, f, h, c, g, e, a.

2. High blood pressure; cigarette smoking; diets high in saturated fats and cholesterol; lack of regular exercise.

3. c.

4. d.

5. d.

6. d.

7. b.

8. b.

9. b.

10. a.

CHAPTER 9

1. f, c, h, g, e, a, d, b.

2. If the victim is unresponsive, turn the person onto the side, keeping the head and neck supported. Care for the ABC. Call for an ambulance. Maintain body temperature. Continue to monitor conscious state and ABC.

3. c.

4. Wearing seat belts including shoulder restraints; wearing approved helmets, eyewear, faceguards, and mouthguards, when appropriate; preventing falls; obeying rules in sports and recreational activities; avoiding inappropriate use of drugs; inspecting work and recreational equipment; thinking and talking about safety.

5. d.

6. d.

7. When the seizure lasts more than a few minutes; when the victim has repeated seizures; when the victim appears to be injured; when you are uncertain about the cause of the seizure; when the victim is pregnant; when the victim is a known diabetic; when the victim is an infant or child; when the seizure takes place in water; when the victim fails to regain consciousness after the seizure.

8. e.

9. c.

10. a.

11. b.

12. d.

CHAPTER 10

1. f, e, b, g, c, a, h, d.

2. Nausea; vomiting; diarrhoea; chest or abdominal pain; breathing difficulty; sweating; loss of consciousness; seizures.

3. The type of substance; the amount of substance; how it entered the body; the victim's size, weight and age.

4. Apply a firm bandage over the bite site. Use a second bandage, starting at the fingers or toes and working up the limb as far as possible. Immobilise the limb with a splint. Help the victim to rest.

5. Wear long-sleeved shirts and long pants. Tuck pant legs into socks or boots. Tuck shirt into pants. Wear light-coloured clothing. Use a rubber band or tape the area where pants and socks meet so nothing can get under clothing. Stay in the middle of trails and avoid underbrush and tall grass. Wear hiking boots. Avoid areas populated with snakes. If you see a snake, look for others. Walk back on the same path. Inspect carefully for insects or ticks after being outdoors. If you are outdoors for a long time, check yourself several times during the day, especially in hairy areas of the body. Spray pets that go outdoors with repellent if you are in a grassy or wooded area or if the area is infested with insects or ticks.

6. Keep all repellents out of the reach of children. Never spray permethrin on your skin or a child's skin. Never use repellents on children's hands. Use repellents sparingly. Wash repellent-treated skin after coming indoors. If you suspect you are having a reaction to a repellent, wash treated skin immediately and call your doctor.

7. Wash the area thoroughly with large amounts of water. Call the Poisons Information Centre number for advice. Continue to flush the area until ambulance personnel arrive.

8. c.

9. e.

10. a.

11. d.

12 The area around the sting site becomes red or swollen. Your friend feels nauseated, dizzy, or weak; or vomits; or experiences breathing difficulty.

CHAPTER 11

1. b, f, a, c, d, e.

2. Heat, chemicals, electricity, and radiation.

3. Superficial, partial-thickness, full-thickness.

4. c.

5. e.

6. c.

7. c, e, d, a, b.

8. Pale; sweating heavily; feeling weak, nauseated, dizzy.

9. You could have worn lightweight clothing that allowed the air to pass through and a hat; have taken frequent breaks; and have drunk water often.

10. She could have you rest comfortably and give you cool water to drink slowly.

11. White, waxy, cold fingers that lack feeling .

12. Cover the affected areas, handling them gently. Do not rub. Warm the areas gently by soaking them in water no warmer than 36–38°C. Test the water. If it is uncomfortable to the touch, it is too warm. Do not let the affected areas touch the bottom or sides of the container. When the affected areas look red and feel warm, bandage them with a dry, sterile dressing, and seek professional medical attention.

CHAPTER 12

1. b, d, a, c.

2. b, c, d, a.

3. Pain and soreness persisting in the wound; swelling and redness; warmth around the area; pus; fever; swelling and tenderness in lymph glands.

4. d.

5. d.

6. a.

7. e.

8. c.

9. a.

10. a.

11. You should not put pressure over the depressed area. Control bleeding by applying pressure around the area of the injury.

CHAPTER 13

1. To absorb blood and other fluids and to provide a barrier against infection.

2. d.

3. a.

4. e.

5. Hold dressings in place. Apply pressure to control bleeding. Protect a wound from dirt and infection. Provide support to the injured part.

6. d.

7. c.

8. d.

9. d.

10. b.

CHAPTER 14

1. h, b, f, c, a, i, k, d, j, g, e.

2. Splint only if you can do it without causing more pain and discomfort to the victim. Splint an injury in the position you find it. Splint the injured area and the joint above and below the injury site. Check for proper circulation before and after splinting.

3. A fall from a height greater than the victim's height; any diving mishap; a person found unconscious for unknown reasons; any injury involving severe blunt force to the head or trunk; any injury that penetrates the head or trunk; a motor vehicle crash involving a driver or passengers not wearing safety belts; any person thrown from a motor vehicle; any injury in which a victim's helmet is broken; lightning strike.

4. Changes in the level of consciousness; severe pain or pressure in the head, neck, or back; tingling or loss of sensation in the extremities; partial or complete loss of movement of any body part; unusual bumps or depressions on the head or spine; blood or other fluids in the ears or nose; profuse external bleeding of the head, neck or back; seizures; impaired breathing or vision as a result of injury; nausea or vomiting; persistent headache; loss of balance; bruising of the head, especially around the eyes and behind the ears.

5. d.

6. d.

7. b.

8. e.

9. d.

10. Call an ambulance if you suspect a serious injury; monitor the ABC; control bleeding; minimise shock; support or immobilise the injured part; rest the injured part.

11. Injured leg appears noticeably shorter than the other leg; injured leg is turned outward; severe pain; inability to move the leg.

CHAPTER 15

1. False.

2. True.

3. b.

4. d.

CHAPTER 16

1. b.

2. d.

3. a.

4. b.

5. a.

CHAPTER 17

1. Move a victim only if there is immediate danger such as a fire, lack of oxygen, risk of drowning, risk of explosion, collapsing structure, or uncontrollable traffic hazards.

2. Assisted walk; two-person assisted walk; two-handed seat carry; four-handed seat carry; fore and aft carry; chair lift; arm drag; clothes drag; wheelchair lift; stretcher moves.

3. Bend at the knees and hips and lift with your legs, not your back; keep back straight and head erect; keep centre of gravity low and feet spread about shoulder width apart, with one foot slightly forward.

4. c.

CHAPTER 18

1. b.

2. May last 10 to 16 hours or more for a first delivery, or 10 hours or less for later deliveries.

3. b.

4. a.

5. c.

6 a.

7. d.

8. c.

9. a.

CHAPTER 19

1. f, c, d, e, a, h, b, g.

2. Difficulty breathing; chest pain; altered level of consciousness; moist or flushed skin; mood changes; nausea; vomiting; sweating; chills; fever; headache; dizziness; rapid pulse; rapid breathing; restlessness; excitement; irritability; talkativeness; hallucinations; confusion; slurred speech; poor co-ordination; trembling.

3. Alcohol; nicotine; caffeine; aspirin; laxatives; sleeping pills; diet pills.

4. Use common sense. Keep prescriptions in their appropriate containers. Clearly label all medications including when, how, and how often they should be taken. Dispose correctly of all left-over prescriptions. Never take another person's prescription or even one prescribed for you at a previous time.

5. Survey the scene to be sure it is safe. Do a primary survey and care for any life-threatening conditions. Call the local Poisons Information Centre or your local emergency number. Question the victim or bystanders. Find out what substance was taken, how much was taken, and when it was taken. Help maintain normal body temperature. Withdraw if the victim suddenly becomes violent or threatening. If you suspect someone has used a designer drug, tell ambulance personnel.

6. b, c, a, d.

7. c.

8. e.

9. Containers; drug paraphernalia; symptoms and signs of other medical problems.

CHAPTER 20

1. Buy and eat products that are low in saturated fat and cholesterol. Use unsaturated oils and fats for cooking and eating. Eat less salt by removing the salt shaker from the table and adding less salt when cooking. Include more fibre in your diet by eating more fruits, vegetables, and grains.

2. Exercise regularly. Develop hobbies. Avoid foods containing stimulants such as caffeine. Do relaxation exercises. Set realistic, attainable goals.

3. Lung cancer and cardiovascular (heart) disease.

4. Limit your drinks to one per hour. Have non-alcoholic beverages available. Do not drink before a party. Avoid drinking when angry or depressed. Eat plenty of food before and while drinking. Avoid salty foods. Do not play drinking games.

5. Develop and draw an escape plan with two exits from each room if possible. Plan where everyone will meet after leaving the building. Designate who should call the fire department and from which phone outside the burning building.

6. Know the fire evacuation procedure and the location of the nearest fire extinguisher and first aid kit. Wear recommended safety gear and follow safety procedures.

7. Know and follow rules recommended for the activity. Wear appropriate protective gear. Wear reflective clothing, when appropriate. Make sure your equipment is in good working order. Take lessons and learn how to participate safely in a new activity. Compete at a skill level appropriate for your skills and physical condition.

8. Walk or ride a bike instead of driving. Take the stairs instead of lifts or escalators. Pedal an exercise bike while watching TV, listening to music, or reading.

9. Wear a seat belt.

10. For example, walk; jog; run; bike; swim; hike; cross-country ski.

11. e.

12. c.

13. Refer to the list on pages 354–355.

14. Check this with your instructor.

FIRST AID AND DISEASE TRANSMISSION

Introduction

A disease which can be passed, or transmitted, from one person to another is called a communicable, or infectious, disease. Many diseases can be passed from one person to another, some more easily than others. It is natural to have concerns about disease transmission if you have to provide care in an emergency situation. These concerns have increased over the past few years as a result of the high level of public awareness of AIDS. This appendix presents basic information about how infections occur and the potential for disease transmission during first aid care. It also explains how you can protect yourself and others against disease transmission while giving first aid care.

How Infections Occur

Infection is a condition caused by disease-producing micro-organisms. When the body is invaded by these micro-organisms, the disease process begins. Most infections are caused by bacteria and viruses.

Bacteria are single-celled micro-organisms present throughout our environment. Bacteria do not depend on another organism for life and can live outside the body. Relatively few bacteria infect humans, but those which do can cause serious disease, such as tetanus. It is difficult for the body to fight a bacterial infection. Physicians may prescribe antibiotics which either kill the bacteria or weaken them enough that the body can overcome their effects.

Unlike bacteria, viruses are dependent on another organism to live. Once in the body, they are difficult to eliminate because few medications are effective in fighting viral infections. The body's immune system is the primary defence against them. Viruses cause many diseases, including the common cold.

How Diseases Can be Transmitted During First Aid Care

Your body has a natural defence system which protects it against disease—the skin and the immune system. However, in situations which require first aid care, communicable diseases can be transmitted by:

- contact (touching)
- breathing
- bites

Contact

Contact transmission occurs when one touches an infected person or a contaminated object. Micro-organisms in a person's blood and other body fluids can enter another person's body through breaks or cuts in the skin or through the membranes of the eyes or mouth, causing infection. Direct contact with blood or other body fluids carries the greatest risk of infection. Infections transmitted by blood are referred to as blood-borne infections.

Infection can also be transmitted by contact with objects which have been contaminated with the blood or other body fluids of an infected person. Even though your intact skin protects you from diseases transmitted by contact, sharp objects handled carelessly can pierce your skin and transmit infection to you. Therefore, be extremely careful when handling potentially contaminated objects and avoid touching blood with your bare hands unless absolutely necessary.

Breathing

Infections transmitted through air are called airborne infections. You can become infected if you breathe in droplets which become airborne when someone who has an infection, such as a cold or flu, sneezes. You are at no greater risk of such an infection when giving first aid than when associating with family, friends or colleagues, or when in public places.

Bites

An animal, such as a dog or possum, or an insect, such as a tick, can transmit disease through a bite. Rabies and Lyme disease are transmitted in this way. A human bite can also transmit disease. Providing first aid care rarely involves the danger of being bitten by an animal or a person. Therefore, in an emergency situation, contracting a disease through a bite is rare.

Specific Communicable Diseases

Some communicable diseases, such as the common cold, are more easily transmitted than others. Although it does cause minor discomfort for the sufferer, the common cold is short-lived and rarely has serious consequences. Other diseases, such as hepatitis B and HIV infection, are far more dangerous. Hepatitis B is a serious liver disease which can last for months. A person infected with HIV (human immunodeficiency virus), who eventually develops AIDS (acquired immune deficiency syndrome), can become a victim of many infections which have fatal consequences.

However, these serious diseases are not easily transmitted. They are not spread through casual contact. For instance, the principal ways people become infected with HIV include sexual contact—through semen or vaginal fluid; blood-to-blood contact—through sharing needles or syringes with an infected person; and mother-to-child contact—before, during, or just after birth, or, rarely, through breast milk. The virus does not live in a dry environment for more than a few hours, and is killed by alcohol, chlorine bleach, and other common disinfectants. Once it is killed, you cannot reactivate the virus by adding water.

The risk of infection by HIV through any other means is extremely low. In a first aid situation in which the rescuer comes into contact with a person's blood, there is a higher risk of infection with other diseases, such as hepatitis B, than with HIV.

You may be concerned about disease transmission via saliva if you have to give expired air resuscitation. Saliva is not known to transmit HIV and the risk is only theoretical.

If you are in a situation in which you might be called upon to give first aid frequently, especially where expired air resuscitation is likely to be required, you should consider using a resuscitation mask. Using a resuscitation mask allows you to give EAR without mouth-to-mouth contact. If you wish to carry and use a resuscitation face mask, you will need to attend a CPR revision and recertification course every year to maintain your skills.

How to Reduce the Risk of Infection

Remember that you are most likely to give first aid to yourself or someone you know, such as a family member, whose health status you may know. One of the easiest steps you can take to prevent infection while giving first aid is to maintain good personal hygiene practices, such as handwashing before and immediately after giving care.

In addition, because germs can enter the body through breaks in the skin, you should always try to take precautions to prevent direct contact with a person's body fluids when giving first aid.

To reduce the risk of infection while you are giving care, you should:

- avoid touching or being splashed by body fluids when possible.

- place an effective barrier between you and the victim's body fluids. Ideally, you should use disposable latex gloves whenever possible. In an emergency when gloves are not available and you have to control bleeding, ask the victim to help you by applying direct pressure, or place a dressing or other clean, dry cloth between your hand and the wound.

- cover any cuts, scrapes, or skin conditions you may have by wearing protective clothing such as disposable latex gloves.

- wash your hands thoroughly with soap and water immediately after providing care, even if you wore gloves. Use a utility or rest room sink, not one in a food preparation area.

- avoid eating, drinking and touching your mouth, nose, or eyes while providing care or before washing your hands.

- avoid touching objects which may be contaminated with blood or other body fluids.

- avoid handling any personal items, such as a pen or comb, while providing care or before washing your hands.

- be prepared with an adequately stocked first aid kit which includes ready-to-use antiseptic wipes and disposable latex gloves.

The precautions listed above are part of widely accepted practices. If you take appropriate safety measures, risk of infection is minimal. Always give first aid care in ways which protect you and the victim from disease transmission. Use protective barriers which are appropriate to the emergency, and wash your hands thoroughly as soon as possible after giving first aid care.

LEGAL INFORMATION

The following information is intended as a guide only, and to answer commonly asked questions. It is also hoped that it will assist in resolving doubts or suspicions about the possibility of legal action which may suppress a first aider's natural desire to render assistance.

Legal Implications of First Aid

You should be aware of four legal considerations related to first aid: consent, duty of care, negligence, and recording.

Consent

Australian law is based on the premise that all people have control over their own bodies. If a person is touched or in fear of being touched without consenting to it, that person can bring a charge of assault or battery. Therefore, before you start helping a victim, you should ask for and receive the victim's consent for you to give first aid. In an emergency where a victim is unconscious or bleeding seriously and unable to communicate, the law assumes the injured person would give consent. This consent applies only to conditions that imperil the life or future health of the person.

If the victim is a minor, obtain the consent of a parent or guardian if possible. In a life-threatening situation without a parent or guardian present to give consent, you can assume consent and give first aid.

Duty of Care

Australian law does not impose a duty on any person to render assistance unless you already owe a "duty of care" to the person injured. You may owe a duty of care to a person, however, if you are responsible for the injured person. You also take on a duty of care once you begin giving first aid in an emergency. An employee whose job responsibilities include giving first aid also has a duty of care for first aid to someone in the workplace.

Once you begin giving first aid, you have a duty of care to do everything reasonable in the circumstances. You cannot abandon the victim once you have begun, because you now have taken on this duty. You can, of course, let a medical practitioner or other person with better qualifications take over when they arrive at the scene.

When you follow the rules and do so with ordinary skill, you will have met the duty of care required.

Negligence

A person can be guilty of negligence only if all four of the following factors are established:

1. The first aider owed a duty of care to the victim.
2. The first aider breached the standard of care required by that duty.
3. The victim sustained damage.
4. The victim's damage was caused by the first aider's breach of the standard of care.

First aiders with basic first aid training could be expected to:

- use reasonable care in assessing the priorities of the situation based on their training, and take steps to call for medical assistance
- keep the victim stabilised until professional help is available
- follow established protocols
- follow the guidelines in this Manual
- not misrepresent themselves or take undue risks

In the unlikely event that a first aider was sued, the court would look at all of the circumstances to determine what was "reasonable" in the particular situation.

The concept of reasonableness is so basic in law that it is difficult to define it precisely. Reasonableness certainly relates to the reasons one has for making decisions and taking action (or failing to take action). The evidence of professionals would probably be considered, and this Manual reviewed to identify the rules that should have been followed.

A court might look at some of the following questions:

- What did the first aider know at the time about the problem?
- What should the first aider have discovered by asking questions and having a thorough look?
- What were the important questions to ask and signs to observe?
- What are the rules in this Manual for managing the problem that was assessed?

For example, consider a situation in which the first aider gives cardiopulmonary resuscitation (CPR) in an emergency (see Chapter 4). A reasonable and prudent rescuer would be expected to check the victim's response, airway, breathing, and circulation before starting CPR. A reasonable and prudent rescuer would not start CPR on a person who had merely fainted. A reasonable and prudent rescuer is not expected to perform miracles: common sense and a reasonable degree of skill are all that the law would require under such emergency circumstances.

Moreover, a person who needs CPR is unconscious, non-breathing, and pulseless. This victim will die if appropriate emergency medical care, including CPR, is not given. If CPR fails to restore life, the victim will be no worse off than before. A victim who survives, however, will have nothing to complain about, even if the CPR caused some physical injury such as broken ribs. The only alternative was death. Of course, whenever the first aid procedure does carry a risk of injury, as is the case with CPR, only a first aider with the correct level of skill and training should attempt it.

With reasonableness as the main standard for judging actions, we are not aware of any documented case in Australia, Canada, or America where any first aider has been successfully sued after giving emergency first aid.

Recording

In case of any later dispute, a first aider should make a record at the time of the injury. This record should describe what was known about the problem and what was done. In the workplace, Senior and Occupational first aiders must keep a record of every incident. The particular forms to use and the details to record vary from State to State, according to State laws. Even in emergencies outside the workplace, the first aider should write at least a note about any first aid given.

Be careful with how you write this record, because it could be used one day as a legal document in court. Records should be clear and concise. They should be accurate and factual, reflecting your observations only and not opinions or attempts at medical conclusions.

Employers want to ensure that first aid has been given appropriately, because they have legal liability when a first aider gives assistance as an employment responsibility. Give the employer a copy of any first aid report. Follow any applicable industrial laws or guidelines supplied by the employer.

Follow these general guidelines for preparing a first aid report:

1. Write only in ink.

2. Sign and date the record and any alterations to it.

3. Do not use correction fluid to correct mistakes. Cross out any incorrect entry, leaving it legible still; initial the correction.

4. Keep the information in the record confidential.

GLOSSARY
Pronunciation Guide

Abrasion: An open wound in which the skin has been rubbed or scraped away; often called a graze.

Abdomen: The middle part of the body, situated between the chest and the pelvis, containing organs such as the stomach, liver, and spleen.

Abscess *(ab-sess)*: A collection of pus in a tissue cavity following infection.

Absorbed poison: A poison that enters the body through the skin or mucous membranes.

Addiction: The compulsive need to use a substance. An addicted user initially suffers mental, physical, social and emotional distress after stopping.

Airway: The pathway for air from the mouth and nose to the lungs.

Airway obstruction: Partial or complete blockage of the airway which either prevents or makes it difficult for air to reach a person's lungs.

Alimentary *(al-i-men-ta-ry)* **canal:** The long passage through which food passes and is digested and absorbed; it extends from the mouth to the anus.

Allergy: A disorder in which the body becomes over-sensitive to a particular substance; different allergies affect different tissues and may have local or general effects.

Alveoli *(al-vee-o-ly)*: The air sacs of the lungs in which the exchange of oxygen and carbon dioxide takes place.

Amnesia *(am-nee-zee-a)*: A total or partial loss of memory often caused by a concussion or other head injury.

Amniotic sac *(im-nee-ot-ic)*: A fluid-filled sac that encloses and protects the developing foetus in the uterus; commonly called the bag of waters.

Amputation: An injury in which an appendage, such as a finger or toe, arm or leg, has been completely severed from the body.

Analgesics *(an-al-gee-ziks)*: Drugs used for the relief of pain.

Anaphylaxis *(a-naf-il-ak-sis)*: A severe allergic reaction; a form of shock.

Aneurysm *(an-yoo-riz-m)*: A weakness in the wall of a blood vessel which may rupture.

Angina *(an-jy-na)*: A condition which occurs when the coronary arteries become seriously narrowed by disease and the supply of oxygenated blood to the heart becomes insufficient for the increased oxygen needed during activity. It is characterised by pain or pressure in the chest which is relieved by rest and/or medication.

Angulated *(ang-gyu-lay-ted)*: Sharply bent.

Ankle drag: An emergency move in which you pull the victim away from a danger by the legs.

Antibiotic: A substance used to block the growth of certain micro-organisms or kill them.

Antibody: A disease-fighting protein that helps protect the body against specific infections.

Anticoagulant *(anti-co-ag-yu-lant)*: A substance or drug that stops or reduces the coagulation, or clotting, of the blood; used to prevent blood clots within the body.

Antidote: A substance given to counteract the effects of a poison.

Antiseptic: A substance which helps to limit the growth and spread of micro-organisms in and around a wound.

Antivenom: An antiserum containing antibodies against specific poisons in the venom of snakes, spiders, or scorpions; used in treatment of bites or stings (formerly known as antivenene).

Appendicitis: Inflammation of the appendix causing abdominal pain.

Arteries: Large blood vessels that carry oxygen- rich blood from the heart to all parts of the body.

Arthritis: An inflammatory condition of the joints causing pain and swelling.

Asepsis *(ay-sep-sis)*: Protection against infection by using sterile techniques in wound cleaning and other procedures.

Aspiration: The contamination of the air passages of the lungs with foreign material such as blood, vomit, broken teeth, or other foreign bodies.

Assisted walk: A planned move in which you support and assist the victim to walk.

Asthma *(ass-ma)*: A condition in which the air passages become narrowed by muscle spasm, swelling of mucous membranes, and increased mucus production.

Atherosclerosis *(ath-e-ro-scle-ro-sis)*: Condition in which blood vessels are narrowed by the build-up of cholesterol and other deposits.

Aura: An unusual sensation or feeling which a victim may experience before an epileptic seizure; it may be a visual hallucination; a strange sound, taste, or smell; an urgent need to get to safety.

Automatic external defibrillator *(dee-fib-ril-a-tor)* **(AED):** A device used to monitor heart rhythms and administer an electric shock to cardiac arrest victims in an attempt to restore normal heart rhythm.

Avulsion: An injury in which a portion of the skin and sometimes other soft tissue is partially or completely torn away.

Bacteria: A group of micro-organisms capable of causing infection.

Bandage: Material used to wrap or cover a part of the body, commonly used to hold a dressing or splint in place.

Bile: A yellow-green secretion of the liver that is stored in the gallbladder and released to help the body digest and absorb fat.

Birth canal: The passageway from the uterus to the vaginal opening through which a baby passes at birth.

Bladder: A sac-shaped organ in the pelvis in which urine is stored until released.

Blood clot: A coagulated mass formed by the clotting of blood.

Blood pressure: The pressure exerted on the artery walls by the circulating volume of blood.

Blood volume: The total amount of blood circulating within the body.

Body mechanics: The principles for moving and lifting in ways that prevent straining your body or putting yourself at risk of injury.

Body splinting: Using a body part to support an injured one, such as using an uninjured leg to support an injured one.

Bone: A dense, hard tissue that forms the skeleton.

Booster shot: A smaller dose of a vaccine given to help maintain the antibodies produced as a result of an initial immunisation.

BPC dressing: A machine-compressed sterile combine dressing stitched to a bandage, used for controlling bleeding to a large area; commonly used by defence personnel and also known as mines or field dressings. (BPC refers to British Pharmacopoeia Codex, an international published standard for drugs and bandages.)

Brain: The centre of the nervous system that controls all body functions.

Breathing emergency: Emergency in which breathing is so impaired that life is threatened.

Breech delivery: The delivery of a baby with feet or buttocks first.

Bronchi (brong-kee): The large passages through which air passes to and from the lungs.

Burn: An injury to the skin or other body tissues caused by heat, chemicals, electricity, or radiation.

Calipering: The method of locating the position on the chest for chest compressions, found by locating the notches at the upper and lower ends of the sternum with the index fingers of both hands and exten-ding the thumbs an equal distance to meet in the middle of the sternum.

Capillaries (ca-pil-er-eez): Tiny blood vessels linking arteries and veins that transfer oxygen and other nutrients from the blood to all body cells and remove waste products.

Carbon dioxide: A colourless, odourless gas that is a waste product of respiration.

Cardiac arrest: Condition in which the heart has stopped or is too weak to pump effectively enough to provide a palpable pulse.

Cardiopulmonary (car-dee-o-pul-mon-ry) resuscitation (re-sus-i-tay-shon) (CPR): The technique combining expired air resuscitation and external chest compressions for a victim whose breathing and heart have stopped.

Cardiovascular (car-dee-o-vask-yoo-lar) disease: Disease of the heart and blood vessels; commonly known as heart disease.

Cardiovascular fitness: A healthy condition of the heart and blood vessels, attained through diet, exercise, and other good habits, in which cardiovascular disease is less likely.

Carotid (ca-rot-id) arteries: Major blood vessels that supply blood to the head and neck.

Cells: The basic units of all living tissue.

Cerebral compression: A condition of increased pressure inside the skull that compresses brain tissue and disrupts functioning.

Cervix: The upper part of the birth canal, between the vagina and the uterus.

Chair lift: A planned move in which two first aiders carry the victim in a chair.

Chest: The upper part of the trunk, containing the heart, major blood vessels, and lungs; also called the thorax.

Childbirth: The process of a baby being born, starting with the onset of labour.

Choking: Airway obstruction caused by a foreign body or swollen tissues.

Cholesterol: A fatty substance made by the body and found in certain foods. Too much cholesterol in the blood can cause fatty deposits on artery walls which may restrict or block blood flow.

Circulatory: Relating to the movement of blood through the heart and blood vessels.

Clavicle (klav-i-kl): See collarbone.

Closed wound: A wound in which soft tissue damage occurs beneath unbroken skin.

Clothes drag: An emergency move in which you pull the victim away from a danger by clothing gathered behind the neck.

Clotting: The process by which blood thickens at a wound site to seal an opening in a blood vessel and stop bleeding.

Collarbone: A horizontal bone that connects with the sternum and the shoulder; also called the clavicle.

Combine dressing: A dressing made up of layers of gauze and cotton wool, used when bulk is needed for controlling bleeding or for absorbing discharge from a wound.

Concussion: A temporary impairment of brain function, usually without permanent damage to the brain, resulting from a shaking or jarring impact to the head.

Congestive heart failure: A condition in which the heart is weak and functions poorly because of chronic heart disease or old age.

Consent: Permission given by the victim to the first aider.

Contusion (kon-tyu-sion): A closed wound caused by force to the body; also called a bruise.

Coronary arteries: Blood vessels which supply the heart muscle with oxygen-rich blood.

Coronary (co-ron-ry) thrombosis (throm-bo-sis): A clot which blocks a coronary artery.

Corrosive: Having the power or tendency to destroy or eat away, sometimes through chemical action.

Critical burn: Any burn that is potentially life-threatening, disabling or disfiguring; a burn requiring medical attention.

Crowning: The time in labour when the baby's head shows at the opening of the vagina.

Cryogenic (cry-o-jen-ic) burn: A cold burn that results from contact with a substance such as liquid oxygen, liquid nitrogen, or snow and ice; similar to frostbite.

Cyanosis (sy-a-no-sis): A bluish discolouration of the skin, tongue and lining of the mouth.

Cyclone: A severe tropical storm system characterised by high to extreme winds and often heavy rain.

Deformity: A change in shape from the normal.

Dehydration *(de-hy-dray-shon)*: Excessive loss of water from the body tissues which leads to a disturbance in the balance of essential electrolytes; may follow any condition in which there is rapid depletion of body fluids.

Delivery: The part of the childbirth process when the baby emerges from the birth canal.

Dependency: The desire to continually use a substance.

Depressants: Substances which affect the central nervous system to slow down physical and mental activity and alleviate anxiety.

Dermis: The thick layer of living tissue that lies beneath the epidermis.

Designer drug: A potent and illegal street drug formed from a medicinal substance whose chemical composition has been modified ("designed").

Diabetes *(dy-a-bee-teez)*: Diabetes mellitus is a condition in which the body does not produce enough insulin.

Diabetic emergency: A condition in which a person becomes ill because of an imbalance of insulin.

Diaphragm *(dy-a-fram)*: A dome-shaped muscle that aids breathing and separates the chest from the abdomen.

Direct pressure: The pressure applied by hand on a wound to control bleeding.

Disease transmission: The transfer of disease.

Disease: An abnormal condition of the body that impairs normal function of cells, tissues or body systems.

Disinfectant: A chemical used to destroy harmful micro-organisms; it is stronger than an antiseptic and is not safe for use on human skin.

Dislocation: The displacement of a bone from its normal position at a joint.

Dressing: A pad placed directly on a wound to absorb blood and other body fluids and to provide a barrier against infection.

Drowning: Death by suffocation when submerged in water or other liquid.

Drug: Any substance other than food which affects the functions of the body.

Electrolytes *(e-lec-tro-lites)*: Elements or compounds found in blood and tissue fluids, e.g. potassium, sodium, and chloride. Proper quantities and a balance among them are essential for normal metabolism and function.

Embedded object: An object which remains fixed in a wound.

Embolism *(em-bo-liz-m)*: A piece of foreign material or tissue which travels through the bloodstream and blocks a blood vessel.

Embolus *(em-bo-lus)*: Air or fatty deposit which travels in the circulatory system, eventually lodging in and blocking a small blood vessel.

Emergency: A situation requiring immediate action.

Emergency action principles: Four steps to guide your actions in any emergency.

Emergency moves: Methods for quickly moving a victim to safety.

Envenomation *(en-ven-om-ay-shon)*: The injection of venom by a snake, spider, or other animal to kill or immobilise its prey or enemy.

Epidermis *(ep-i-der-mis)*: The outer layer of skin.

Epiglottis *(ep-i-glot-is)*: A small flap of tissue which covers the windpipe when food or liquids are swallowed.

Epilepsy *(ep-i-lep-see)*: A chronic condition characterised by seizures, which usually can be controlled by medication.

Exhale: To breathe air out of the lungs.

Expired air resuscitation (EAR): The technique of ventilating the lungs of a non-breathing victim.

External bleeding: Visible bleeding.

Extremities: The arms and legs, hands and feet.

Face mask: A rigid or semi-rigid device which covers the victim's mouth and nose to provide an airtight seal during expired air resuscitation.

Fainting: A loss of consciousness resulting from a temporary reduction of blood flow to the brain.

Femoral *(fem-o-ral)* **arteries:** The large arteries that supply the legs with oxygen-rich blood.

Femur *(fee-mur)*: The thighbone.

Fibre: A dietary substance found in some foods, notably fruit and vegetables, that contributes to good health.

Finger sweep: A technique used to remove foreign material from a victim's mouth.

First aid: Immediate care given to a victim of injury or sudden illness until more advanced care can be provided.

First aider: A person trained in first aid, who voluntarily gives first aid when needed.

Flash flood: Flood which results from surface water run-off after heavy rains; often with fast-rising water levels and swift currents.

Fore-and-aft carry: An emergency move in which two first aiders carry a victim away from a danger by lifting the victim under the arms and by the legs.

Forearm: The upper extremity from the elbow to the wrist.

Fracture: A break or disruption in bone tissue.

Frostbite: A serious condition in which body tissues freeze, commonly at the extremities, in the fingers, toes, ears, and nose.

Full-thickness burn: A burn injury involving both layers of skin and underlying tissues; skin may be charred.

Genitals: The external reproductive organs.

Germs: Disease-producing micro-organisms.

Haemophilia *(hee-mo-fil-ee-a)*: A disease more common in males caused by a lack of one or more clotting factors in the blood. Excessive bleeding internally and externally may follow minor trauma and may also occur spontaneously in the absence of trauma.

Haemorrhage *(hem-o-rage)*: A loss of a large amount of blood in a short period of time.

Hallucinogens *(hal-oo-sin-o-jenz)*: Substances which affect mood, sensation, thought, emotion and self-awareness; alter perceptions of time and space and produce delusions.

Hanging: The accidental or intentional suspension of the body's weight by something wrapped around the neck.

Hazardous material: Any substance, including liquids and gasses, used in the home or work place which can cause injury or illness if spilled or improperly handled

Heart: A fist-sized muscular organ which pumps blood throughout the body.

Heart attack: Damage which occurs to the heart muscle when blood supply in the coronary arteries is blocked and heart tissue does not receive enough oxygen-rich blood; also called myocardial infarction.

Heat exhaustion: A form of shock due to depletion of body fluids resulting from exposure to a hot environment.

Heat stroke: A life-threatening condition that develops when the body's temperature regulating and cooling mechanisms are overwhelmed and body systems begin to fail.

Hormone: A substance that circulates in body fluids and has a specific effect on cell activity.

Hostage: A person held involuntarily, usually by someone committing a criminal act.

Humerus *(hyu-me-rus)*: The bone of the upper arm.

Hyperglycaemia *(hy-per-gly-see-mee-a)*: A greater than normal amount of sugar in the bloodstream.

Hyperventilation *(hy-per-ven-til-ay-shon)*: A condition in which a person develops a carbon dioxide and oxygen imbalance in the body related to an altered pattern of breathing.

Hypoglycaemia *(hy-po-gly-see-mee-a)*: A less than normal amount of sugar in the bloodstream.

Hypothermia *(hy-po-ther-mee-a)*: A life-threatening condition in which the body's warming mechanisms fail to maintain normal body temperature and the entire body cools to 35°C or lower.

Immobilisation: The use of a splint or other method to keep an injured body part from moving.

Immune system: The body system that protects against infection.

Immunisation *(im-yoo-ny-zay-shon)*: The introduction of a specific substance into the body which builds resistance to an infection.

Infection: Condition caused by disease-producing micro-organisms in the body.

Ingested poison: A poison that is swallowed.

Inhalants *(in-hay-lants)*: Substances (gases or fumes) inhaled into the body to produce an effect.

Inhale: To breathe air into the lungs.

Inhaled poison: A poison breathed into the lungs.

Injected poison: A poison which enters the body through a bite, sting, or hypodermic needle.

Injection: The placing of a substance into the body through a bite, a sting, or a hypodermic needle.

Injury: Damage that occurs when the body is subjected to an external force such as a blow, a fall, or a collision.

Insulin *(in-su-lin)*: A hormone that enables the body to use sugar for energy; frequently used to treat diabetes.

Insulin-dependent diabetes: A type of diabetes that occurs when the body produces little or no insulin.

Internal bleeding: Bleeding inside the body.

Involuntary: Without conscious control or direction.

Ischaemia *(iss-kee-mee-a)*: A decreased supply of oxygen-rich blood to a body organ or part, often marked by pain and organ failure.

Jaw support: The technique of supporting the jaw at the point of the chin in a way which avoids any pressure on the soft tissues of the neck.

Jaw thrust: The technique of moving the jaw forward to open the airway by applying forward pressure behind the angle of the jaw.

Joint: A structure where two or more bones are joined.

Labour: The birth process beginning with the first contraction and lasting through delivery and stabilisation of the mother after delivery of the placenta.

Laceration *(lass-e-ray-shon)*: A jagged cut of the skin and possibly other soft tissue, usually from a sharp object.

Large intestine: Part of the alimentary canal where water and some minerals are absorbed from the digested material entering from the small intestine, and where waste products are prepared for elimination.

Ligament: A fibrous band that holds bones together at a joint.

Liver: A large abdominal organ that has many functions; when injured, it can bleed severely.

Lower leg: The lower extremity between the knee and the ankle.

Lungs: A pair of organs in the chest which provide the mechanism for taking oxygen in and removing carbon dioxide during breathing.

Lyme disease: An illness transmitted by a certain kind of infected tick.

Lymph *(limf)*: A fluid containing white cells that flows through body tissues to help the body fight infection.

Major incident: A situation in which several victims need care or abnormal environmental conditions complicate first aid management.

Medical emergency: A sudden illness requiring immediate medical attention.

Medication: A drug given to prevent or correct the effects of a disease or condition or otherwise enhance mental or physical welfare.

Membrane: A thin sheet of tissue that covers a structure or lines a cavity such as the mouth or nose.

Meningitis *(men-in-jy-tis)*: Infection or inflammation of the membranes covering the brain or spinal cord.

Micro-organism: A bacteria, virus, or other microscopic organism that may enter the body. Those that cause an infection or disease are commonly called germs.

Migraine: A recurring, usually severe type of headache which may last for hours or days.

Miscarriage: The spontaneous loss of a foetus before the 28th week of pregnancy, usually due to an abnormality of the foetus; also called a spontaneous abortion.

Muscle: A fibrous tissue that lengthens and shortens to create movement.

Muscular cramps: Painful spasms of skeletal muscles following exercise or work in warm or moderate temperatures, usually involving the calf and abdominal muscles.

Musculoskeletal *(musk-yoo-lo-skel-e-tal)*: Relating to the muscles and the skeleton.

Myocardial *(my-o-car-dee-al)* **infarction:** Damage which occurs to the heart muscle when blood supply in the coronary arteries is blocked; called heart attack.

Narcotics: Powerful depressant substances used to relieve anxiety and pain.

Narrow bandage: A triangular bandage folded to form a long, narrow strip.

Near-drowning: A situation in which a person who has been submerged in water survives.

Nerve: A part of the nervous system which carries impulses to and from the brain and all body parts.

Nutrients: Substances that provide nourishment, normally consumed as part of the diet to provide energy and material for growth.

Obesity: Weighing 20 percent more than desirable body weight, which increases the risk for certain illnesses.

Oesophagus *(ee-sof-a-guss)*: The tubular structure which carries food and liquids from the mouth into the stomach; also known as the gullet.

Open wound: A wound resulting in a break in the skin surface.

Organ: A group of specialised cells and tissues that work together to do a specific job.

Overdose: A situation in which a person takes enough of a substance that it has toxic (poisonous) or fatal effects.

Oxygen: A tasteless, colourless, odourless gas, which is essential to maintain life.

Pain: An unpleasant sensation caused by noxious stimulation of sensory nerve endings, often occurring as a symptom of infection or other disorders.

Pancreas *(pang-kree-as)*: An organ in the abdomen, lying behind the stomach, which makes insulin for the body.

Paramedic *(parra-med-ic)*: Someone certified after successfully completing an approved paramedic training program. Paramedics represent the highest level of ambulance officers.

Partial-thickness burn: A burn injury involving both layers of skin, characterised by red, wet skin and blisters.

Pelvis: The lower part of the trunk containing the intestines, bladder, and reproductive organs.

Personal flotation device (PFD): A buoyant device such as a cushion or life-jacket; designed to be held or worn to keep a person afloat.

Pharynx *(farrinks)*: A part of the airway formed by the back of the nose and throat.

Pistol grip position: A position of the hand on the victim's jaw to support the jaw during expired air resuscitation.

Placenta *(pla-sen-ta)*: The organ attached to the uterus and to the unborn child via the umbilical cord, for delivering nutrients to the baby in the uterus.

Plasma *(plaz-ma)*: The liquid part of blood.

Platelets *(plate-lets)*: Structures in the blood made up of cell fragments; essential for blood clotting.

Pleural *(plu-ral)* **cavity:** The space between the lungs and the chest wall.

Pneumothorax *(new-mo-thor-aks)*: A collection of air or gas in the pleural space that causes the lung to collapse (pneumo = air, thorax = chest).

Poison: Any substance that causes injury, illness, or death when introduced into the body.

Poisons Information Centre (PIC): A specialised reference centre in each capital city which provides information in cases of poisoning or suspected poisoning emergencies.

Pores: Tiny openings in the skin that help regulate body temperature.

Pressure bandage: A bandage applied firmly to create pressure on a wound to aid in controlling bleeding.

Pressure immobilisation technique: Application of a pressure bandage, used as a first aid technique for many bites and stings; it delays venom entering the circulation through the lymphatic system.

Primary survey: A check for life-threatening conditions.

Profuse bleeding: Rapid and heavy bleeding.

Prolapsed cord: A complication of childbirth in which a loop of umbilical cord protrudes through the vagina before the delivery of the baby.

Pulse: The beat felt in arteries near the skin's surface with each contraction of the heart.

Puncture: A wound that results when the skin is pierced with a pointed object such as a nail.

Rabies: A disease caused by a virus transmitted through the saliva of an infected animal.

Radial *(ra-de-al)* **arteries:** Blood vessels near the surface of the skin at the wrist, where the pulse is commonly taken.

Reassurance: The process of assuring a victim that help is on the way and that you will not leave the person alone; reassurance can help alleviate pain.

Red blood cells: The solid component of blood that transports oxygen and carbon dioxide.

Regurgitation *(ree-gur-ji-tay-shon)*: The passive flow of stomach contents into the mouth and airway, where it may be aspirated into the lungs; it is silent and may not be noticed by the first aider.

Reproductive organs: Male and female organs with reproductive functions, including internal organs and the genitals.

Residual current devices (RCDs): Devices installed in appropriate places in the home to prevent accidental electrocution; sometimes called safety switches.

Respiration: The breathing process of the body that takes in oxygen and eliminates carbon dioxide and other waste gases.

Respiratory arrest: Condition in which there is cessation of breathing.

Respiratory distress: Condition in which breathing is difficult.

Rib cage: The cage of bones formed by the 12 pairs of ribs, the sternum, and the spine.

Risk factors: Conditions or behaviours which increase the chance that a person will develop a disease.

Rupture: A tear or break in an organ or body tissue; to tear or break.

Saturated fat: A dietary substance found in some foods, such as meat and milk products, which in excessive quantities contributes to cardiovascular disease.

Scald: A burn caused by exposure of the skin to a hot liquid or vapour.

Scapula *(skap-yoo-la)*: See shoulder blade.

Seat carry: A planned move by which two first aiders make a seat of their hands and arms for carrying the victim.

Secondary survey: A check for injuries or conditions that could become life-threatening if not cared for.

Seizure: A disorder in the brain's electrical activity, marked by loss of consciousness and often uncontrollable muscle movement; may occur in an infant or child as a result of a sudden high temperature; often called a convulsion.

Shock: The failure of the circulatory system to provide adequate oxygen-rich blood to all parts of the body.

Shoulder blade: A large, flat, triangular bone at the back of the shoulder in the upper part of the back; also called the scapula.

Shoulder separation: Dislocation of the shoulder in which the shoulder blade is separated from the collarbone.

Signs: Details observed about a sick or injured person using the five senses.

Skeletal muscles: Muscles that attach to bones.

Skin: The tough, supple membrane that covers the entire surface of the body.

Skull: The bony structure of the head.

Sling: A bandage used to hold, support, or immobilise a body part.

Small intestine: Part of the alimentary canal where digested food substances from the stomach are absorbed into the blood.

Soft tissue: Body structures that include the layers of skin, fat, and muscles.

Spinal column: The column of vertebrae extending from the base of the skull to the tip of the tailbone (coccyx).

Spinal cord: A bundle of nerves extending from the brain at the base of the skull to the lower back, protected by the spinal column.

Spine: A series of bones (vertebrae) that surrounds and protects the spinal cord; also called the backbone.

Spleen: An organ in the abdomen; one of its functions is to store blood.

Splint: A commercial or improvised device used to immobilise an injured or fractured body part.

Spontaneous pneumothorax *(new-mo-thor-aks)*: A pneumothorax that occurs without any injury to the chest wall, caused by an internal rupture of lung tissue, following a violent bout of coughing, severe asthma attack, serious lung infection, or rupture of a cyst on the surface of the lung.

Sprain: The stretching and tearing of ligaments and other soft tissue structures at a joint.

Sterile: Free from living micro-organisms.

Sternum: The long, flat bone in the middle of the front of the rib cage; also called the breastbone.

Stimulants: Substances which affect the central nervous system to speed up physical and mental activity.

Stomach: The major organ of digestion, where partly processed food and liquid are broken down into substances the body can use.

Strain: The stretching and tearing of muscles and tendons.

Strangulation: The accidental or intentional squeezing of the neck and windpipe which obstructs a person's air supply.

Stress: A general response of the body to demands upon it; uncontrolled stress over time can have unhealthy effects on the body.

Stretcher: Any of several different devices for lifting and carrying a victim, typically with a frame on which the person lies while two or more first aiders hold on to the frame or poles along the sides.

Stroke: A disruption of blood flow to a part of the brain which causes permanent damage, usually caused by a blood clot or bleeding vessel; also called a cerebrovascular accident (CVA).

Substance abuse: The deliberate, excessive use of a substance without regard to health concerns or accepted medical practices.

Substance misuse: The use of a substance for unintended purposes or for intended purposes but in improper amounts or doses.

Sucking chest wound: An injury in which the chest cavity is punctured allowing air to pass freely in and out of the chest cavity.

Suffocation: The accidental or intentional cutting off of a person's air supply by an external object.

Superficial burn: A burn injury involving only the top layer of skin, characterised by red, dry skin.

Symptoms: Sensations felt by the sick or injured person which are described to the first aider or health professional.

Target heart rate: The heart rate maintained by continuous and vigorous exercise which gives the heart a healthy workout.

Tendon: A fibrous band that attaches muscle to bone.

Tension pneumothorax: A type of pneumothorax that develops following a rupture of the chest wall or lung tissue when air collects in the pleural space and cannot get out.

Tetanus *(tet-a-nuss)*: An acute infectious disease of the nervous system which is potentially fatal.

Thigh: The lower extremity between the pelvis and the knee.

Thrombus: A blood clot attached to the wall of a vein or artery which can block blood flow.

Tissue: A collection of similar cells that act together to perform specific body functions.

Tolerance: A condition which occurs when a user of a substance has to increase the dose and frequency of use to obtain the same desired effect.

oxaemia *(tok-see-mee-a)* of pregnancy: A condition a woman may experience in late pregnancy which may lead to seizures; also called eclampsia.

Trachea *(tra-kee-a):* The tube from the upper airway to the lungs; also called the windpipe.

Traction splint: A mechanical device or manual technique that reduces the deformity of a leg fracture by stretching the muscles to prevent the leg from shortening.

Transient ischaemic *(iss-kee-mic)* attack (TIA): A temporary disruption of blood flow to the brain; sometimes called a mini-stroke.

Trauma: A wound or injury caused by violent force; the force or mechanism, such as a fall, pressure, or shock, that causes such an injury.

Triage *(tree-arj):* The process of assessing multiple victims to determine who should receive care first

Trunk: The part of the body containing the chest, abdomen, and pelvis.

Ulcer: A usually painful crater-like sore in the stomach or other tissue resulting from an infection or other harmful condition.

Umbilical cord *(um-bil-i-cal):* The cord-like structure attaching the child to the placenta while the baby is in the uterus and for a short time after delivery.

Upper arm: The upper extremity from the shoulder to the elbow.

Uterus *(yoo-te-russ):* The organ in the woman's pelvis where the baby develops; commonly called the womb.

Varicose veins: Veins that become swollen with pooled blood due to failure of the valves.

Veins: Blood vessels which carry blood low in oxygen from all parts of the body to the heart.

Venom: The poisonous material produced by snakes, scorpions, spiders, and other animals for injecting into their prey or enemies.

Ventricular *(ven-trik-yoo-lar)* fibrillation *(fib-ri-lay-shon):* An abnormal heart rhythm occurring when no organised electrical impulse controls heart contractions, causing the heart to fail to pump blood.

Vertebrae *(ver-te-bray):* The 33 bones of the spinal column.

Victim: A person experiencing illness or injury and in need of medical assistance or first aid.

Virus: A disease-producing micro-organism.

Vital organs: Organs whose functions are essential to life, including the brain, heart, and lungs.

Vital signs: Important information about the victim's condition from checking breathing, pulse, and skin characteristics.

Voluntary: With conscious control or direction.

Withdrawal: The condition produced when an addicted person stops using or abusing a substance.

Wound: An injury to the skin which sometimes involves underlying soft tissues.

CREDITS

Position of photographs and illustrations on the page: t = top; b = bottom; l = left; r = right; c = centre

Photographs

All photographs in this manual were produced by Jerry Galea Photography, with the exception of the following:
Page 4: The Royal Flying Doctor Service. 7: American Red Cross. 26: American Red Cross. 54: Stephen Cullen. 66: tr, Stephen Cullen. 78: t (inset), Stephen Cullen. 79: t (inset), b (inset), Stephen Cullen. 80: inset, Stephen Cullen. 81: inset, Stephen Cullen. 84: American Red Cross. 86 & 87: American Red Cross. 100: American Red Cross. 132: Marketing and Media Department — Australian Red Cross, SA. 145: American Red Cross. 152: r, American Red Cross. 153: American Red Cross. 162: tl, cl, Victorian College of Agriculture & Horticulture Ltd., Burnely, Vic.; bl, Royal Botanic Gardens, Melbourne. 164 & 165: Steven Wilson. 166: r, Michael Gray. 167: Mike Tyler. 168: tl, br, American Red Cross; cl, bl, Mike Tyler. 169: cl, cr, br, American Red Cross; tr, Mike Tyler; bl, Surf Life Saving, Qld. 170: c, Mike Tyler. 171: t, Surf Life Saving, Qld; c, American Red Cross; b, ANT Photo Library. 172: American Red Cross. 174: t, American Red Cross. 183: American Red Cross. 185: American Red Cross. 187: b, American Red Cross. 188: American Red Cross. 192: American Red Cross. 204–207: American Red Cross. 208: r, American Red Cross. 209: cr, br, American Red Cross. 216: t, American Red Cross. 217: American Red Cross. 218: r, American Red Cross. 219: American Red Cross. 257: American Red Cross. 259: t, American Red Cross. 269: cl, American Red Cross. 271: American Red Cross. 273: American Red Cross. 274: tr, cr, American Red Cross. 289: American Red Cross. 295: Police Department, Vic. 298: Emergency Management Australia. 299: Emergency Management Australia. 300: t, Emergency Management Australia; b, Country Fire Authority, Vic. 304: American Red Cross. 326: Bert Vander Mark. 327: Bert Vander Mark. 337: cl, cr, bl, American Red Cross. 339: cl, Custom Medical Stock Photo, Inc.; cr, American Red Cross. 341: American Red Cross. 353: Quit Campaign. 357: American Red Cross.

Illustrations

All illustrations in this manual were produced by Rolin Graphics, with the exception of the following:
Page 15: American Red Cross. 16: tl, cl, American Red Cross. 17: tl, American Red Cross. 19: b, American Red Cross. 21: American Red Cross. 22: American Red Cross. 23: American Red Cross. 24: t, American Red Cross. 33: b, American Red Cross. 52: American Red Cross. 60: bl, br, American Red Cross. 61: bl, American Red Cross. 64: b, American Red Cross. 65: cl, American Red Cross. 98: American Red Cross. 99: American Red Cross. 115: Larry Nolte. 117: Larry Nolte. 129: American Red Cross. 146: American Red Cross. 147: American Red Cross. 148: American Red Cross. 159: tl, tr, cr, American Red Cross. 183: American Red Cross. 186: Larry Nolte. 189: American Red Cross. 203: American REd Cross. 204–207: American Red Cross. 210: American Red Cross. 211: b, American Red Cross. 212: American Red Cross. 213: Amerian Red Cross. 217: American Red Cross. 218: American Red Cross. 253: American Red Cross. 254: American Red Cross. 255: American Red Cross. 256: American Red Cross. 258: American Red Cross. 260: American Red Cross. 262: American Red Cross. 263: American Red Cross. 265: American Red Cross. 266: t, American Red Cross. 267: American Red Cross. 268: American Red Cross. 270: American Red Cross. 271: American Red Cross. 272: American Red Cross. 311: American Red Cross. 325: American Red Cross. 328: American Red Cross. 353: CSIRO, Division of Human Nutrition. 355: t, American Red Cross. 356: tr, Larry Nolte.

INDEX